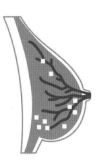

ATLAS OF
BREAST
PATHOLOGY

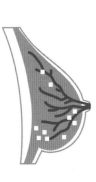

ATLAS OF BREAST PATHOLOGY

Steven G. Silverberg, MD
Professor of Pathology
University of Maryland School of Medicine
Director of Anatomic Pathology
University of Maryland Medical Center
Baltimore, Maryland

W.B. SAUNDERS COMPANY
An Imprint of Elsevier Science
Philadelphia ■ London ■ New York ■ St. Louis ■ Sydney ■ Toronto

W.B. SAUNDERS COMPANY
An Imprint of Elsevier Science

The Curtis Center
Independence Square West
Philadelphia, Pennsylvania 19106

Library of Congress Cataloging-in-Publication Data

Silverberg, Steven G.,

Atlas of breast pathology / Steven G. Silverberg

p. cm.

Includes index.

ISBN 0–7216–9557–4

1. Breast—Pathophysiology—Atlases. 2. Breast—Cancer—Pathophysiology—Atlases.
  3. Breast—Diseases—Diagnosis. I. Title.

RC280.B8 S4973 2002

618.1′9—dc21   2002019195

Acquisitions Editor: Natasha Andjelkovic
Project Manager: Agnes Hunt Byrne
Production Manager: Peter Faber
Illustration Specialist: Lisa Lambert

ATLAS OF BREAST PATHOLOGY   ISBN 0–7216–9557–4

Printed in China.

Last digit is the print number: 9   8   7   6   5   4   3   2   1

To Kiyoe

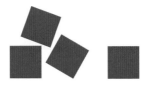

CONTRIBUTORS

Sue A. Bartow, MD ■ Associate Professor, Laboratory Medicine and Pathology, University of Minnesota School of Medicine, Minneapolis, Minnesota
Normal Anatomy and Physiologic Changes

Wendie A. Berg, MD, PhD ■ Associate Professor, Director of Breast Imaging, Department of Radiology and Greenebaum Cancer Center, University of Maryland School of Medicine, Baltimore, Maryland
Radiologic Techniques and Core Needle Breast Biopsy

Ira J. Bleiweiss, MD ■ Associate Professor, Mt. Sinai School of Medicine of New York University; Associate Attending Pathologist, Mt. Sinai Medical Center, New York, New York
Intraductal Papillary Lesions

Andra R. Frost, MD ■ Associate Professor, Department of Pathology, University of Alabama at Birmingham, Birmingham, Alabama
Atypical Lobular Hyperplasia, Lobular Carcinoma In Situ, and Infiltrating Lobular Carcinoma

Nancy S. Hardt, MD ■ Professor of Pathology and Obstetrics and Gynecology, University of Florida, Gainesville, Florida
Iatrogenic Lesions of the Breast

Syed A. Hoda, MD ■ Associate Professor of Clinical Pathology, Weill Medical College of Cornell University; Associate Attending Pathologist, New York Presbyterian Hospital-Weill Cornell Center, New York, New York
Stromal and Vascular Tumors

Olga B. Ioffe, MD ■ Assistant Professor, University of Maryland School of Medicine; Staff Pathologist; University of Maryland Medical Center, Baltimore, Maryland
Ductal Carcinoma In Situ and Atypical Ductal Hyperplasia; Infiltrating Carcinoma: Infiltrating Duct Carcinoma Not Otherwise Specified and Prognostic Factors Other Than Histologic Type; Infiltrating Carcinoma: Histologic Types Other Than Infiltrating Duct Carcinoma Not Otherwise Specified

Mirka W. Jones, MD ■ Associate Professor of Pathology, University of Pittsburgh School of Medicine; Staff Pathologist, Magee Womens Hospital of University of Pittsburgh Medical Center, Pittsburgh, Pennsylvania
Nipple Adenoma/Subareolar Papillomatosis and Benign Adnexal/Salivary Gland Type Tumors

Dhruv Kumar, MD ■ Attending Pathologist, Department of Pathology, Washington Hospital Center, Washington, D.C.
Radiologic Techniques and Core Needle Breast Biopsy

Shahla Masood, MD ■ Professor and Associate Chair, Department of Pathology, University of Florida; Director, The Breast Health Center, Chief of Pathology, Shands Jacksonville, Jacksonville, Florida
Fine-Needle Aspiration Cytology

Harold A. Oberman, MD ■ Professor Emeritus, Department of Pathology, University of Michigan Medical School, University of Michigan Health System, Ann Arbor, Michigan
Fibroadenomas, Adenomas, Cystosarcomas, and Hamartomas

Arthur S. Patchefsky, MD ■ Clinical Professor of Pathology, Jefferson Medical College of Thomas Jefferson University; Clinical Professor of Pathology, Hahnemann-MCP School of Medicine; Chairman and Senior Member, Department of Pathology, Fox Chase Cancer Center, Philadelphia, Pennsylvania
Nonproliferative and Benign Proliferative Epithelial Lesions

Steven G. Silverberg, MD ■ Professor and Director of Anatomic Pathology, Department of Pathology, University of Maryland Medical Center, Baltimore, Maryland
Ductal Carcinoma In Situ and Atypical Ductal Hyperplasia; Infiltrating Carcinoma: Infiltrating Duct Carcinoma Not Otherwise Specified and Prognostic Factors Other Than Histologic Type; Infiltrating Carcinoma: Histologic Types Other Than Infiltrating Duct Carcinoma Not Otherwise Specified

Eric S. Wargotz, MD ■ Clinical Professor of Pathology, George Washington University School of Medicine, Washington, D.C.; Chief of Pathology and Laboratory Director, Doctor's Community Hospital, Lanham, Maryland
Inflammatory, Infectious, and Other Non-Neoplastic Lesions

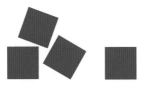

PREFACE

The concept of an atlas of breast pathology has been evolving for almost a decade and finally entered the preparation stage as the twentieth century drew to a close. What was planned, and, I hope, achieved, was to create a pictorial representation of the major, and many minor, mammary lesions encountered by the general pathologist, with the illustration legends serving as the major component of the text. Because familiarity with both the radiographic appearances and the cytopathologic features of breast lesions is essential to the modern practice of breast surgical pathology, chapters are included on these subjects. Equally important in the communication between the pathologist and the other clinical members of the breast cancer management team (and, ultimately, the patient) is the often confusing arena of prognostic markers, the current panoply of which is discussed in detail.

Atlas of Breast Pathology can be used as a quick reference for specific subjects, as well as serving as a primer of breast pathology for both pathology residents and nonpathologist physicians who are active in diagnosing, treating, and counseling patients with breast diseases.

As is usually true with works of this sort, I am indebted to a multitude of people who have contributed to my interest in breast pathology in the long run and to this book in the short run. Among the former are Drs. Fred Stewart and Bill Shelley (both deceased), and Drs. Saul Kay, Claude Gompel, and Bob McDivitt. The latter include all of the chapter authors, with particular thanks to Dr. Olga Ioffe, who provided invaluable advice as well as contributing to three major chapters; W.B. Saunders personnel, with special thanks to Marc Strauss, Natasha Andjelkovic, and Peter Faber; the many pathologists around the world who have referred cases to me over the years for consultation, pictures of some of which appear within these pages. Finally, as with past efforts, the completion of this work was aided immeasurably by the patience, advice, and understanding of my wife, Kiyoe.

STEVEN G. SILVERBERG, MD

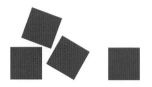

CONTENTS

■ **CHAPTER 1**

Radiologic Techniques and Core Needle Breast Biopsy................. 1
Wendie A. Berg
Dhruv Kumar

■ **CHAPTER 2**

Normal Anatomy and Physiologic Changes.......................... 19
Sue A. Bartow

■ **CHAPTER 3**

Inflammatory, Infectious, and Other Non-Neoplastic Lesions............ 26
Eric S. Wargotz

■ **CHAPTER 4**

Fibroadenomas, Adenomas, Cystosarcomas, and Hamartomas......... 39
Harold A. Oberman

■ **CHAPTER 5**

Nipple Adenoma/Subareolar Papillomatosis and Benign Adnexal/
Salivary Gland Type Tumors 49
Mirka W. Jones

■ **CHAPTER 6**

Nonproliferative and Benign Proliferative Epithelial Lesions............. 57
Arthur S. Patchefsky

■ **CHAPTER 7**

Intraductal Papillary Lesions 67
Ira J. Bleiweiss

■ **CHAPTER 8**

Ductal Carcinoma In Situ and Atypical Ductal Hyperplasia 77
Olga B. Ioffe
Steven G. Silverberg

■ **CHAPTER 9**

Atypical Lobular Hyperplasia, Lobular Carcinoma In Situ, and
Infiltrating Lobular Carcinoma 100
Andra R. Frost

■ **CHAPTER 10**

Infiltrating Carcinoma: Infiltrating Duct Carcinoma Not Otherwise
Specified and Prognostic Factors Other Than Histologic Type.......... 117
Olga B. Ioffe
Steven G. Silverberg

■ **CHAPTER 11**

Infiltrating Carcinoma: Histologic Types Other Than Infiltrating Duct
Carcinoma Not Otherwise Specified 139
Steven G. Silverberg
Olga B. Ioffe

■ **CHAPTER 12**

Stromal and Vascular Tumors..................................... 153
Syed A. Hoda

■ **CHAPTER 13**

Iatrogenic Lesions of the Breast.................................. 163
Nancy S. Hardt

■ **CHAPTER 14**

Fine-Needle Aspiration Cytology 179
Shahla Masood

Index.. 201

CHAPTER 1

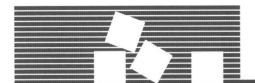

Radiologic Techniques and Core Needle Breast Biopsy

Wendie A. Berg
Dhruv Kumar

More than 180,000 cases of breast cancer are diagnosed each year, and roughly 1.2 million breast biopsies are performed. Mammography depicts approximately 90% of cancers; however, in dense breast tissue, up to 25% of cancers may be mammographically occult. Clinical breast evaluation and, increasingly, ultrasonography remain important adjuncts to annual screening mammography. Monthly routine breast self-examination should begin by age 20. A baseline mammogram is recommended between ages 35 and 40, with mammographic screening annually thereafter. Ultrasonography is the primary method of imaging evaluation of palpable masses in women under the age of 30, the age group in which fibroadenomas account for the vast majority of lesions. Ultrasonography is also widely used to evaluate masses or focal densities seen mammographically. Far beyond differentiating cysts from solid masses, ultrasonography is used to guide biopsy, characterize lesions, and even detect additional foci of cancer.[1]

With widespread mammographic screening, >50% of breast cancer is detected at stage 0 or stage I, when it is most curable. Typically, cancer manifests mammographically as either a developing density or clustered microcalcifications. The vast majority of ductal carcinoma in situ (DCIS)[2] and atypical ductal hyperplasia (ADH)[3, 4] present as clustered microcalcifications. A branching or ductal pattern of calcifications is more typical of high-grade DCIS, while a fine granular or amorphous cluster of calcifications is more common with low-grade DCIS.[5] The typical low-grade invasive cancer is a spiculated mass, while higher-grade lesions tend to have indistinct or even rarely, well-defined borders.[6] Invasive lobular carcinoma tends to be more subtle mammographically, often presenting as asymmetrical density or architectural distortion[7], and lobular carcinoma in situ (LCIS) is typically mammographically occult.[8–10]

Unfortunately, tremendous overlap occurs in the mammographic appearance of breast cancer and benign breast conditions, particularly fibrocystic changes. Only 15% to 35% of lesions recommended for biopsy prove malignant. Historically, open surgical biopsy was necessary to establish the histopathologic identity of mammographic abnormalities. Presently several options are available for preoperative diagnosis, ranging from fine-needle aspiration (FNA), to large (14-gauge) core needle biopsy (CNB), and vacuum-assisted core biopsy (e.g., the 11-gauge Mammotome [Ethicon Endosurgery, Cincinnati, OH]), and even larger devices (e.g., ABBI [Advanced Breast Biopsy Instrument, US Surgical, Norwalk, CT]). The latter is not discussed because valid clinical indications for the relatively more invasive ABBI procedure have not been forthcoming. Needle localization is still needed to direct excision of nonpalpable abnormalities, and radiography or ultrasonography of the specimen must confirm inclusion of the targeted abnormality in the excised tissue. If a reliable diagnosis of invasive or in situ carcinoma is achieved preoperatively, the initial surgery is usually therapeutic and includes axillary lymph node sampling when appropriate. Thus it is the task of radiologists, pathologists, and breast surgeons to achieve an accurate preoperative diagnosis. Our review of some histopathologic and imaging issues is directed toward that goal.

Fine-needle aspiration can be diagnostic, but it has several limitations. For nonpalpable lesions, the insufficient sample rate averaged 34% across academic institutions participating in the recent Radiation Diagnosis Oncology Group V trial.[11] Among insufficient samples, 10% proved malignant. Although some benign lesions can be reliably diagnosed as benign, a specific diagnosis is not usually achieved, leaving unanswered the question of whether a lesion has been adequately sampled. Cytologic "atypia" is not diagnostic: about 45% of such lesions prove malignant. One cannot reliably distinguish infiltrating from in situ carcinoma on the basis of FNA: the information from FNA is insufficient on which to base therapeutic surgery decisions such as the need for lymph node sampling.

1

FNA remains appropriate for lesions too small for definitive sonographic characterization as simple cysts and for complicated cysts, though these lesions can usually be followed.[12] Cytology may only be warranted in evaluating bloody aspirates.[13, 14]

Recently, initial diagnosis by large core needle breast biopsy has all but replaced surgical excision and FNA in many institutions. CNB is less invasive and nearly as accurate in diagnosis as excision. Most mass lesions can be visualized under ultrasound and adequately sampled with a 14-gauge automated biopsy gun; after five passes, an accurate diagnosis is achieved in over 99% of such lesions.[15] Microcalcifications are more problematic, as they can be associated with fibrocystic changes or other benign causes adjacent to or interspersed with cancer[16]; obtaining more (usually >10) specimens with larger, 11-gauge vacuum-assisted probes has improved the accuracy of core needle biopsy of cancers presenting only as microcalcifications, although underestimation of the severity is still possible. In one series evaluating 14-gauge automated biopsy guns, 30% of cancers presenting as calcifications were diagnosed only as atypical ductal hyperplasia on CNB, and another 7% yielded only benign results.[17] Over half of lesions showing ADH on CNB prove malignant at excision.[18, 19] Our experience suggests that an accurate diagnosis is achieved in 94% of lesions presenting as microcalcifications when a vacuum-assisted 11-gauge probe is used (3% miss rate and 3% cancelled cases due to posterior location, thin breast, or poor lesion conspicuity). Underestimation persists even with larger probes, with 6 of 46 lesions (13%) diagnosed as ADH on 11-gauge vacuum-assisted CNB proving to be malignant, and 10 of 89 (11%) initial DCIS diagnoses yielding invasive disease at excision in one recent study.[20] Thus any lesion showing ADH on core biopsy should be excised.

Knowledge of a variety of issues is critical to appropriate patient management using initial diagnosis by CNB. Most important is the recognition that the lesion has been adequately sampled; this requires communication between the radiologist, who should describe the imaging appearance and give likely diagnoses, and the pathologist, who must help determine whether or not microscopic findings correlate with the described imaging appearance of the lesion. Joint review of lesions is recommended. Discordance of imaging and histopathologic findings should prompt repeat biopsy. If microcalcifications are targeted, they must be seen both at specimen radiography and histopathology. A mammographically or sonographically discrete lesion should have a discrete correlate under the microscope: a diagnosis of "benign breast tissue" is not acceptable.[21] "Focal fibrosis" is an especially problematic category, and the tissue must be bordered by fat both mammographically and at histopathology for "focal fibrosis" to be accepted as a definitive diagnosis on CNB. We found that in 32% of specimens showing focal fibrosis, the lesion had been missed.[22] The clinical team managing the patient needs to understand histopathologic issues germane to CNB sampling. The most clinically important of these issues is the potential for underestimation of disease by CNB (see previous discussion).

Several unresolved issues remain with the use of CNB and patient management.[23] Atypical lobular hyperplasia (ALH) and LCIS represent a continuum of what has more recently been described as "lobular neoplasia," and typically there is no discrete mammographic correlate. Thus, if lobular neoplasia is the only finding at core biopsy, the lesion is likely to have been missed. Although infiltrating carcinomas can show adjacent foci of lobular neoplasia, the isolated finding of lobular neoplasia on CNB is usually incidental. When targeted calcifications were sampled yielding benign results and ALH or LCIS was also seen on core biopsy, we found that 3 of 13 patients (23%) with residual calcifications had ADH at excision and 1 of 13 patients (8%) had DCIS at excision.[24] Additional study is needed to determine appropriate patient management in this context.

The diagnosis of radial scar on core needle biopsy is made challenging by the lack of the entire lesion in the sample, with the result that overall architecture may be difficult to appreciate. Further, there is an association between radial scar and a spectrum of lesions from ADH to tubular carcinoma, with 25% to 31% of cases showing adjacent carcinoma.[25, 26] Mammographically, radial scars are usually spiculated masses that may have central lucency. The difficulty in diagnosis, mammographically suspicious appearance, and association with more worrisome lesions together result in a recommendation for excision of any lesion suspicious for a radial scar on CNB in most centers. Direct excision is preferred.

Papillary lesions are considered by some clinicians to be problematic on core biopsy. In our experience, 10% to 20% of lesions yielding benign papilloma on CNB had adjacent ADH or carcinoma at excision. Indeed, Ciatto and coworkers demonstrated a threefold increased risk of cancer ipsilateral to an excisional diagnosis of papilloma (single or multiple), and therefore papilloma should at least be considered a high-risk lesion.[27]

Mammogram
    Abnormal (85%–90% of cancers)
        Mass or focal density ⟶ Ultrasound (US)-guided CNB
        Suspicious microcalcifications ⟶ Stereotactic 11-gauge vacuum-assisted biopsy
    Negative, palpable mass (10%–15% of cancers) ⟶ CNB with or without US guidance versus excision

Histopathology of CNB
    Nonspecific benign breast tissue ⟶ Repeat biopsy
    Specific benign breast tissue ⟶ Mammographic, clinical follow-up
    ALH or LCIS ⟶ ?Excise
    Atypical ductal hyperplasia ⟶ Excise
    Malignant ⟶ Therapeutic, definitive surgery

Figure 1–1. Diagnosis of breast disease. From 85% to 90% of breast cancer is detectable mammographically and suited to image-guided core needle biopsy (CNB). If the lesion is visible sonographically, ultrasound-guided CNB is more comfortable for the patient and a 14-gauge automated biopsy gun is used. Nearly all lesions presenting as microcalcifications can be well sampled with stereotactic mammographic guidance using 11-gauge vacuum-assisted probes. Definitive diagnosis of palpable lesions is also readily achieved by CNB although negative imaging study results should not preclude excision of a clinically suspicious mass. Initial diagnosis by CNB facilitates surgical planning. Usually a single surgical procedure achieves complete excision and clear margins. Axillary nodal sampling can also be performed at the initial surgery if the lesion is known to be an infiltrating cancer. Unlike fine needle aspiration, CNB can readily distinguish between in situ and infiltrating tumors. A specific diagnosis of lymphoma or metastatic disease to the breast is also possible with CNB. Underestimation of disease remains problematic in about 5% of CNBs, so any result of atypical ductal hyperplasia merits excision. Management after CNB diagnosis of ALH or LCIS remains controversial.[24]

Consider Direct Excision
Mammographically suspect radial scar
Very small (<1 cm) spiculated mass if no axillary nodal sampling is needed
Small (<2 cm) focus of calcifications typical of DCIS
Not visible sonographically, technically not feasible stereotactically
    Extremely posterior at chest wall
    Very subtle calcifications lacking sufficient conspicuity
    Compressed breast thickness <15 mm

Figure 1–2. Lesions to consider for direct excision. Certain lesions are not ideally suited for diagnosis by core needle biopsy (CNB) and should be considered for diagnostic surgical biopsy. Mammographically, radial scars are spiculated masses that tend to have central lucency. Histopathologically, radial scar lesions are difficult to diagnose without the entire lesion and because they can be associated with early cancers, excision is the rule.[25] In a patient with a lesion that is mammographically typical for a small cancer and for which axillary nodal sampling is not performed, CNB adds an unnecessary procedure because the diagnostic surgical procedure is usually therapeutic as well. Certain lesions cannot be adequately visualized or positioned for CNB and require needle localization and excision. The biopsy gun with the shortest throw has an excursion of 15 mm on firing, making extremely thin breasts unsuitable candidates for stereotactic biopsy.

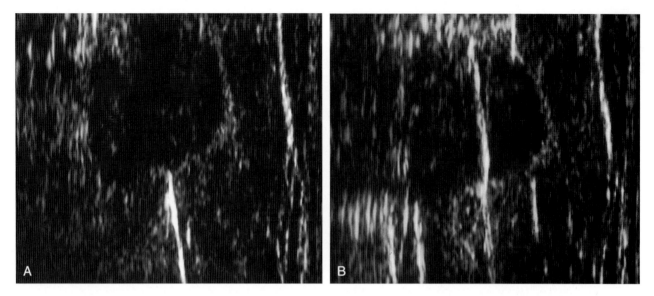

Figure 1–3. Ultrasonographically guided core needle biopsy. Using sterile technique and after infiltration of the skin and subcutaneous tissues with 1% lidocaine, a small skin incision is made and the 14-gauge automated biopsy gun is inserted under direct sonographic visualization. *A,* Prefire image demonstrates the tip of the biopsy gun at the edge of the lesion. The needle is inserted parallel to and along the long axis of the transducer to maximize conspicuity. *B,* Postfire image demonstrates needle traversing lesion with tip just through it. Typically, automated biopsy guns have a throw of 15 to 22 mm. The inner chamber advances, immediately followed by an outer cutting needle. The samples average 15 to 22 mm in length and 1.5 to 2 mm in width. Obtaining five samples ensures adequate sampling in >99% of mass lesions.[15]

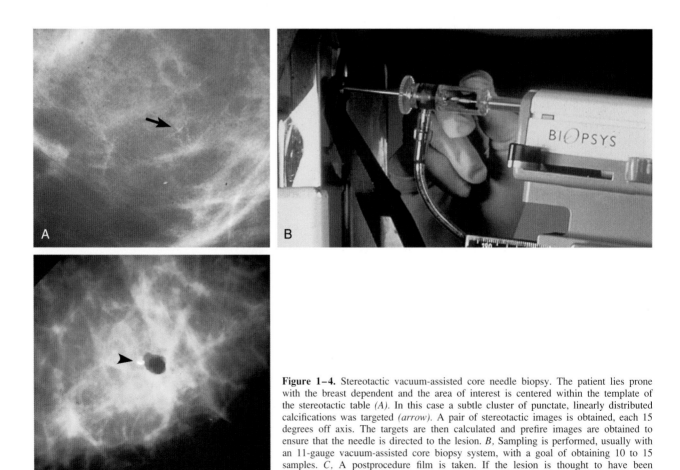

Figure 1–4. Stereotactic vacuum-assisted core needle biopsy. The patient lies prone with the breast dependent and the area of interest is centered within the template of the stereotactic table *(A).* In this case a subtle cluster of punctate, linearly distributed calcifications was targeted *(arrow).* A pair of stereotactic images is obtained, each 15 degrees off axis. The targets are then calculated and prefire images are obtained to ensure that the needle is directed to the lesion. *B,* Sampling is performed, usually with an 11-gauge vacuum-assisted core biopsy system, with a goal of obtaining 10 to 15 samples. *C,* A postprocedure film is taken. If the lesion is thought to have been removed or nearly removed, a small clip *(arrowhead)* is placed through the probe to mark the site for possible subsequent needle localization and excision.

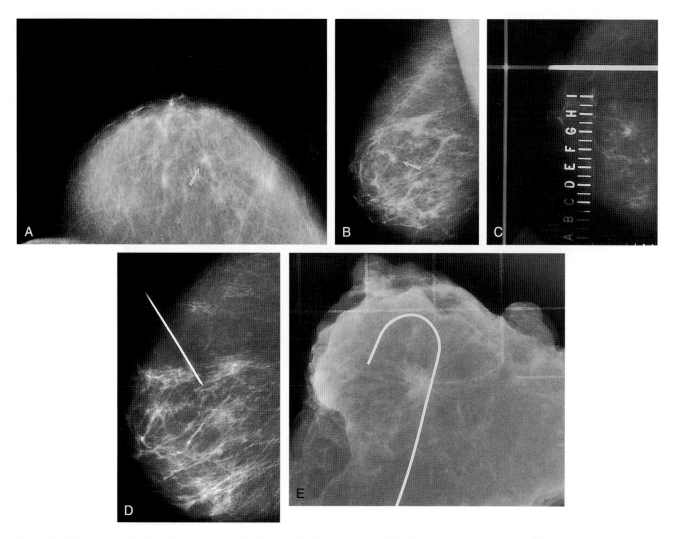

Figure 1–5. Needle localization of a mammographic abnormality. Initial craniocaudal *(A)* and mediolateral oblique *(B)* (or more commonly true lateral) mammographic views are reviewed to identify the approach with the shortest distance from the skin to the lesion. Arrows point to a subtle spiculated mass in the upper mid left breast, highly suspicious for cancer. *C,* The lesion is centered with the template grid opening of the paddle on the upper breast. The mass is seen at coordinates 2–G *(arrow)*. Based on the distance measured from a true lateral mammographic film, a 5-cm hook-wire needle is advanced into the lesion with the breast compressed. Mammograms are then obtained while the patient's breast is still compressed and in the perpendicular true lateral projection *(D)* to ensure that the needle tip is at or just beyond the lesion *(arrow)*. Blue dye is sometimes instilled through the needle, the hook wire is deployed, and films are sent with the patient to the operating room. *E,* A magnification specimen radiograph is then obtained to ensure removal of the targeted lesion. Typically the lesion is circled on the specimen radiograph, and the specimen radiograph is sent with the specimen to pathology. Use of a grid box facilitates communication with the pathologist as to the precise location of the area(s) of interest in the specimen. Histopathology revealed a 3-mm infiltrating ductal (tubular) carcinoma.

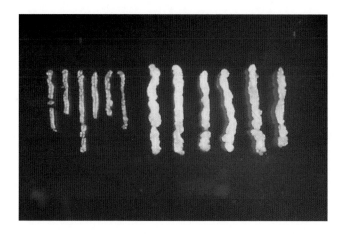

Figure 1–6. Core needle biopsy specimens. Typical samples from 14-gauge automated guns are seen on the left and those from 11-gauge vacuum-assisted guns on the right. An average of five times more material is sampled per specimen with the 11-gauge system.[28]

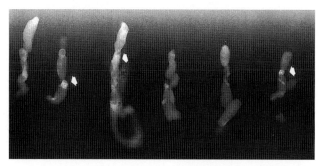

Figure 1–7. Specimen radiograph of microcalcifications in 11-gauge core biopsy specimens taken from the same patient as Figure 1–4. It is critical to document successful retrieval of calcifications (from calcified lesions) to ensure adequate sampling. Obtaining a minimum of 10 specimens has been shown to result in retrieval of calcifications in 95% of lesions.[29] If no calcifications are obtained, repeat biopsy is mandatory. Specimens containing the calcifications *(arrows)* can be inked with vital dyes to facilitate identification for the pathologist.[22]

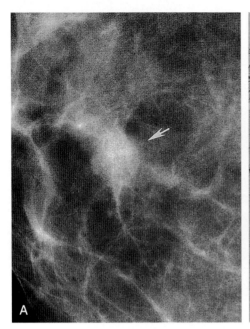 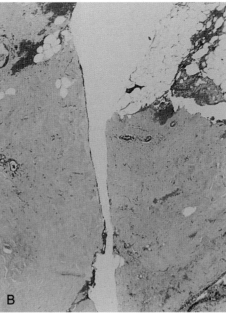

Figure 1–8. Focal fibrosis on core needle biopsy (CNB). *A,* Mammogram shows a partially circumscribed, partially indistinct indeterminate mass *(arrow),* not visible on ultrasonography. *B,* 14-gauge CNB specimens show focal dense fibrosis bordered by fat *(right).* Mammographically and histopathologically, this is a discrete lesion bordered by fat, and mammographically the lesion is of low suspicion for cancer. As such, this is an acceptable result and can be followed. In this case, the lesion has proven to be stable for 4 years of mammographic follow-up.

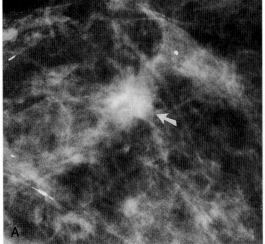 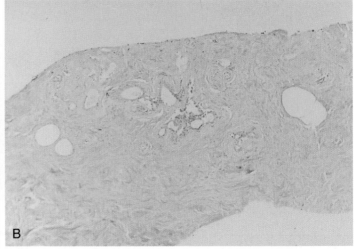

Figure 1–9. Lack of mammographic-histopathologic concordance. *A,* A new, highly suspicious, spiculated mass was noted on mammographic screening *(arrow).* A vague hypoechoic mass was seen on ultrasound in the proper location. *B,* 14-gauge core needle biopsy (CNB) specimens showed normal breast tissue with no discrete lesion evident *(right).* As such, repeat stereotactically guided CNB was performed yielding infiltrating ductal carcinoma. It is critical that both the radiologist and pathologist have a clear sense of what results are acceptable and correlate the mammographic and histopathologic results.

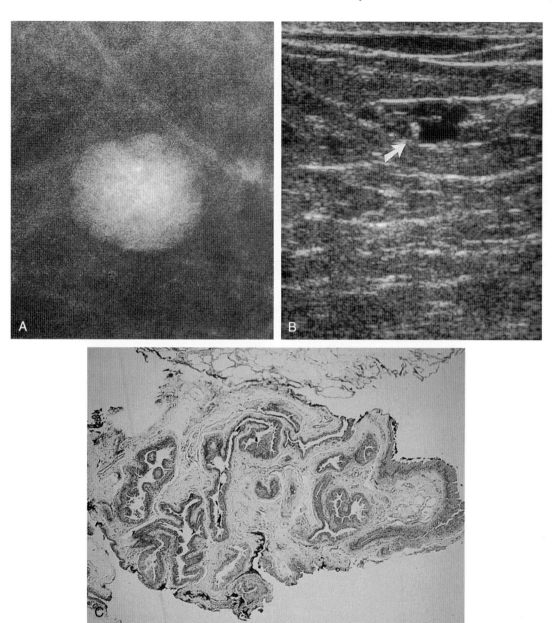

Figure 1–10. Focal apocrine metaplasia. *A,* Mammographically, a new, indeterminate, microlobulated mass was identified. *B,* Sonographically, tiny cystic areas were seen within the lesion. A single calcification was also evident *(arrow).* Because this does not meet the criteria for a simple cyst, core needle biopsy (CNB) was performed. *C,* A discrete focus of cystically dilated acini lined by apocrine metaplastic epithelium was found at histopathology. The presence of tiny cystic spaces at ultrasonography should suggest the diagnosis of microcysts or focal apocrine metaplasia. The pathologist should recognize focal apocrine metaplasia as a discrete process accounting for the microlobulated mass at imaging. Such lesions often resolve or diminish after CNB.[30]

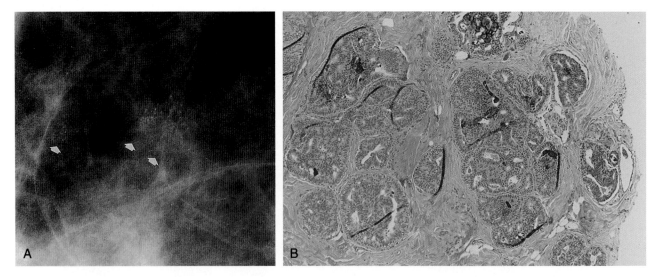

Figure 1–11. Atypical ductal hyperplasia (ADH) on core needle biopsy (CNB): underestimation of disease. *A,* ADH and ductal carcinoma in situ (DCIS) usually manifest mammographically as clustered microcalcifications *(arrows).* *B,* On CNB, this was interpreted as ADH versus DCIS with microcalcifications. Several ductal profiles are seen. The epithelial cells are monomorphic and form "Roman bridges." However, many of the spaces between proliferating cells are not round, but irregular, precluding a diagnosis of cribriform DCIS and favoring ADH. Distinction of these entities on the basis of the few ducts sampled with CNB can be difficult, and the area sampled may not be representative of the most severely involved ducts. As such, any lesion yielding ADH on core needle biopsy must be excised. From 0 to 20% of lesions diagnosed as ADH on 11-gauge vacuum-assisted CNB and 50% of those found on 14-gauge CNB prove malignant at excision.[18, 19]

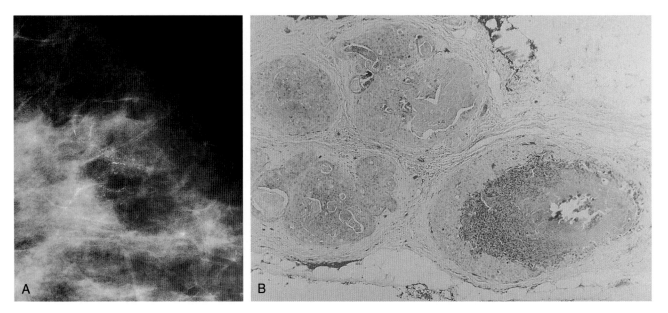

Figure 1–12. Ductal carcinoma in situ (DCIS). *A,* Mammographically, fine branching and linear calcifications that appear to be oriented along ducts are highly suspicious for DCIS. Definitive management is excision, followed by radiation to the breast if the breast is conserved. Direct excision is appropriate for small (<2 cm) foci typical of DCIS. Unfortunately, most calcifications due to DCIS are round or mildly pleomorphic and appear mammographically very similar to fibrocystic changes and other benign conditions; core needle biopsy (CNB) is reasonable for the vast majority of such lesions. Initial diagnosis by CNB is appropriate in planning surgery when mastectomy or wide excision is needed. *B,* Histopathologically, CNB specimens obtained with an 11-gauge probe show several ducts distended with high-grade DCIS with comedo necrosis, confirmed at mastectomy. When 10 or more samples are obtained with an 11-gauge probe, 5% to 11% of lesions prove to have an infiltrating component at excision that was not sampled at CNB[20, 31]; when CNB is performed with a 14-gauge automated biopsy gun, 19% to 20% prove to have an infiltrating component.[18, 32]

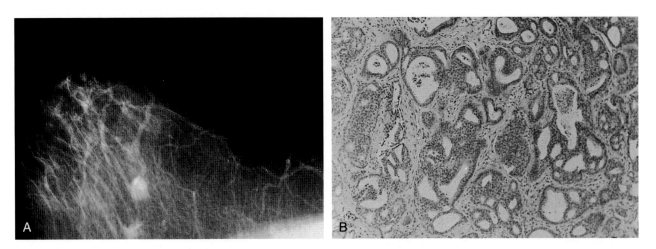

Figure 1–13. Infiltrating ductal (cribriform) carcinoma. *A,* Two new masses were noted mammographically. The more anterior of these has partially circumscribed, partially indistinct borders and is indeterminate. The more posterior of the masses appears spiculated, highly suspicious for cancer. These could not be clearly visualized on ultrasonography. The more posterior mass was inaccessible to stereotactic biopsy. The more anterior mass was sampled with 14-gauge core needle biopsy (CNB) under stereotactic guidance. *B,* Histopathology of CNB specimens was initially interpreted as atypical ductal hyperplasia. Both lesions were excised and both showed infiltrating ductal (cribriform) carcinoma.

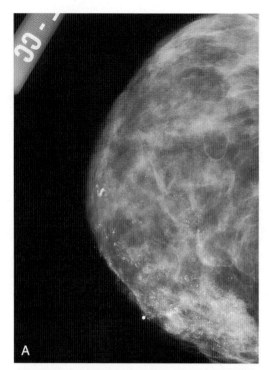

Figure 1–14. Infiltrating ductal carcinoma with an extensive intraductal component. *A,* Craniocaudal mammogram in this 37-year-old woman shows a broad area of fine and pleomorphic calcifications in a segmental (duct and its branches) distribution, highly suspicious for ductal carcinoma in situ (DCIS). The radiopaque marker denotes a palpable mass. *B,* Ultrasonography of the palpable abnormality reveals an indistinctly marginated hypoechoic mass containing a few echogenic calcifications. The presence of a mass or focal density in association with suspicious calcifications suggests the presence of an infiltrating component, and core needle biopsy (CNB) sampling should be directed to that area. Sonographically guided CNB confirmed infiltrating and intraductal carcinoma, and the patient immediately underwent mastectomy and axillary lymph node dissection. *C,* At excision, a 1-cm infiltrating tumor was identified with an extensive intraductal component involving the entire inner breast.

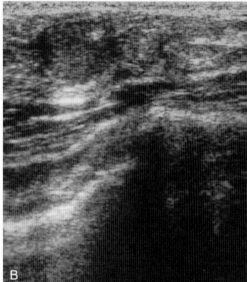

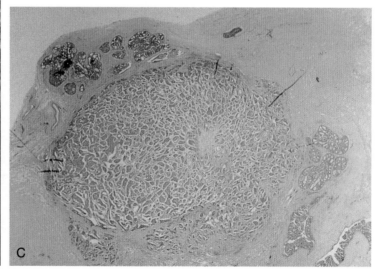

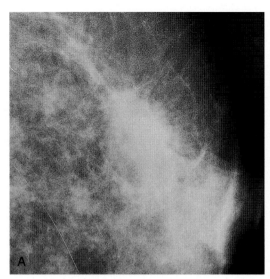

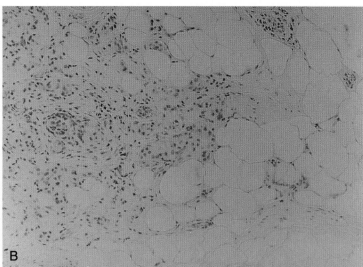

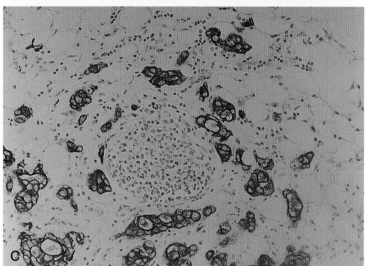

Figure 1–15. Infiltrating ductal carcinoma on core biopsy. *A,* Mammogram revealed a new, spiculated, highly suspicious mass in this 53-year-old woman with a history of contralateral cancer 3 years earlier. *B,* Histopathology reveals nests of monomorphic ductal cells infiltrating fat. Distinction of in situ carcinoma involving sclerosing adenosis from infiltrating well-differentiated carcinoma can be challenging on CNB. *C,* Cytokeratin stain nicely demonstrates nests of tumor cells surrounding fat spaces, compatible with infiltrating ductal carcinoma. Excision was interpreted as ductal carcinoma in situ (DCIS) involving sclerosing adenosis with foci of microinvasion. For highly suspicious masses, CNB provides the diagnosis before surgery, so a single definitive surgery is performed together with axillary lymph node sampling. With direct excisional biopsy, margins are involved with tumor in over half of cases. When the diagnosis is established preoperatively by CNB, clear margins are achieved at surgery in from 92% to 100% of cases.[33]

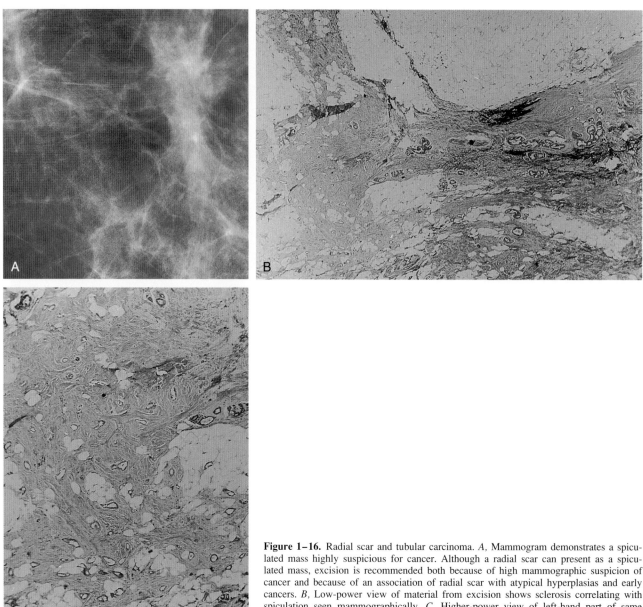

Figure 1–16. Radial scar and tubular carcinoma. *A,* Mammogram demonstrates a spiculated mass highly suspicious for cancer. Although a radial scar can present as a spiculated mass, excision is recommended both because of high mammographic suspicion of cancer and because of an association of radial scar with atypical hyperplasias and early cancers. *B,* Low-power view of material from excision shows sclerosis correlating with spiculation seen mammographically. *C,* Higher-power view of left-hand part of same lesion shows 2-mm focus of tubular carcinoma. The rate of carcinoma associated with radial scars and radial sclerosing lesions has been 25% to 28% in several series; tubular carcinoma frequently coexists with such lesions.[25, 26]

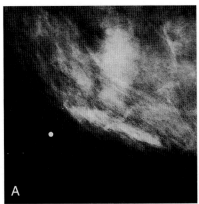

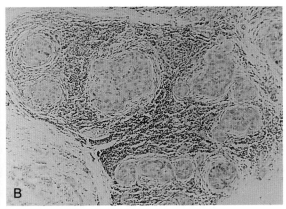

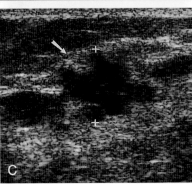

Figure 1–17. Value of image guidance for core needle biopsy (CNB) of palpable lesions. *A,* Mammogram shows vague area of increased density in a rather tubular pattern corresponding to area of palpable abnormality marked with a radiopaque marker. *B,* Blind CNB performed in the surgeon's office revealed cancerization of lobules. This diagnosis implies a ductal carcinoma involving the acini rather than lobular carcinoma in situ. As such, excision is needed. Staining with E-cadherin can be used to confirm the ductal origin of the lesion.[34, 35] *C,* Ultrasonography performed preoperatively revealed an irregular hypoechoic mass with adjacent, more circumscribed tubular masses. Sonographically, the central mass *(arrow)* was considered the most suspicious and proved to be an infiltrating ductal carcinoma. Adjacent tubular masses were due to ductal carcinoma in situ (DCIS).

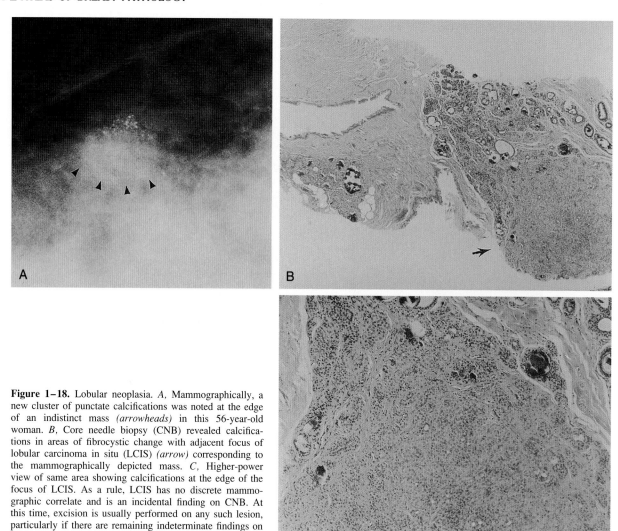

Figure 1–18. Lobular neoplasia. *A,* Mammographically, a new cluster of punctate calcifications was noted at the edge of an indistinct mass *(arrowheads)* in this 56-year-old woman. *B,* Core needle biopsy (CNB) revealed calcifications in areas of fibrocystic change with adjacent focus of lobular carcinoma in situ (LCIS) *(arrow)* corresponding to the mammographically depicted mass. *C,* Higher-power view of same area showing calcifications at the edge of the focus of LCIS. As a rule, LCIS has no discrete mammographic correlate and is an incidental finding on CNB. At this time, excision is usually performed on any such lesion, particularly if there are remaining indeterminate findings on mammography. The above findings were confirmed at excision.

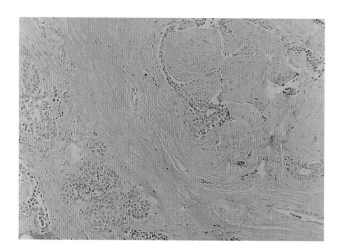

Figure 1–19. Lobular carcinoma in situ (LCIS) in a fibroadenoma. Areas of lobular neoplasia are evident within and adjacent to this fibroadenoma on core needle biopsy. It is doubtful that excision is necessary for such a lesion, although additional studies are needed. Clearly any other lesions in either breast need to be viewed with greater suspicion. LCIS was confirmed at excision, as this patient had a synchronous retroareolar infiltrating lobular carcinoma and elected mastectomy.

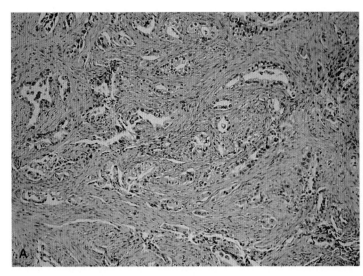

Figure 1–20. Lung cancer metastatic to breast. Mammographically, a new indistinctly marginated mass was noted, suspicious for cancer. *A,* Core needle biopsy (CNB) showed an adenocarcinoma with clear cells, likely metastatic from lung or kidney. *B,* Following the CNB results, a chest radiograph was obtained, revealing the patient's primary tumor in the left midlung *(arrowheads).* As a result, the patient underwent chemotherapy directly and avoided unnecessary surgery.

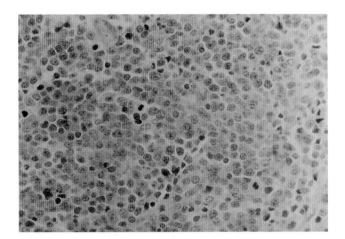

Figure 1–21. Lymphoma involving breast. Core needle biopsy (CNB) can also establish the diagnosis of lymphoma involving the breast, as in this case. If such a diagnosis is suspected, the specimens should be kept on gauze moistened with saline, and not placed in formalin, for transport to pathology. Fixing part of the tissue in B5 for morphologic detail and freezing additional core specimens for molecular studies can then be done if warranted. Again, the patient underwent chemotherapy based on results of CNB and was spared unnecessary surgery.

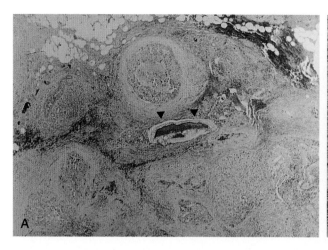
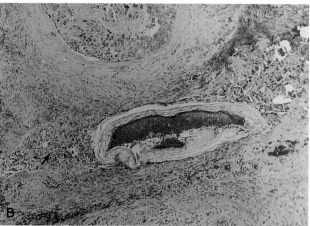

Figure 1–22. Epithelial displacement by core needle biopsy (CNB). Small fragments of tumor and epithelium are displaced by any needle procedure, including CNB, in about a quarter of cases.[36, 37] *A,* Diagnosis of ductal carcinoma in situ (DCIS) had been made in this case by CNB. A small focus of skin is noted along the needle track *(arrowheads). B,* Higher-power view shows small tumor cell nests also displaced *(arrow),* which could be mistaken for evidence of infiltration. Except for the potential to upgrade a lesion, the clinical significance of such epithelial displacement is not known. Epidermal inclusion cysts can also result. It is likely that radiation will treat any cells displaced along the needle track, but this remains unproven. If radiation is not to be given, excision of the needle track has been recommended.[38]

References

1. Berg WA, Gilbreath PL: Multicentric and multifocal cancer: Whole-breast US in preoperative evaluation. Radiology 214:59–66, 2000.
2. Dershaw DD, Abramson A, Kinne DW: Ductal carcinoma in situ: Mammographic findings and clinical implications. Radiology 170:411–415, 1989.
3. Helvie MA, Hessler C, Frank TS, Ikeda DM: Atypical hyperplasia of the breast: Mammographic appearance and histologic correlation. Radiology 179:759–764, 1991.
4. Stomper PC, Cholewinski SP, Penetrante RB, et al: Atypical hyperplasia: Frequency and mammographic and pathologic relationships in excisional biopsies guided with mammography and clinical examination. Radiology 189:667–671, 1993.
5. Stomper PC, Connolly JL: Ductal carcinoma in situ of the breast: Correlation between mammographic calcification and tumor subtype. AJR Am J Roentgenol 159:483–485, 1992.
6. Lamb PM, Perry NM, Vinnicombe SJ, Wells CA: Correlation between ultrasound characteristics, mammographic findings and histological grade in patients with invasive ductal carcinoma of the breast. Clin Radiol 55:40–44, 2000.
7. Hilleren DJ, Andersson IT, Lindholm K, Linell FS: Invasive lobular carcinoma: Mammographic findings in a 10-year experience [see comments]. Radiology 178:149–154, 1991.
8. Pope TL Jr, Fechner RE, Wilhelm MC, et al: Lobular carcinoma in situ of the breast: Mammographic features. Radiology 168:63–66, 1988.
9. Beute BJ, Kalisher L, Hutter RV: Lobular carcinoma in situ of the breast: Clinical, pathologic, and mammographic features. AJR Am J Roentgenol 157:257–265, 1991.
10. Carson W, Sanchez-Forgach E, Stomper P, et al: Lobular carcinoma in situ: Observation without surgery as an appropriate therapy. Ann Surg Oncol 1:141–146, 1994.
11. Pisano ED, Fajardo LL, Tsimikas J, et al: Rate of insufficient samples for fine-needle aspiration for nonpalpable breast lesions in a multicenter clinical trial: The Radiologic Diagnostic Oncology Group 5 Study. The RDOG5 investigators. Cancer 82:679–688, 1988.
12. Venta LA, Kim JP, Pelloski CE, Morrow M: Management of complex breast cysts. AJR Am J Roentgenol 173:1331–1336, 1999.
13. Ciatto S, Cariaggi P, Bulgaresi P: The value of routine cytologic examination of breast cyst fluids. Acta Cytol 31:301–304, 1987.
14. Hindle WH, Arias RD, Florentine B, Whang J: Lack of utility in clinical practice of cytologic examination of nonbloody cyst fluid from palpable breast cysts. Am J Obstet Gynecol 182:1300–1305, 2000.
15. Liberman L, Feng TL, Dershaw DD, et al: US-guided core breast biopsy: Use and cost-effectiveness. Radiology 208:717–723, 1998.
16. Berg WA: When is core breast biopsy or fine-needle aspiration not enough? Radiology 198:313–315, 1996.
17. Liberman L, Dershaw DD, Glassman J, et al: Analysis of cancers not diagnosed at stereotaxic core breast biopsy. Radiology 203:151–157, 1997.
18. Jackman RJ, Nowels KW, Shepard MJ, et al: Stereotaxic large-core needle biopsy of 450 nonpalpable breast lesions with surgical correlation in lesions with cancer or atypical hyperplasia. Radiology 193:91–95, 1994.
19. Liberman L, Cohen MA, Dershaw DD, et al: Atypical ductal hyperplasia diagnosed at stereotaxic core biopsy of breast lesions: An indication for surgical biopsy [see comments]. AJR Am J Roentgenol 164:1111–1113, 1995.
20. Burak WE Jr, Owens KE, Tighe MB, et al: Vacuum-assisted stereotactic breast biopsy: Histologic underestimation of malignant lesions. Arch Surg 135:700–703, 2000.
21. Berg WA, Hruban RH, Kumar D, et al: Lessons from mammographic-histopathologic correlation of large core breast biopsies. Radiographics 16:1111–1130, 1996.
22. Berg WA, Jaeger B, Campassi C, Kumar D: Predictive value of specimen radiography for core needle biopsy of noncalcified breast masses. AJR Am J Roentgenol 171:1671–1678, 1998.
23. Gundry KR, Berg WA: Treatment issues and core needle breast biopsy: Clinical context (perspective). AJR Am J Roentgenol 171:41–49, 1998.
24. Berg WA, Mrose HE, Ioffe OB: Atypical lobular hyperplasia or lobular carcinoma in situ on core needle breast biopsy. Radiology 218:503–509, 2001.
25. Frouge C, Tristant H, Guinebretiere JM, et al: Mammographic lesions suggestive of radial scars: Microscopic findings in 40 cases. Radiology 195:623–625, 1995.
26. Hassell P, Klein-Parker H, Worth A, Poon P: Radial sclerosing lesions of the breast: Mammographic and pathologic correlation. Can Assoc Radiol J 50:370–375, 1999.
27. Ciatto S, Andreoli C, Cirillo A, et al: The risk of breast cancer

subsequent to histologic diagnosis of benign intraductal papilloma: Follow-up study of 339 cases. Tumori 77:41–43, 1991.

28. Berg WA, Krebs TL, Campassi C, et al: Evaluation of 14- and 11-gauge directional, vacuum-assisted biopsy probes and 14-gauge biopsy guns in a breast parenchymal model. Radiology 205:203–208, 1997.

29. Jackman RJ, Burbank F, Parker SH, et al: Atypical ductal hyperplasia diagnosed at stereotactic breast biopsy: Improved reliability with 14-gauge, directional, vacuum-assisted biopsy. Radiology 204:485–488, 1997.

30. Warner JK, Kumar D, Berg WA: Apocrine metaplasia: Mammographic and sonographic appearances. AJR Am J Roentgenol 170:1375–1379, 1998.

31. Liberman L, Smolkin JH, Dershaw DD, et al: Calcification retrieval at stereotactic, 11-gauge, directional, vacuum-assisted breast biopsy. Radiology 208:251–260, 1998.

32. Parker SH, Burbank F, Jackman RJ, et al: Percutaneous large-core breast biopsy: A multi-institutional study. Radiology 193:359–364, 1994.

33. Yim JH, Barton P, Weber B, et al: Mammographically detected breast cancer: Benefits of stereotactic core versus wire localization biopsy. Ann Surg 223:688–697; discussion, 697–700, 1996.

34. Moll R, Mitze M, Frixen UH, Birchmeier W: Differential loss of E-cadherin expression in infiltrating ductal and lobular breast carcinomas. Am J Pathol 143:1731–1742, 1993.

35. Ioffe O, Silverberg SG, Simsir A: Lobular lesions of the breast: Immunohistochemical profile and comparison with ductal proliferations [abstract]. Mod Pathol 13:23A, 2000.

36. Youngson BJ, Liberman L, Rosen PP: Displacement of carcinomatous epithelium in surgical breast specimens following stereotaxic core biopsy. Am J Clin Pathol 103:598–602, 1995.

37. Diaz LK, Wiley EL, Venta LA: Are malignant cells displaced by large-gauge needle core biopsy of the breast? AJR Am J Roentgenol 173:1303–1313, 1999.

38. Chao C, Torosian MH, Boraas MC, et al: Local recurrence of breast cancer in the stereotactic core needle biopsy site: Case reports and review of the literature. The Breast J 7:124–127, 2001.

CHAPTER 2

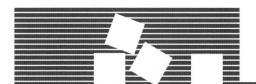

Normal Anatomy and Physiologic Changes

Sue A. Bartow

INTRODUCTION

The human mammary gland was once thought to actively develop during puberty under the influence of estrogen and other growth hormones, but once fully developed, it entered a "resting" state unless stimulated by the hormones of pregnancy. Following pregnancy and lactation, the gland was thought to again enter a resting state until menopause. After menopause, the gland was known to become less firm and more dependent, but little more was known about the involutional aging process. With the technology of radiographic imaging and its utility for detecting cancers in the breast came the impetus to learn more about the normal anatomy and physiology of the mammary gland. During the 1970s, Sefton Wellings and John Wolfe and their colleagues produced a remarkable body of work detailing the subgross anatomy of the female breast and its variations in the population, along with correlative studies of radiographic features of the organ.[1, 2] In the 1980s, other investigators described the histologic features of cyclical changes that occur in the breast with ovarian hormonal periodicity and distinguished those changes from the abnormal alterations observed by pathologists.[3] The combined information derived from these studies defined the functional unit of the adult female breast from which the majority of both benign and malignant lesions arise as the terminal duct lobular unit.

The objectives of this chapter are to illustrate, through the use of gross photographs, radiographs, and photomicrographs, features of the normal female breast during postnatal development, the menstrual cycle and pregnancy, and after the menopause. Morphologic features are related to the hormonal milieu. It has become clear that the human mammary gland is functionally dynamic not only during development and pregnancy but throughout the reproductive life of the woman. This has profound implications for the genesis of neoplasia in the breast. Thus it remains relevant to understand the spectrum of normal anatomy and physiology as a background for mastering the pathology of the breast.

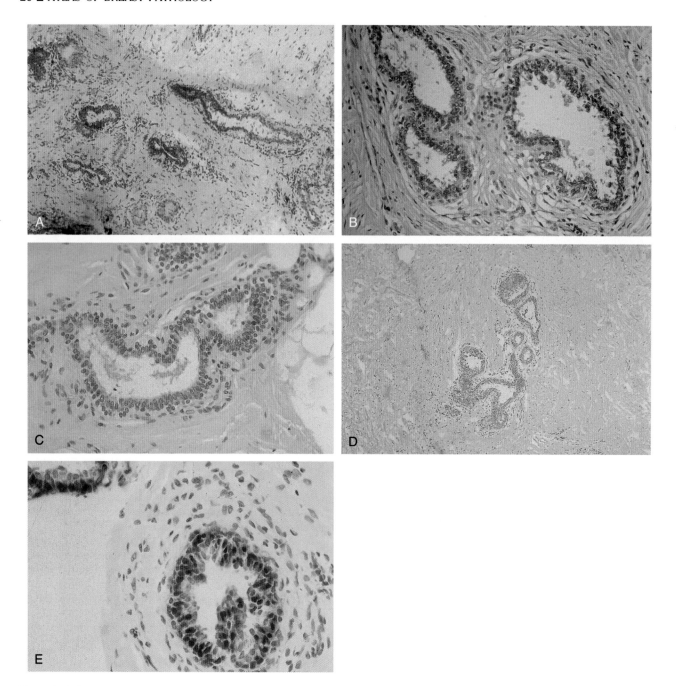

Figure 2–1. Developmental stages of the female breast. *A,* The infantile breast bud is composed of a small amount of cellular stroma within which are dispersed small, round to elongated duct structures. In the newborn, these may have cytologic features of secretory activity (presumably due to maternal hormones). Shown is a section of breast tissue from a 17-week-old infant. Occasional luminal epithelial cells may show faint positivity for estrogen receptor as well as evidence of cell cycling by immunostaining with antibodies such as proliferating cell nuclear antigen (PCNA). This architectural structure with occasional positive nuclear staining for estrogen receptor protein and PCNA continues into the early childhood years. Staining for progesterone receptor protein is negative in the breast tissue of infants and young girls. *B,* Breast tissue in older, but still premenarchal girls (5 to 8 years) shows increasing amounts of stroma separating the small branching ducts. Shown is a breast duct from a 7-year-old girl stained for the presence of estrogen receptor protein. The duct epithelial cell nuclei show positivity for estrogen receptor protein; they may also begin to show faint nuclear positivity for progesterone receptor protein as well as faint PCNA staining in occasional luminal epithelial cells. *C,* Perimenarchal breast tissue shows early formation of small complex ducts suggesting beginning "lobule" formation and some snouts on luminal epithelial cells, such as seen in this example from a 14-year-old girl. *D,* Progesterone receptor protein positivity is detected in this stage of development in the early lobule formation and terminal ducts in 15% to 20% of cells. Estrogen receptor staining in nuclei becomes negative. *E,* Cells positive for PCNA are also present in a distribution similar to that seen for progesterone receptor protein.

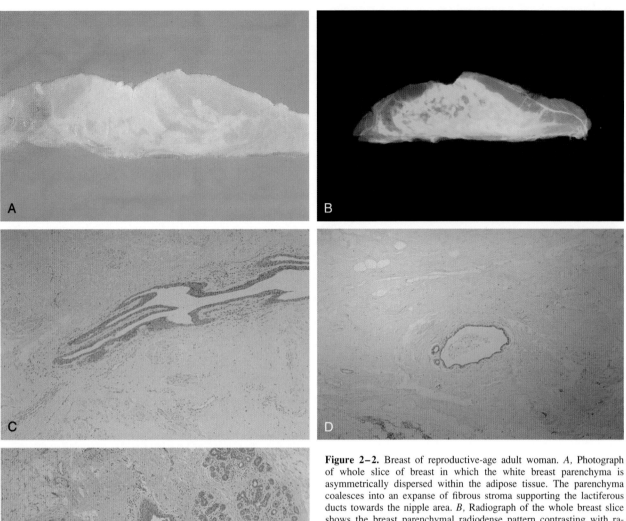

Figure 2–2. Breast of reproductive-age adult woman. *A,* Photograph of whole slice of breast in which the white breast parenchyma is asymmetrically dispersed within the adipose tissue. The parenchyma coalesces into an expanse of fibrous stroma supporting the lactiferous ducts towards the nipple area. *B,* Radiograph of the whole breast slice shows the breast parenchymal radiodense pattern contrasting with radiolucent adipose tissue. *C,* Histology of the large ducts under the nipple and areola. These lactiferous ducts are lined by columnar epithelium. Immediately under the nipple, this epithelium transforms to a squamous type and is continuous with the surface epithelium of the nipple. *D,* As the glandular components branch peripherally from the lactiferous ducts, they continue to be encased in fibrous connective tissue. The layered epithelial lining is that of cuboidal type epithelium. *E,* Intermediate-size ducts continue to branch peripherally into multiple terminal duct/lobular units. The amount of fibrous stroma surrounding the glandular elements is variable. The terminal duct/lobular units are formed only after the onset of menarche as a result of the synergy of estrogen and progesterone.

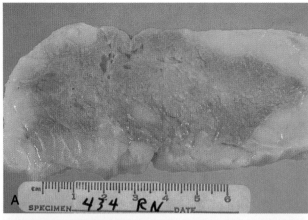

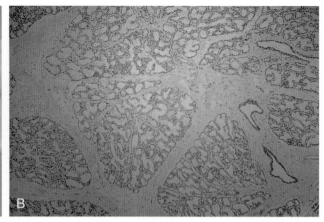

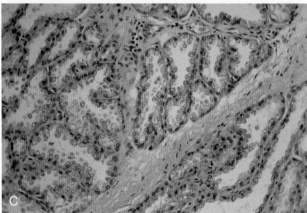

Figure 2–3. Term pregnant breast. *A,* Gross photograph of whole breast in a term pregnant woman. The usual white fibrous appearance and consistency of the breast parenchyma is transformed to a tan color and softer consistency. Dilated lactiferous ducts are apparent in the subareolar area. *B,* Photomicrograph of term pregnant breast tissue. There is a marked increase in number and complexity of the terminal ductules resulting in physiologic hyperplasia of the terminal duct/lobular units. *C,* A portion of a terminal duct/lobular unit in term pregnancy shows the transformation of the ductules into complex structures with hyperplastic lining cells showing evidence of secretory activity and papillary infolding. In the later stages of pregnancy, there is loss of staining of the terminal duct epithelial cells for estrogen and progesterone receptor protein, as well as loss of evidence of cell cycling by PCNA staining.[4]

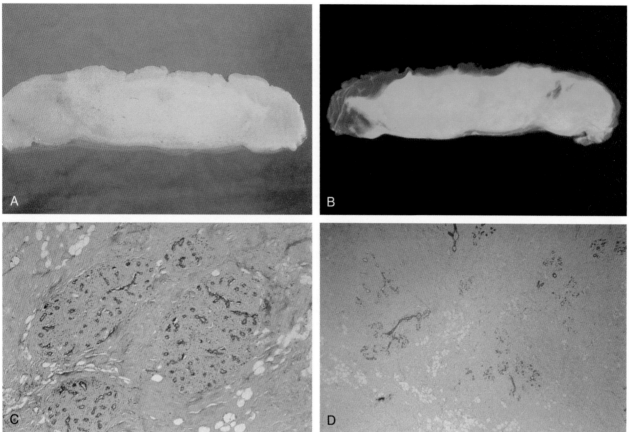

Figure 2–4. Dense breast tissue of young women. *A,* Gross photograph of a slice of whole breast of a 19-year-old woman. Eighty percent of women in the United States 20 years of age and younger have a majority of their breast tissue composed of dense fibrous parenchyma as opposed to adipose tissue. This varies to some extent according to body habitus. Young, obese women have a larger component of adipose tissue in the breast. *B,* The corresponding radiograph of the breast in *A* shows the dense parenchymal pattern that can mask tumors in the breast, making the use of mammography in many situations of limited utility. *C,* Photomicrograph of dense breast in a young woman shows confluent connective tissue and extralobular stroma that appears to be continuous with similarly dense intralobular stroma. This abundance of connective tissue correlates with an apparent decrease in size and number of the terminal ductules. This is typical of the follicular phase of the menstrual cycle. During the luteal phase, the intralobular stroma typically becomes much less dense and the terminal ductules more open and numerous. *D,* Photomicrograph of the breast tissue in a young woman after tamoxifen therapy and oophorectomy. In women who have undergone oophorectomy and/or functional eradication of the ovarian hormonal cycling, there may be an extreme degree of increase in the fibrous connective tissue component relative to adipose tissue with concomitant morphologic obliteration of the terminal duct/lobular unit epithelial structures.

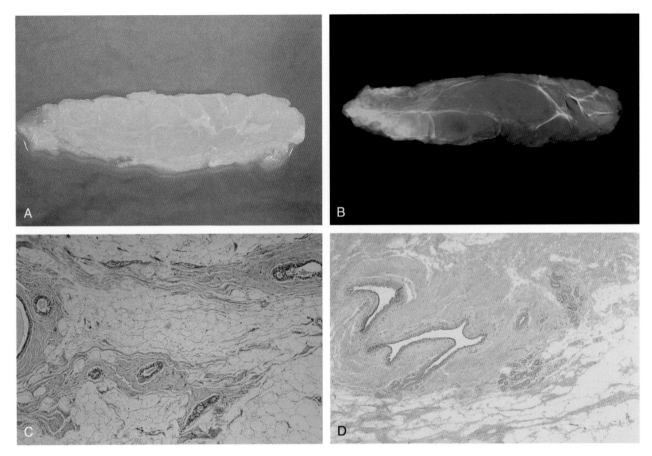

Figure 2–5. *A,* Whole slice of breast from an elderly woman. Eighty percent of women past the age of 65 have breast tissue that is composed of 80% adipose tissue as opposed to dense parenchyma. The remaining parenchyma is widely dispersed in small fibrous strands. *B,* Radiograph of atrophic breast tissue corresponding to whole slice of breast seen in *A.* Once the breast has become predominantly fatty, it is strikingly more amenable to detection of abnormalities by mammogram. *C,* Photomicrograph of postmenopausal, atrophic breast tissue. The terminal duct/lobular units, which formed at the onset of puberty, to a large extent have involuted. The remaining extralobular ducts continue to be surrounded by fibrous connective tissue and may become mildly cystically dilated. *D,* The slings of fibrous connective tissue around the dilated ducts in atrophic breast may result in a "ductal" pattern radiographically.

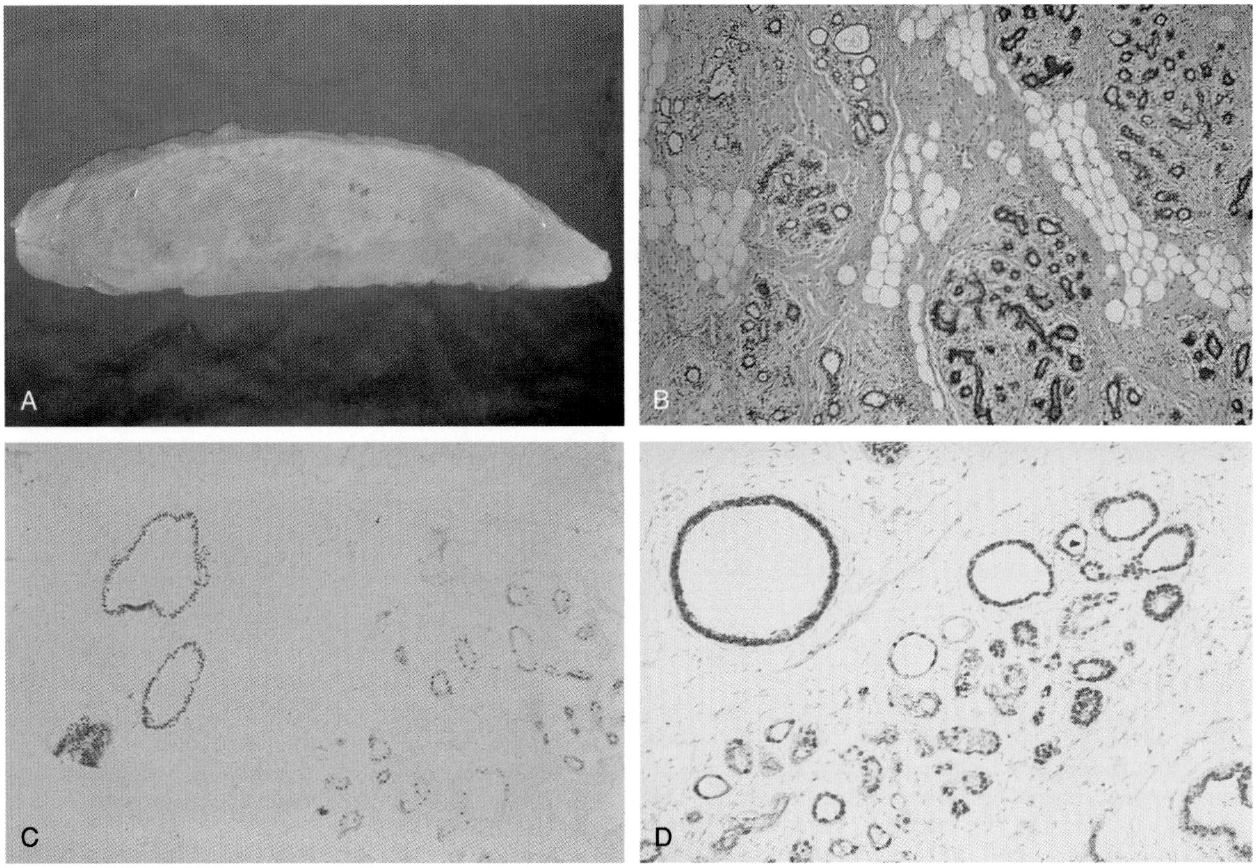

Figure 2–6. Spectrum of minimal change within "normal" breast. *A,* Whole slice of breast tissue in a woman who was clinically entirely lacking in symptoms or signs of breast disease. Small cysts are scattered throughout the breast. This finding may be present in up to 70% of women in the United States.[5] *B,* Photomicrograph of terminal duct/lobular units showing a spectrum of normal to minimal early dilatation of the terminal duct/lobular units. Although this could be construed as early fibrocystic change, it is commonly present in adult women and should not be diagnosed as fibrocystic change of clinical significance. *C, D,* Photomicrographs of breast tissue stained for estrogen receptor protein. A spectrum ranges from small, normal terminal duct/lobular unit structures to those that are minimally cystic. There is usually strong staining for estrogen and progesterone receptor protein in terminal ductules that show early cystic dilatation.[4] In contrast, the relatively normal small ductules show only sparse cells with nuclear staining for estrogen receptor protein.

References

1. Wellings SR, Jensen HM, Marcum RG: An atlas of subgross pathology of the human breast with special reference to possible precancerous lesions. J Natl Cancer Inst 55:231–273, 1975.
2. Wellings SR, Wolfe JN: Correlative studies of the histological and radiographic appearance of the breast parenchyma. Radiology 129:299–306, 1978.
3. Longacre TA, Bartow SB: A correlative morphologic study of human breast and endometrium in the menstrual cycle. Am J Surg Pathol 10:382–393, 1986.
4. Bartow SA: Use of the autopsy to study ontogeny and expression of the estrogen receptor gene in human breast. J Mammary Gland Biol Neoplasia 3:37–48, 1998.
5. Bartow SA, Pathak DR, Black WC, Key CR: Prevalence of benign, atypical, and malignant breast lesions in populations at different risk for breast cancer: A forensic autopsy study. Cancer 60:2751–2760, 1987.

CHAPTER 3

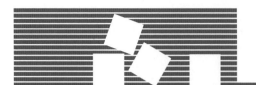

Inflammatory, Infectious, and Other Non-Neoplastic Lesions

Eric S. Wargotz

INTRODUCTION

The amalgam of disorders under this category is broad, many are rare, and they include processes specific to the mammary gland (including various forms of mastitis and duct ectasia, mammary fat necrosis, mammary infarct, lymphocytic mastitis, and granulomatous lobular mastitis), as well as systemic autoimmune and infectious diseases presenting as one or multiple mammary lesions. These systemic disorders include sarcoidosis, amyloidosis, collagen vascular diseases, and others. Infectious diseases include those caused by mycobacterial, fungal, and parasitic organisms. Diagnosis of all these disorders is reliably made only with tissue examination, and the treatment of most is surgical.

Non-neoplastic lesions of the breast most often present clinically as one or more palpable masses or as foci of increased density on a mammogram, raising a suspicion for malignancy and prompting their excision. Once the presence of mammary cancer has been excluded, the benign mammary pathology present may represent a rare view of an undiagnosed systemic disease that is either autoimmune or infectious in nature.

Acknowledgment

I wish to thank the many contributors to the Armed Forces Institute of Pathology and the residents and staff of the George Washington University, Department of Pathology for the contribution of some of the figures. Special thanks go to Drs. Steven G. Silverberg, Stanley Robboy, and Henry J. Norris for access to their material and to my associate, James N. Elliott, for his generous additional service during preparation of this chapter.

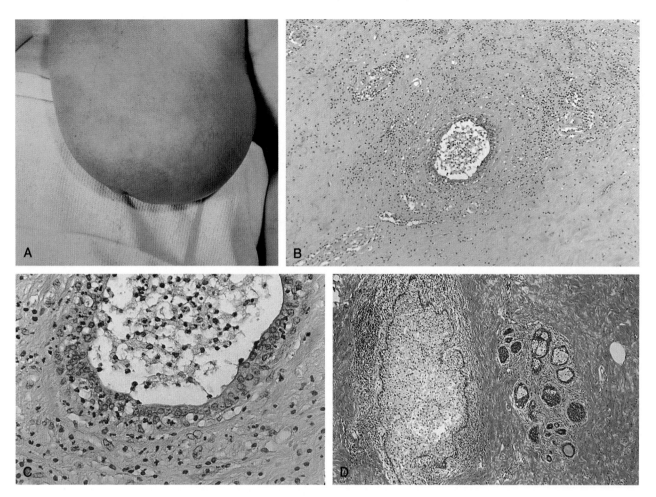

Figure 3–1. Acute mastitis.[1, 2] This condition most commonly occurs in women who are lactating (puerperal mastitis) secondary to a dry, irritated, and cracked nipple-areola complex with subsequent development of an acute bacterial infection, usually *Staphylococcus aureus,* resulting in erythema and exquisite tenderness of the mammary skin *(A).* It may be mistaken clinically for inflammatory carcinoma. Depending on the duration of infection, the mammary stroma may demonstrate edema, increased fibrosis, or both with a moderate to marked mixed inflammatory infiltrate dominated by neutrophils *(B).* Given the portal of entry via the ductal system, it is not surprising that the infiltrate is centered on ducts and lobules, filling them, infiltrating duct walls, and extending into the surrounding stroma *(C).* Antibiotic treatment is usually effective if diagnosis is made early. If left untreated, microabscesses *(D).* may lead to clinically apparent abscesses, fistulas, and persistent infection with sepsis.

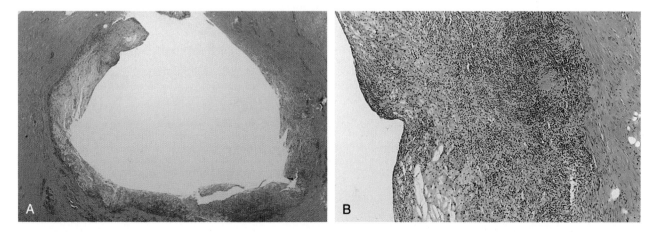

Figure 3–2. Subareolar abscess.[3–5] Occurring predominantly in women of reproductive age without a predilection for lactating women, subareolar abscess develops as a result of squamous metaplasia of one or more lactiferous ducts with subsequent obstruction by cellular material, distention, and rupture *(A).* Keratin debris within the stroma results in inflammation and fibrosis followed by bacterial infection *(B).* Actinomycotic infection is the most common etiology, occurring in lactating women in the postpartum period. Sinus tracts frequently develop, and surgical intervention is often required to control persistent disease.

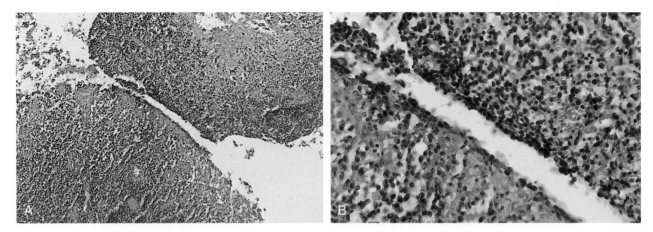

Figure 3–3. Plasma cell mastitis.[6] This unusual form of mastitis develops almost exclusively in parous women, may occur anywhere in the breast, and characteristically produces persistent nipple discharge and nipple retraction. These features coupled with the presence of a firm mass underlying erythematous, often tender skin usually result in a clinical diagnosis of carcinoma. The monotonous appearing infiltrate surrounds and infiltrates ducts, frequently resulting in a markedly attenuated ductal lining or its complete loss *(A)*. Neutrophils and lymphocytes are admixed sparsely throughout the marked plasma cell infiltrate *(B)*. Involvement of lobules is not uncommon. Foreign body giant cells reactive to cellular and lipid material may also be found.

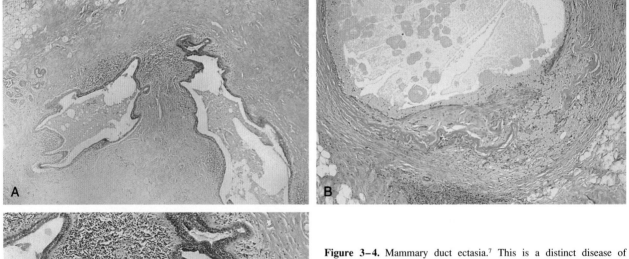

Figure 3–4. Mammary duct ectasia.[7] This is a distinct disease of uncertain pathogenesis identified by the presence of dilated ducts, most often subareolar, with periductal inflammation of variable intensity, periductal fibrosis, and histiocytes within lumens, within walls, and around ducts *(A)*. Stasis of duct contents is generally believed to result in the histologic findings. Women of all ages may be affected, and parity does not appear to be a factor. Mammary duct ectasia is usually subclinical in its early stages but may present with nipple discharge and vague, ill-defined tenderness. As the disease progresses, with resolution of intense inflammation and the development of marked fibrosis, palpable and often mammographically detected lesions are identified. The abundant histiocytes in mammary duct ectasia help define this disease entity and are generally of three types. (1) Lipid-containing foam cells ("colostrum cells") may be admixed with granular or amorphous intraluminal material *(B, C)*.

Illustration continued on opposite page

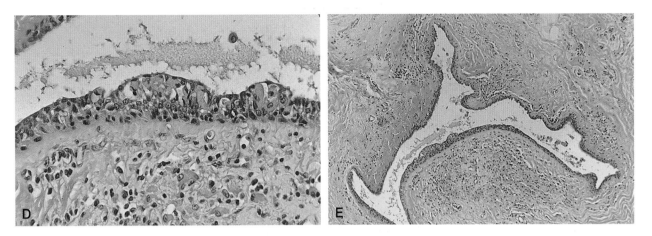

Figure 3–4. *Continued.* (2) Histiocytes with granular eosinophilic cytoplasm are characteristically present admixed with the ductal epithelium and in the surrounding stroma *(D).* (3) Histiocytes with pale amphophilic, yellow- or brown-appearing cytoplasm containing ceroid pigment ("ochrocytes" or "fluorocytes") may be found in the ductal epithelium and in the stroma around ectatic ducts *(E).*

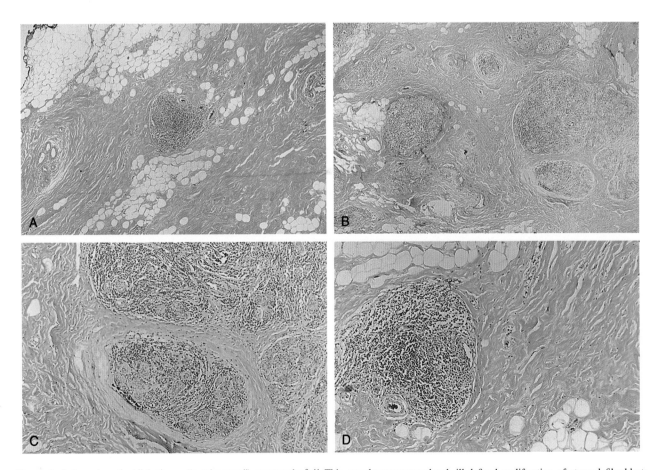

Figure 3–5. Lymphocytic (diabetic, or "autoimmune") mastopathy.[8–11] This grossly nonencapsulated, ill-defined proliferation of stromal fibroblasts and myofibroblasts with keloid-like collagen, lymphocytic perivasculitis, and lymphocytic mastitis (lobulitis dominates) *(A, B)* has been described predominantly in premenopausal women with insulin-dependent diabetes mellitus. Approximately 50% of patients present with bilateral masses. A minority of cases has been described in men and individuals with systemic lupus erythematosus and hypothyroidism. Histologically, proliferative stroma is densely collagenized with foci reminiscent of keloid bands, and lobules are obscured by an intense lymphoid infiltrate *(C, D).* A perivascular lymphoid infiltrate also obscures small blood vessels *(D).* This disease is self-limiting and excision of the nontender mass(es) is adequate treatment.

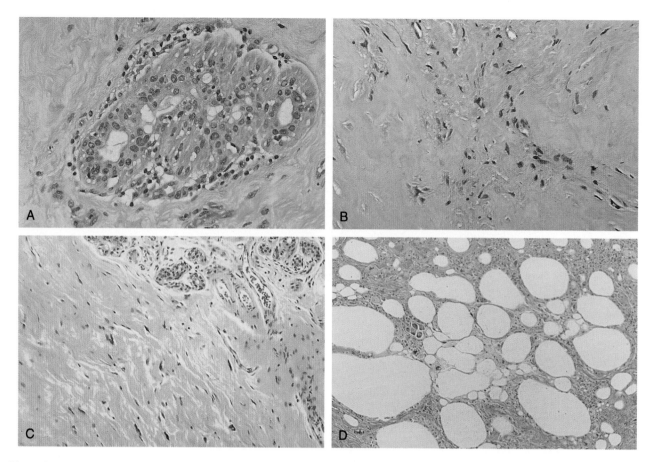

Figure 3–6. Postradiation mastopathy.[12] This condition follows therapeutic radiation of the breast and typically evolves from erythema, inflammation, and atrophy of the mammary skin with subclinical underlying parenchymal changes over a period of months, to clinically apparent diffuse sclerosis and firmness in the following years. Histologic changes typically involve lobules and terminal ducts and consist of increased collagen deposition in the lobular stroma, atrophy and atypical reactive changes of the epithelial lining, and thickened basement membranes *(A)*. Depending on the modes of therapy used, varying degrees of stromal fibrosis *(B)*, some with foci of radiation-induced atypical fibroblasts *(C)*, and fat necrosis are observed *(D)*. The changes are persistent, and excision of densely sclerotic foci may assist in the relief of clinical discomfort.

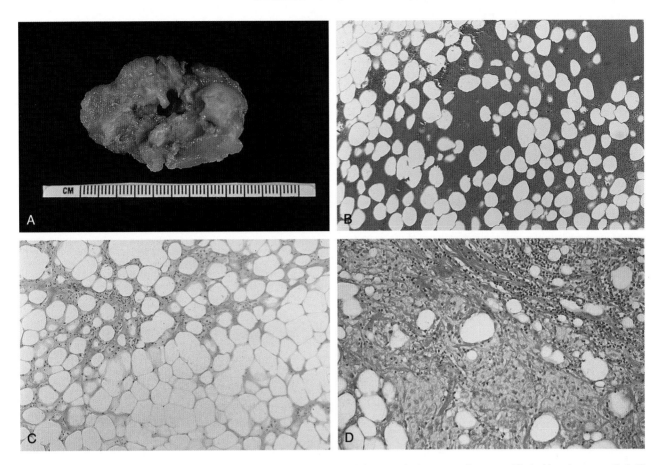

Figure 3–7. Fat necrosis.[13, 14] A traumatic insult precedes the development of fat necrosis; however, often a specific incident is not recalled. The inciting event may be passive and accidental as typically occurs in overweight women and women with large breasts, or it may be attributable to surgery or radiation. Fat necrosis is usually located superficially in the breast and may be fixed to the overlying skin resulting in dimpling that forms a firm palpable mass highly suspicious for carcinoma. Grossly fat necrosis appears relatively well circumscribed, yellow and tan or red with cystic foci *(A)*. Histologically, initial fat cell injury and hemorrhage *(B)* is quickly followed by histiocytic reaction to lipid *(C)* including foreign body type giant cell response *(D)*, a variable inflammatory infiltrate, and eventual fibrotic scarring *(D)*.

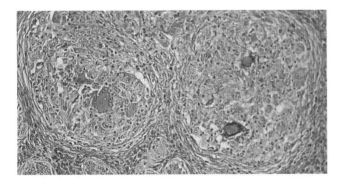

Figure 3–8. Granulomatous ("idiopathic") lobular mastitis.[15, 16] The etiology is unknown; however, a relationship with prior pregnancy has been suggested. The patient usually presents with a tender, palpable hard mass not involving the central or subareolar location. Histologically, the granulomatous inflammation centers in and on lobules with Langhans-type giant cells admixed with plasma cells and lymphocytes. Lobular destruction is present. Foci of fat necrosis, microabscesses, and fibrosis as well as the absence of systemic disease help to distinguish this lesion from sarcoidosis. Organismal special stains are negative. In some patients excision of the lesion is curative, while in others treatment with steroids has been useful to control recurrence.

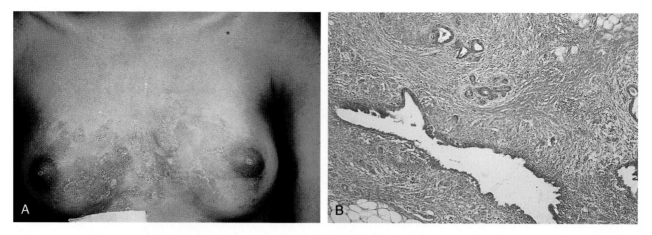

Figure 3–9. Sarcoidosis.[17-19] Patients with breast involvement most often have a known history of systemic involvement by sarcoidosis. Only in rare instances has sarcoidosis presented as a primary lesion of the breast. Clinically, sarcoid involvement of the breast presents as a hard palpable mass or, in some cases, masses with involvement of the overlying skin *(A)*. Histologically, noncaseous granulomatous inflammation containing Langhans-type giant cells is present around ducts and lobules, and destruction of these structures may be seen *(B)*. Unlike granulomatous lobular mastitis, adjacent foci of fat necrosis, abscesses, and reactive fibrosis are absent. Without the use of organismal special stains, it may be impossible to distinguish sarcoidosis from granulomatous inflammation due to tuberculosis or fungal organisms. Sarcoid-type granulomas may be present in association with mammary carcinoma. The ability to control mammary sarcoidosis is related to the effectiveness of therapy in the treatment of the systemic disease.

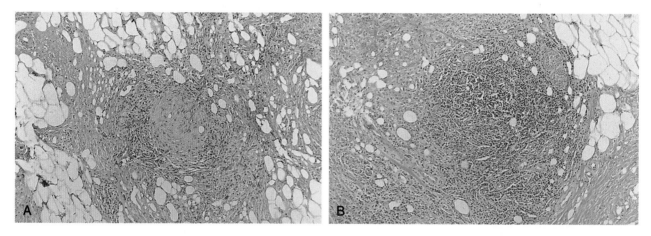

Figure 3–10. Lupus mastitis, Weber-Christian disease, and granulomatous angiopanniculitis.[20-22] These three disorders are rare in the breast and have many common features. All of these recurring lesions develop in a subcutaneous location with involvement of the superficial breast parenchymal tissue, and all have foci of fat necrosis, panniculitis, and a granulomatous component. Common features are shown in *A* and *B* from a case of lupus mastitis. Differentiating features are calcification and immunoglobulin deposits around blood vessels in lupus mastitis; recurrent subcutaneous nodules accompanied clinically by fever, arthralgias, and malaise in Weber-Christian disease; and small blood vessel and capillary perivasculitis in granulomatous angiopanniculitis.

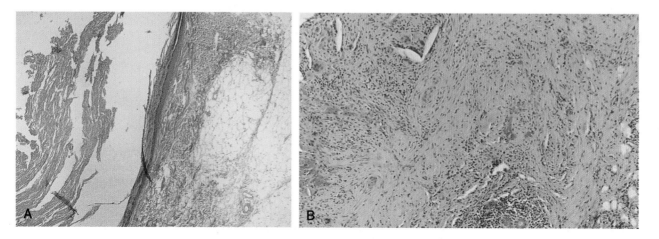

Figure 3–11. Ruptured ducts and inclusion cysts. Although most inclusion cysts are of the epidermal type and occur in association with the mammary skin, mammary ducts, particularly those of the subareolar area, may undergo squamous metaplasia, become obstructed, and form inclusion cysts that are indistinguishable from their epidermal counterparts *(A)*. When inclusion cysts rupture, there is a mixed inflammatory response, and a foreign body granulomatous reaction to the keratin in the stroma results *(B)*.

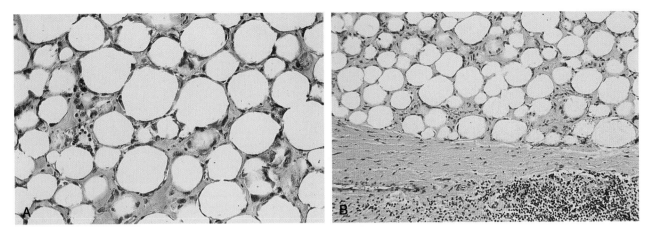

Figure 3–12. Paraffinoma.[23, 24] Injection of paraffin for breast augmentation was not widely used in the United States but remained in favor throughout Asia until silicone was developed and available in the late 1950s and early 1960s. Once injected, the paraffin incites a foreign body giant cell reaction in which a solitary large vacuole occupies much of the giant cell *(A)*. These vacuoles are of relatively uniform appearance, being round and of similar size. Inflammation and fibrosis result in the development of a clinically hard mass *(B)*. Sinus tracts and fistula formation have been reported to result in the discharge of paraffin.

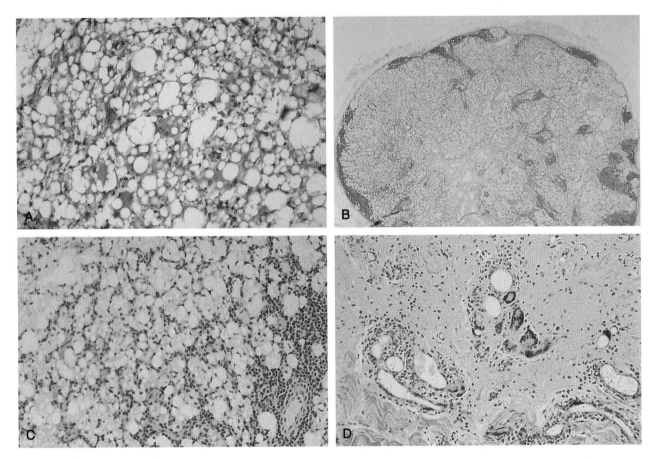

Figure 3–13. Silicone (see also Chapter 13).[24-28] Silicone gel has been used for breast augmentation for nearly 4 decades. Initially it was injected directly into the breast as liquid silicone (dimethylsiloxane) and later the gel was contained in prostheses. Both the injected "free" silicone and leakage of silicone gel from prostheses result in a tissue response sometimes referred to as "silicone mastitis" and "silicone granuloma," consisting of a foreign body giant cell reaction, histiocytic infiltrate, and fat necrosis *(A)*. Unlike the paraffinoma, the spaces created in the giant cells and histiocytes are highly variable in size. The silicone may drain to axillary lymph nodes, and histologically the nodes demonstrate enlargement, marked histiocytic infiltrate containing engulfed silicone, and loss of lymphoid tissue *(B, C)*. Much of the silicone is lost during histologic processing; however, birefringent crystalline material and particulate material may remain, representing silicone itself and additives used in the injectable form and gel *(D)*. Clinically, silicone injections result in a variety of complications including induration and draining sinus tracts, firm masses resulting in deformities, and migration to distant body sites with possible additional sequelae.

Illustration continued on following page

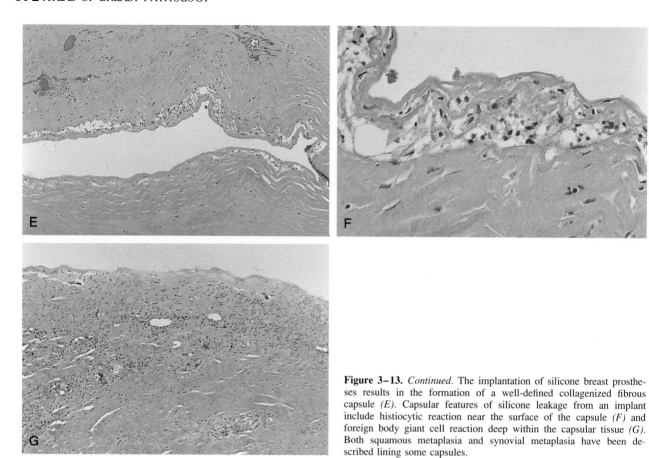

Figure 3–13. *Continued.* The implantation of silicone breast prostheses results in the formation of a well-defined collagenized fibrous capsule *(E).* Capsular features of silicone leakage from an implant include histiocytic reaction near the surface of the capsule *(F)* and foreign body giant cell reaction deep within the capsular tissue *(G).* Both squamous metaplasia and synovial metaplasia have been described lining some capsules.

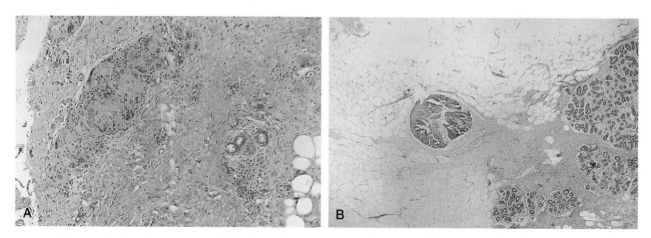

Figure 3–14. Remote suture granuloma. This form of foreign body giant cell reaction is common in the breast subsequent to biopsy or lumpectomy. When a history of prior surgery has not been provided, the finding of a well-formed noncaseous granuloma devoid of foreign material may generate a lengthy list of possible diagnoses *(A).* History should always be sought, particularly when granulomatous inflammation is present. Processing additional tissue may result in the demonstration of calcified remaining suture material *(B).* Well-defined aggregates of multinucleate giant cells with homogeneous finely granular, pink-grey "glassy" appearing cytoplasm embedded within dense fibrotic tissue are typical of remote suture granuloma.

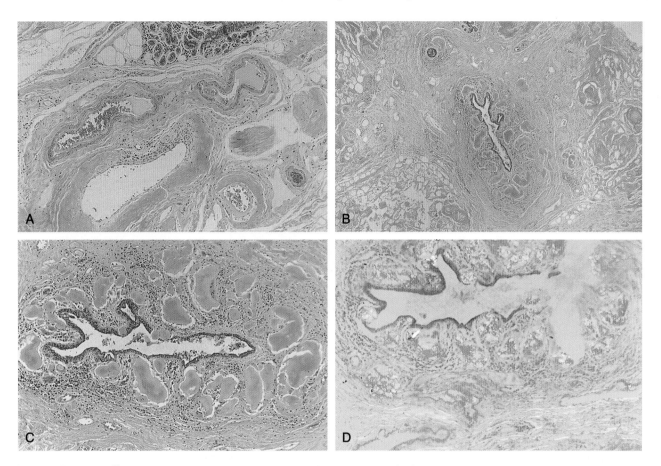

Figure 3–15. Amyloid.[29] Although amyloid may be detected occasionally in the stroma of infiltrating mammary carcinoma, more often its presence is secondary to underlying systemic disease such as systemic primary amyloidosis. In such cases, the amyloid deposits are vascular and perivascular *(A)* as in other organs. Primary amyloid tumor, or "amyloidoma," of the breast is rare. Most of these tumors have been solitary, but cases of multiple and bilateral tumors have been described. Clinically, most patients present with a palpable, hard painless mass. Mammographic calcifications may be present and heighten a clinical suspicion of carcinoma. Total excision is generally curative, but an underlying systemic etiology should be ruled out. The excised mass is usually firm with a grey-white, opalescent or "glassy" cut surface. Histologically, the eosinophilic amyloid is present in the fibrous stroma, fat, blood vessels, and around ducts and lobules *(B, C)*, frequently obliterating them. A lymphoplasmacytic infiltrate of varying intensity may be present and foreign body giant cells are usually present *(B)*. Typical apple-green birefrigence is observed following examination of Congo red–stained sections with polarized light *(D)*.

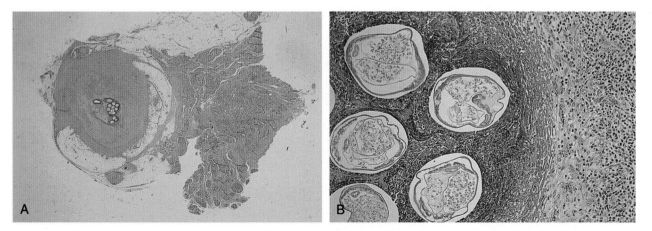

Figure 3–16. Parasites.[30–35] Parasitic infections of the breast are extremely rare and among them, filarial infections are the most common, although cases of *Demodex folliculorum, Loa loa, Schistosoma japonicum, Echinococcus,* and *Taenia* species have been reported. Filariasis involving the breast, most often due to *Wuchereria bancrofti,* usually presents as a solitary, hard, painless, nontender mass fixed to the skin in the upper outer quadrant. Some cases have been reported in patients from Florida; however, most patients are either natives of endemic areas in Africa or individuals who have lived there. Histologically, the granulomatous mass contains adult filarial worms accompanied by a mixed inflammatory infiltrate, including eosinophils *(A, B)*.

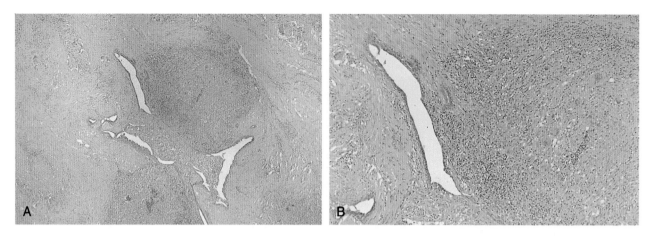

Figure 3–17. Tuberculosis.[36–39] Although tuberculous mastitis has decreased in incidence within the general population of most developed countries, it has been reported in patients with the acquired immunodeficiency syndrome, and in less developed countries it still manifests itself frequently. Atypical mycobacterial infections of the breast are very rare and have been generally associated with prosthestic implants. The clinical presentation of tuberculous mastitis is variable, and it may present as a single, slowly evolving mass; multiple masses; or a diffuse fibrosing process. Nipple discharge is common in all forms. Histologically, the granulomatous inflammation tends to favor ducts over lobules and consists of a mixed inflammatory infiltrate, admixed Langhans giant cells, and periductal fibrosis *(A, B)*. Caseous necrosis and necrosis of the ductal epithelium are frequently present. Acid-fast stains of tissue sections and smears of nipple discharge material may demonstrate organisms; however, culture has been found to be more often diagnostic. Still, in most cases organisms are not demonstrated or recovered, and thus the diagnosis is one of exclusion and patients are treated empirically with appropriate antibiotics.

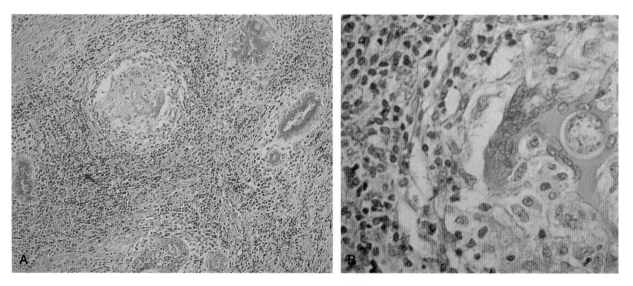

Figure 3–18. Coccidioidomycosis.[40–42] Fungal infections of the breast are exceedingly rare and reported cases include *Histoplasma, Blastomyces, Cryptococcus, Aspergillus,* and *Coccidioides.* Coccidioidomycosis of the breast results in a granulomatous response consisting of foreign body giant cells, Langhans giant cells, mixed inflammatory infiltrate, and fibrosis *(A)*. Giant cells contain the characteristic sporangia *(B)*.

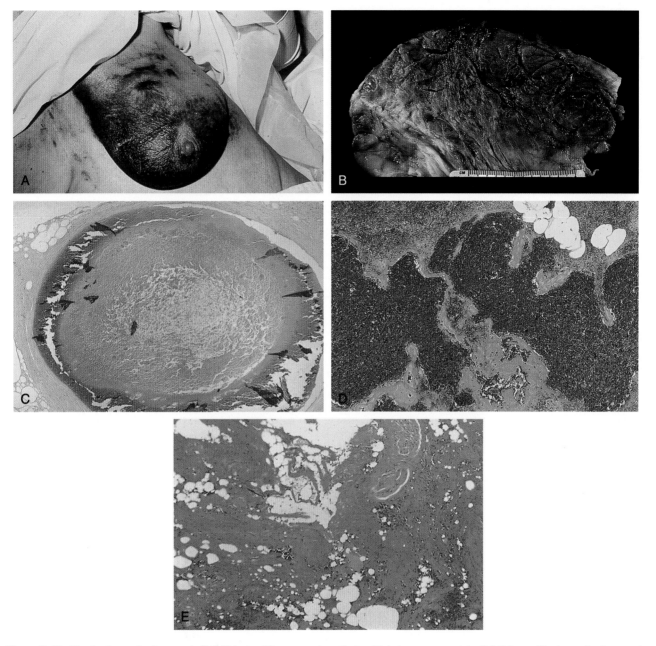

Figure 3–19. Massive hemorrhagic necrosis.[43–49] This condition occurs in patients with heterozygous protein C deficiency. The hemorrhagic necrosis of the breast is usually unilateral and develops within a week of coumarin therapy. The patient develops pain and edema of the breast with the onset of black discoloration and gangrene (A). If there remains any grossly viable portion of the breast, it can be preserved, but all gangrenous tissue requires removal. In many cases, total mastectomy is necessary and on sectioning, the grossly removed breast demonstrates red-brown discoloration with infarction throughout (B). Histologically, thrombi with varying degrees of organization are seen in medium-sized and small blood vessels (C), and hemorrhage and infarction of the mammary tissue occur (D, E). Vasculitis may be present, but it is a secondary development. This is in contrast to thrombophlebitis of the subcutaneous veins of the breast (Mondor's disease) and systemic forms of vasculitis that may present in the breast including giant cell arteritis, Wegener's granulomatosis, and polyarteritis nodosa.

References

1. Eschenbach DA: Acute postpartum infections. Emerg Med Clin North Am 3:87–115, 1985.
2. Rudoy RC, Nelson JD: Breast abscess during the neonatal period: A review. Am J Dis Child 129:1031–1034, 1975.
3. Habif D, Perzin K, Lattes R: Subareolar abscess associated with squamous metaplasia. Am J Surg 119:523–526, 1970.
4. Maier WP, Berger A, Derrick BM: Periareolar abscess in the non-lactating breast. Am J Surg 44:359–361, 1982.
5. Jain BK, Sehgal VN, Jagdish S, et al: Primary actinomycosis of the breast: A clinical review and a case report. J Dermatol 21:497–500, 1994.
6. Parsons WH, Henthorne JC, Clark RL Jr: Plasma cell mastitis. Report of five additional cases. Arch Surg 49:86–89, 1944.
7. Dixon JM, Anderson TJ, Lumsden AB, et al: Mammary duct ectasia. Br J Surg 70:601–603, 1983.
8. Lammie GA, Bobrow LG, Staunton MDM, et al: Sclerosing lymphocytic lobulitis of the breast—evidence for an autoimmune pathogenesis. Histopathology 19:13–20, 1991.

9. Morgan MC, Weaver MG, Crowe JP, Abdul-Karim FW: Diabetic mastopathy: A clinicopathologic study of palpable and nonpalpable breast lesions. Mod Pathol 349–354, 1995.

10. Tomaszewski JE, Brooks JSJ, Hicks D, LiVolsi VA: Diabetic mastopathy: A distinctive clinicopathologic entity. Hum Pathol 23:780–786, 1992.

11. Ely KA, Tse G, Simpson JF, et al: Diabetic mastopathy: A clinicopathologic review. Am J Clin Pathol 113:541–545, 2000.

12. Schnitt SJ, Connolly JL, Harris JR, Cohen RB: Radiation-induced changes in the breast. Hum Pathol 15:545–550, 1984.

13. Bassett LW, Gold RH, Cove HC: Mammographic spectrum of traumatic fat necrosis: The fallibility of "pathognomonic" signs of carcinoma. Am J Roentgenol 130:119–122, 1978.

14. Meyer JE, Silverman P, Gandbhir L: Fat necrosis of the breast. Arch Surg 113:801–805, 1978.

15. Going JJ, Anderson TJ, Wilkinson S, et al: Granulomatous lobular mastitis. J Clin Pathol 40:535–540, 1987.

16. Donn W, Rebbeck P, Wilson C, Gilks CB: Idiopathic granulomatous mastitis. A report of three cases and review of the literature. Arch Pathol Lab Med 118:822–825, 1994.

17. Banik S, Bishop PW, Ormerod LP, O'Brien TEB: Sarcoidosis of the breast. J Clin Pathol 39:446–448, 1986.

18. Fitzgibbons PL, Smiley DF, Kern WH: Sarcoidosis presenting initially as a breast mass: Report of two cases. Hum Pathol 16:851–852, 1985.

19. Oberman HA: Invasive carcinoma of the breast with granulomatous response. Am J Clin Pathol 88:718–721, 1987.

20. Cernea SS, Kihara SM, Sotto MN, Vilela MAC: Lupus mastitis. J Am Acad Dermatol 29:343–346, 1993.

21. Markopoulos CJ, Gogas HJ, Anastassiades OT: Weber-Christian disease with breast involvement. A case report. Breast Dis 7:273–276, 1994.

22. Wargotz ES, Leftkowitz ML: Granulomatous angiopanniculitis of the breast. Hum Pathol 20:1084–1088, 1989.

23. Merckx L, Lamote J, Sacre R: Bilateral ulcerating paraffinoma of the breast in a man. Breast Dis 6:41–44, 1993.

24. Symmers WS: Silicone mastitis in "topless" waitresses and some other varieties of foreign-body mastitis. BMJ 3:19–22, 1968.

25. Hameed MR, Erlandson R, Rosen PP: Capsular synovial-like hyperplasia (CSH) around mammary implants similar to detritic synovitis: A morphologic and immunohistochemical study of 15 cases. Am J Surg Pathol 19:433–438, 1995.

26. Nosanchuk JS: Silicone granuloma of the breast. Arch Surg 97:583–585, 1968.

27. Truong LD, Cartwright J Jr, Goodman MD, Woznick D: Silicone lymphadenopathy associated with augmentation mammoplasty. Am J Surg Pathol 12:484–491, 1988.

28. Barker DE, Retsky MI, Shultz S: "Bleeding" of silicone from bagged breast implants and its clinical relation to fibrous capsule reaction. Plast Reconstr Surg 61:836–841, 1978.

29. Silverman JF, Dabbs DJ, Norris HT, et al: Localized primary (AL) amyloid tumor of the breast. Cytologic, immunohistochemical, and ultrastructural observations. Am J Surg Pathol 10:539–545, 1986.

30. Chen Y, Qun X: Filarial granuloma of the female breast: A histopathological study of 131 cases. Am J Trop Med Hyg 30:1206–1210, 1981.

31. Lang AP, Luchsinger IS, Rawling EG: Filariasis of the breast. Arch Pathol Lab Med 111:757–759, 1987.

32. Ashford RW, Dowse JA, Rogers WN, Powell DEB: Dirofilariasis of the breast. Lancet 1:1198, 1989.

33. Gorman JD, Champaign JL, Sumida FK, Canavan L: Schistosomiasis involving the breast. Radiology 185:423–424, 1992.

34. Kunkel JM, Hawksley CZ: Cysticercosis presenting as a solitary dominant breast mass. Hum Pathol 18:1190–1191, 1987.

35. Vega A, Ortega E, Cavada A, Garijo F: Hydatid cyst of the breast: Mammographic findings. AJR Am J Roentgenol 162:825–826, 1994.

36. Hale JA, Peters GN, Cheek JH: Tuberculosis of the breast: Rare but still extant. Review of the literature and report of an additional case. Am J Surg 150:620–624, 1985.

37. Hartstein M, Leaf HL: Tuberculosis of the breast as a presenting manifestation of AIDS. Clin Infect Dis 15:692–693, 1992.

38. Toranto IR, Malow JB: Atypical mycobacterial periprosthetic infections—diagnosis and treatment. Plast Reconstr Surg 66:226–228, 1980.

39. Lee D, Goldstein EJ, Zarem HA: Localized *Mycobacterium avium-intracellulare* mastitis in an immunocompetent woman with silicone breast implants. Plast Reconstr Surg 95:142–144, 1995.

40. Bocian JJ, Fahmy RN, Michas CA: A rare case of "coccidioidoma" of the breast. Arch Pathol Lab Med 115:1064–1067, 1991.

41. Osborne BM: Granulomatous mastitis caused by histoplasma and mimicking inflammatory breast carcinoma. Hum Pathol 20:47–52, 1989.

42. Seymour EQ: Blastomycosis of the breast. AJR Am J Roentgenol 139:822–823, 1989.

43. Kagan RJ, Glassford GH: Coumadin-induced breast necrosis. Am Surg 47:509–510, 1981.

44. Martin BF, Phillips JD: Gangrene of the female breast with anticoagulant therapy: Report of two cases. Am J Clin Pathol 53:622–626, 1970.

45. Clement PB, Senges H, How AR: Giant cell arteritis of the breast: Case report and review of the literature. Hum Pathol 18:1186–1189, 1987.

46. Dega FJ, Hunder GG: Vasculitis of the breast. Arthritis Rheum 17:973–976, 1974.

47. Tabar L, Dean PB: Mondor's disease: Clinical, mammographic, and pathologic features. Breast 7:18–20, 1982.

48. Jordan JM, Manning M, Allen NB: Wegener's granulomatosis involving the breast. Report of three cases and review of the literature. Am J Med 83:159–164, 1987.

49. Yamashina M, Wilson TK: A mammographic finding in focal polyarteritis nodosa. Br J Radiol 58:91–92, 1985.

CHAPTER 4

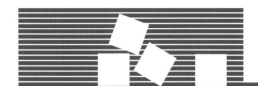

Fibroadenomas, Adenomas, Cystosarcomas, and Hamartomas

Harold A. Oberman

INTRODUCTION

This chapter considers a somewhat heterogeneous group of benign epithelial and periductal stromal tumors whose unifying characteristic is their presentation as a circumscribed mass.

The most common benign mass lesion of the breast is the fibroadenoma. Its histologic growth pattern results from proliferation of both ducts and stroma. Two closely related lesions that are considered concurrently because of their apparent histogenetic relationship are the juvenile fibroadenoma and cystosarcoma phyllodes. The histologic appearance of a fibroadenoma is distinctive. In the typical lesion, the stromal component lacks hypercellularity or cellular atypism, and there is a relatively uniform ratio between stroma and ducts.

The ductal constituents may be compressed and elongated, resulting in an intracanalicular growth pattern, or they may retain their round to oval contour, termed a pericanalicular growth pattern. Such histologic subdivision of these tumors is of questionable value, especially since both patterns often occur in the same tumor. Of greater importance is recognition of the many histologic variations of these patterns.

A variety of benign breast lesions might be considered as adenomas, in that they are circumscribed, may compress adjacent tissue, and are composed of uniform gland-like structures. However, in this setting the designation is particularly problematic. The tubular adenoma, although seemingly fulfilling the criteria of an adenoma, is most likely a variant of a fibroadenoma; the lactating adenoma may represent only an exaggerated area of hyperplasia in a lactating breast; and the ductal adenoma is undoubtedly a variant of an intraductal papilloma.

Cystosarcoma phyllodes has been characterized by a plethora of increasingly complex synonyms. Regardless of the term used for tumors with this growth pattern, it is essential that it convey the pathologist's assessment of histologic malignancy. The benign tumors might well be considered as cellular fibroadenomas, while those with clear-cut malignant characteristics can be termed periductal sarcomas.[1] The distinguishing diagnostic feature of these lesions is their pronounced stromal cellularity. This may vary to a considerable extent in individual tumors so that some areas of tumor may be comparable to a fibroadenoma, while in other areas of tumor the stromal hypercellularity may be remarkable.

In contrast to the stromal proliferation in cystosarcoma phyllodes, the ductal epithelium usually lacks significant proliferative activity. The ducts may be elongated and compressed in a manner exaggerating the pattern of an intracanalicular fibroadenoma. Moreover, the stromal proliferation focally results in invagination of ductal epithelium, producing a papilloma-like appearance. The latter gives the tumor its long-recognized leaflike pattern. Perhaps the most important consideration in assessing prognosis is the adequacy of excision of the tumor. Tumors that involve the margin of surgical removal, even if they have a uniformly benign, albeit cellular, stroma, have a propensity for recurrence.

Hamartomas may consist solely of dense connective tissue that dissects mammary lobules, resulting in attenuation of ducts suggestive of postmenopausal mammary involution or of a gynecomastia-like appearance. Other types of these tumors contain a fibrofatty stroma, resulting in an adenolipomatous appearance. Adenolipomas of the breast are best considered as variants of hamartomas.[2] Occasional hamartomas contain smooth muscle amid the fibrous connective tissue, and another variant pattern is the presence of islands of mature hyaline cartilage in the fibrofatty stroma.

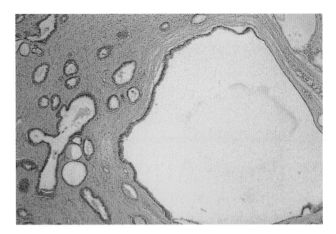

Figure 4–1. Fibrocystic changes in fibroadenoma. Because fibroadenomas are derived from the terminal duct/lobular unit of the breast, it is not surprising that fibrocystic changes often occur in these tumors. Cystically dilated ducts with apocrine metaplasia of the ductal epithelium are seen in this case.

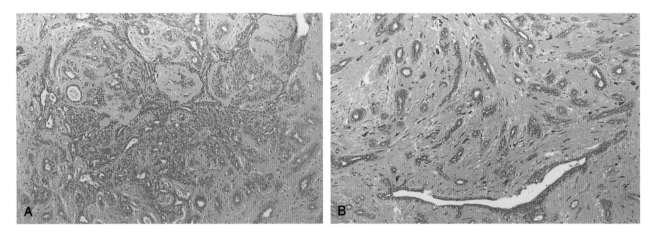

Figure 4–2. Adenosis in fibroadenoma. Adenosis usually involves only a portion of the fibroadenoma, and rarely the entire tumor. *A,* As in adenosis elsewhere in the breast, ducts at the periphery of the lesion are more ectatic than those occurring centrally. Recognition of adenosis is facilitated by noting the presence of both myoepithelium and epithelium in the area of the tumor in question. *B,* With attenuation of the ductal component the growth pattern of adenosis may provoke greater concern, and it may possibly be confused with carcinoma, especially on frozen section.[3]

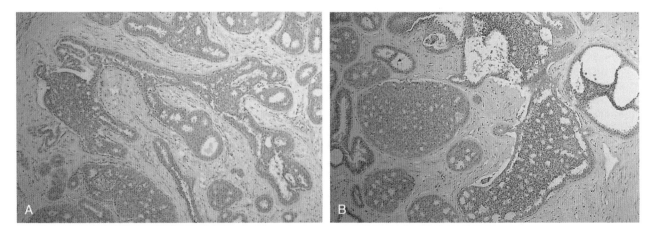

Figure 4–3. Intraductal hyperplasia in fibroadenoma. *A,* Foci of intraductal epithelial proliferation in a fibroadenoma are equivalent to such changes elsewhere in the breast. Histologic criteria for evaluating such areas in the tumor do not differ from those employed elsewhere, although the distinctive pattern of epithelial hyperplasia in the elongated ducts of the fibroadenoma may cause confusion. *B,* The intraductal epithelial proliferation may be associated with ectasia of the involved ducts.

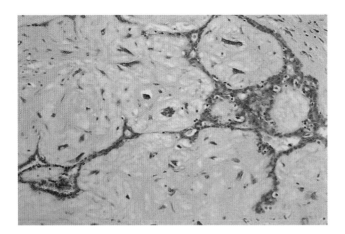

Figure 4–4. Giant cells in fibroadenoma. A peculiar stromal change in these tumors is the presence of multinucleated giant cells. This uncommon finding is comparable to the occasional presence of these benign cells elsewhere in the mammary stroma. They are illustrated only to avoid their mischaracterization as malignant by the unwary observer.

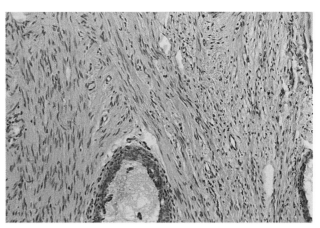

Figure 4–6. Leiomyomatous stroma in fibroadenoma. Smooth muscle is evident in this microscopic field, and its presence was confirmed by a postive stain for muscle actin. Metaplastic change in fibroadenomas is unusual, most often represented by lipomatous foci. Osteochondroid and squamous metaplasia are more commonly seen in cellular periductal stromal tumors (cystosarcomas).

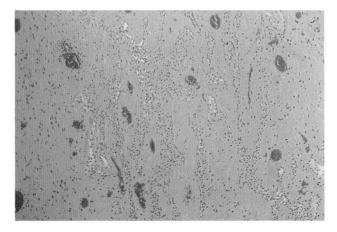

Figure 4–5. Infarct in fibroadenoma. Coagulation necrosis is seen in this section, which usually is associated with a peripheral inflammatory response. Mammary infarcts are more often seen in intraductal papillomas or in hyperplastic lobules of breasts in pregnant or postpartum patients.[4]

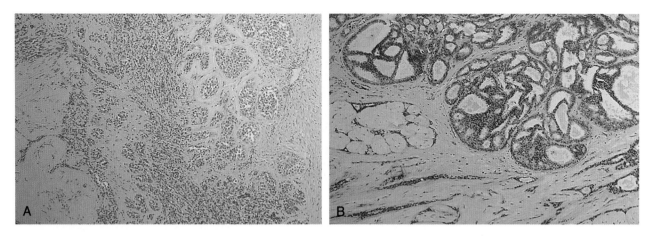

Figure 4–7. Carcinoma in fibroadenoma. Either ductal carcinoma in situ or lobular carcinoma in situ may first be noted in fibroadenomas. The diagnosis of primary noninvasive carcinoma in a fibroadenoma can be made only after excluding the presence of neoplasm elsewhere in the breast, especially in the same quadrant. Lobular carcinoma in situ *(A)* is more common in this situation than is ductal carcinoma in situ *(B)*. Both forms of noninvasive carcinoma have the microscopic characteristics comparable to those seen elsewhere in the breast.

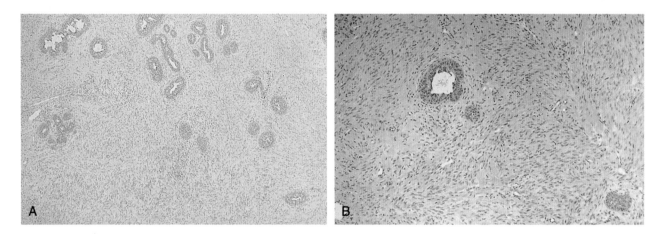

Figure 4–8. Juvenile fibroadenoma. *A,* The predominant microscopic finding is the remarkable stromal cellularity, which contrasts with the cellularity of the ordinary fibroadenoma. Moreover, these tumors lack the fibrotic, or mucinous, stroma of ordinary fibroadenomas. The stromal cells are uniform and lack increased mitotic activity. *B,* In contrast to cystosarcomas, there is absence of cellular atypism of the stromal component and a uniform relation between ducts and stroma without evidence of stromal overgrowth.

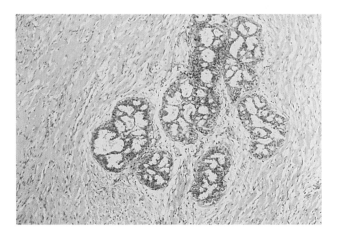

Figure 4–9. Juvenile fibroadenoma. Intraductal epithelial proliferation may be a prominent feature, and the myoepithelial layer is prominent. Such epithelial proliferation is characteristic of juvenile fibroadenomas, and is less common in cystosarcoma phyllodes.

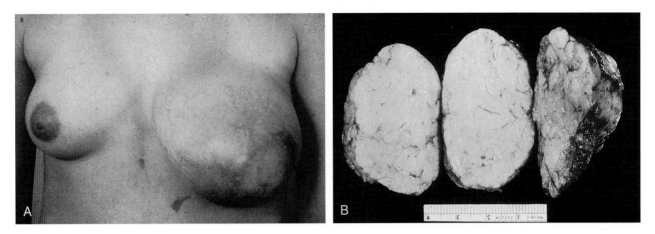

Figure 4–10. Juvenile fibroadenoma. *A,* The rapid growth of the tumor may result in marked asymmetry of the breasts as in this young patient. This is especially remarkable in patients who may be at the age of menarche and who otherwise have only early breast development. In contrast, physiologic, or "virginal" hypertrophy results in bilateral breast enlargement. *B,* The juvenile fibroadenoma removed from this patient is sharply circumscribed, and slitlike spaces are visible on its cut surface.

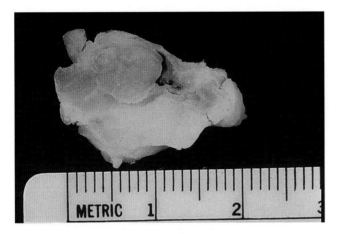

Figure 4–11. Tubular adenoma. These tumors are characteristically sharply circumscribed and tan.

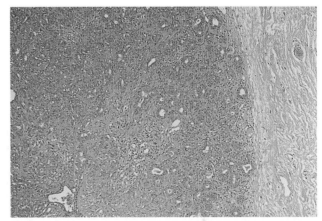

Figure 4–12. Tubular adenomas are distinguished by their circumscription and the uniformity of their tubular component. They differ from tubular carcinoma by the haphazard arrangement in the latter of oval to angulated ducts and by the absence of a myoepithelial layer surrounding ducts in tubular carcinoma.

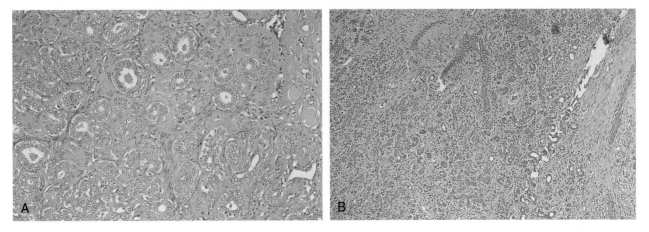

Figure 4–13. Tubular adenoma. *A,* These tumors have a homogeneous microscopic appearance, consisting of a circumscribed collection of ducts of relatively uniform size and shape. The ducts are lined by epithelium and surrounding myoepithelium, and the epithelial cells lack atypism or significant mitotic activity. Cytoplasmic vacuolation of the epithelial cells is not prominent, although eosinophilic secretion may be present in occasional duct lumens. The tumor is distinguished from a fibroadenoma by the relative paucity of stroma and the prominence and uniformity of its ductal component. *B,* Occasional compressed and elongated ducts are often seen in these tumors, suggesting the intracanalicular pattern of a fibroadenoma. It is likely that thorough sampling of these tumors would reveal such foci more frequently, supporting the close relation of the two tumors.

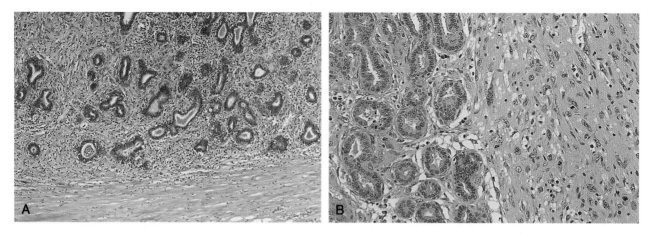

Figure 4–14. Malignant change in tubular adenoma. *A,* This 10-cm-diameter mass manifested rapid clinical growth and had the epithelial pattern of a tubular adenoma, but the stromal proliferation between the uniform ducts had histologic changes of malignancy. *B,* A proliferation of spindle cells, manifesting cellular pleomorphism and increased mitotic activity, was present in some areas of the tumor. If one accepts the likelihood that cystosarcoma phyllodes arises in a preexisting fibroadenoma, a possibility reinforced by the frequent history in these patients of rapid increase in size of a preexisting stable mass, the same association would be appropriate for a tubular adenoma.

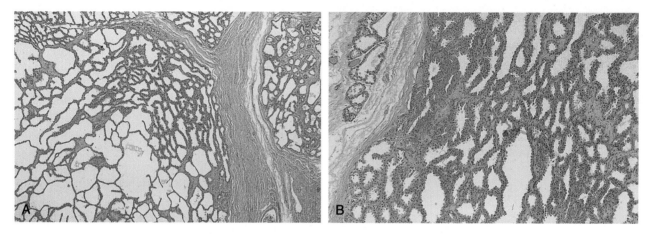

Figure 4–15. Lactational adenoma. These tumors present in pregnant or postpartum women as freely mobile masses that characteristically are tan or yellow. On occasion they may be multifocal. It is debatable whether they should be considered as a true adenoma or rather as a localized area of lobular hyperplasia in a gestational breast. *A,* The lesions consist of enlarged lobules with ectatic acini. Especially in postpartum patients, visible secretion may be absent. *B,* The acini are lined by cells with abundant, often vacuolated, cytoplasm that results in a hobnailed appearance.

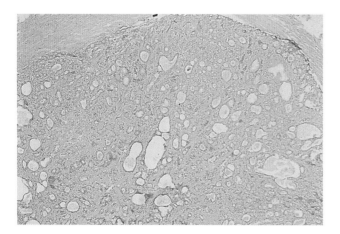

Figure 4–16. Ductal adenoma. These relatively common lesions occur as discrete gray to white nodules that likely are related to intraductal papillomas.[5] The proliferation is sharply circumscribed, and the ducts at the periphery are lined by both epithelium and myoepithelium, have a clearly defined basement membrane, and lack cellular pleomorphism or prominent mitotic activity.

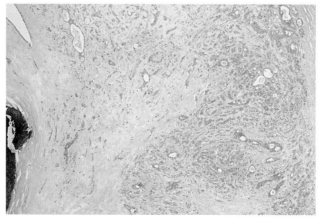

Figure 4–17. Ductal adenoma. Central sclerosis is characteristic of these tumors, occasionally, as in this tumor, with associated calcification. The periphery of the tumor is to the right.

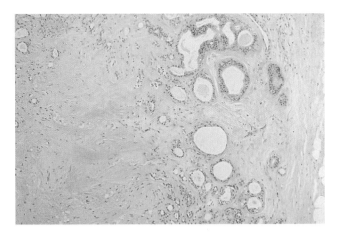

Figure 4–18. Ductal adenoma. Focal apocrine metaplasia of ductal epithelium and ductal attenuation is present in the sclerotic center of this tumor.

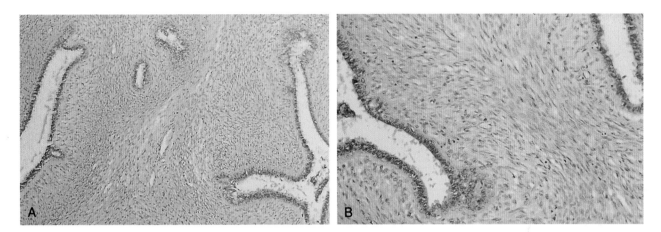

Figure 4–19. Benign cystosarcoma phyllodes. *A,* This figure illustrates the stromal cellularity that is the distinguishing diagnostic feature of these lesions. This feature may vary within individual tumors, necessitating thorough sampling before one provides a final microscopic interpretation. *B,* The stromal cells in benign tumors lack cellular pleomorphism. The diagnosis of malignancy is based on the degree of stromal abnormality, which is evidenced by atypism and increased mitotic activity as well as stromal overgrowth, the latter implying absence of epithelial structures in a low-power (×40) microscopic field. Mitotic activity may be focally evident in benign tumors, as is seen in this figure, especially adjacent to ducts.

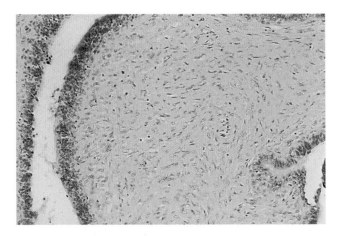

Figure 4–20. Benign cystosarcoma phyllodes. In contrast to the stromal proliferation, the ductal epithelium usually lacks significant proliferative activity. In most instances, the ducts are elongated and compressed in a manner exaggerating the pattern of an intracanalicular fibroadenoma. This appearance may result in grossly recognizable slits and in the characteristic leaflike growth pattern that gives the tumor its name.

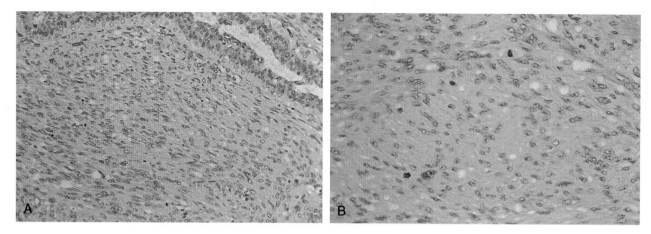

Figure 4–21. Malignant cystosarcoma phyllodes. *A* and *B,* Malignancy in this neoplasm is denoted by cellular crowding, atypism, and increased mitotic activity, especially at the periphery of the tumor.[6] Ductal epithelial abnormality is absent.

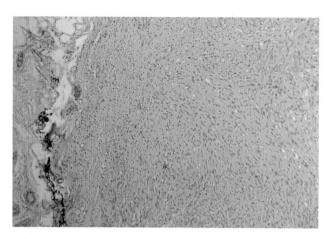

Figure 4–22. Malignant cystosarcoma phyllodes. Stromal overgrowth at the periphery of this tumor is indicative of malignancy. Also note the proximity of the inked margin of excision to the border of the neoplasm. A uninvolved breast margin of at least 1 cm is desirable.

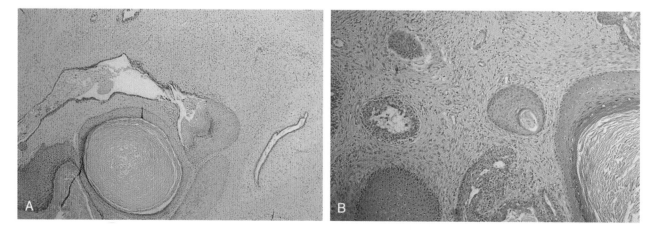

Figure 4–23. Metaplasia in cystosarcoma phyllodes. Squamous metaplasia of ductal epithelium may be associated with formation of abundant keratin, resulting in a distinctive growth pattern that has been likened to that of a cholesteatoma. Squamous metaplasia may occur in both benign *(A)* and malignant *(B)* neoplasms. In *B* the stromal atypism indicates the malignancy of the tumor.

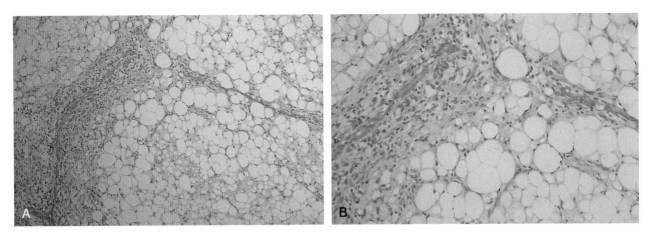

Figure 4–24. Stromal metaplasia in cystosarcoma phyllodes. *A,* In this benign tumor the nucleated lipocytic metaplasia is suggestive of a well-diffentiated liposarcoma. Small islands of mature fat may occur in these tumors, as they do in fibroadenomas.[7] *B,* Stromal cells immediately adjacent to the ductal component usually lack adipose differentiation. Even tumors with a pleomorphic liposarcomatous stroma, with high-grade histologic findings, are associated with an excellent prognosis if they are completely removed with adequate margins.

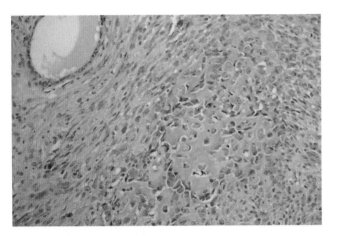

Figure 4–25. Stromal metaplasia in cystosarcoma phyllodes. Osteoid metaplasia in association with changes of stromal malignancy. Osteoid and chondroid metaplasia may also be seen and, on rare occasion, may be a prominent feature of the tumor. Isolated examples of leiomyosarcoma or rhabdomyosarcoma, seemingly presenting as a component of a cystosarcoma, have also been reported. Such metaplastic change has been noted in both benign and malignant tumors.

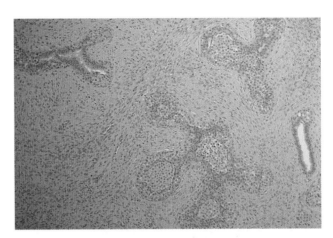

Figure 4–27. Carcinoma in cystosarcoma phyllodes. Lobular carcinoma in situ (LCIS) presents in this uncommon setting. The significance of LCIS or ductal carcinoma in situ (DCIS) in these tumors is comparable to epithelial neoplastic change in a fibroadenoma.

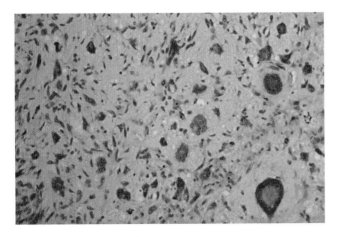

Figure 4–26. Malignant cystosarcoma phyllodes. Multinucleated giant cells are seen in the stroma of a malignant tumor.

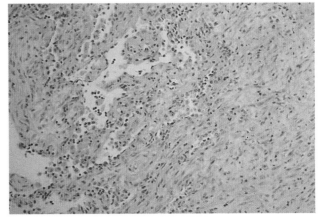

Figure 4–28. Metastatic cystosarcoma phyllodes involving lung. These tumors spread hematogenously, and metastatic involvement of axillary lymph nodes is extremely unusual. Metastases may consist solely of the neoplastic stromal component of the tumor or, less often, may contain both ducts and stroma.

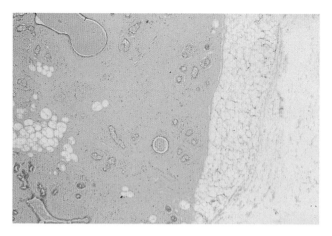

Figure 4–29. Hamartoma. This sharply circumscribed tumor manifests abundant hyalinizing fibrosis that separates the ducts, and also has a small central area of fat. The radiographic picture may indicate greater circumscription than may be apparent on gross examination. Attenuation of ducts due to the fibrosis may result in a microscopic pattern suggestive of postmenopausal mammary involution or a gynecomastia-like appearance.

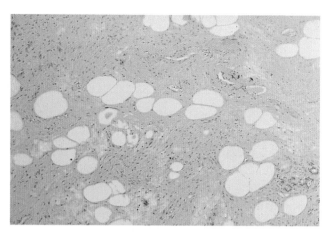

Figure 4–31. Hamartoma. This tumor is composed of smooth muscle and fat surrounding separated ducts.

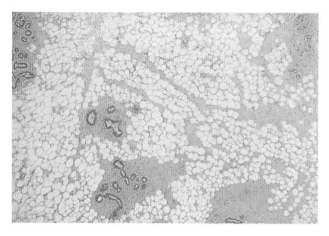

Figure 4–30. Hamartoma. An adenolipomatous pattern results in a tumor that may be clinically difficult to distinguish. Adenolipomas of the breast are best considered as variants of hamartomas. The recognition of this growth pattern is abetted by appreciating that fat is absent from intralobular connective tissue and also is an unusual constituent of fibroadenomas.

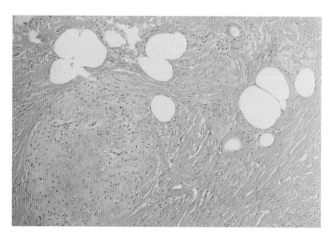

Figure 4–32. Hamartoma. Islands of mature hyaline cartilage, as well as mature fat and fibrous tissue, constitute this tumor.

References

1. Rosen PP, Oberman HA: Tumors of the breast. In Atlas of Tumor Pathology, Series 3, Fascicle 7. Washington, DC, Armed Forces Institute of Pathology, 1993.
2. Oberman HA: Hamartomas and hamartoma variants of the breast. Semin Diag Path 6:135–145, 1989.
3. Oberman HA: Benign lesions of breast confused with carcinoma. In McDivitt R, Oberman HA, Ozello L (eds): The Breast. New York, Williams & Wilkins, 1984, pp 1–33.
4. Flint A, Oberman HA: Infarction and squamous metaplasia of intraductal papilloma. A benign breast lesion that may simulate carcinoma. Hum Pathol 15:764–767, 1984.
5. Lammie GA, Millis RR: Ductal adenoma of the breast—a review of fifteen cases. Hum Pathol 20:903–908, 1989.
6. Moffat CJC, Pinder SE, Dixon AR, et al: Phyllodes tumours of the breast: A clinciopathological review of thirty-two cases. Histopathology 27:205–218, 1995.
7. Rosen PP, Romain K, Liberman L: Mammary cystosarcoma with mature adipose stromal differentiation (lipophyllodes tumor) arising in a lipomatous hamartoma. Arch Pathol Lab Med 118:91–94, 1994.

CHAPTER 5

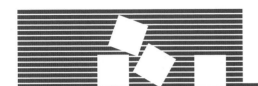

Nipple Adenoma/Subareolar Papillomatosis and Benign Adnexal/ Salivary Gland Type Tumors

Mirka W. Jones

INTRODUCTION

The nipple consists of elastic tissue containing large collecting ducts, bundles of smooth muscle, and sensory nerves. It is elevated and surrounded by the areola. The stratified squamous epithelium overlying the nipple and areola contains numerous apocrine and sebaceous glands, and at the periphery of the areola, hair follicles. Tumors of the nipple are rare and originate from the collecting ducts, from surrounding smooth muscle, or from the adnexal structures of the overlying skin.

Nipple duct adenoma (NDA) or subareolar papillomatosis usually presents as a subareolar mass that can be associated with nipple discharge, ulceration, and pain.[1-5] Although at low power an NDA shows a vague nodular architecture, the margins are ill-defined with irregular ductal structures extending into the surrounding breast tissue. The ducts in NDA are lined by epithelial and myoepithelial cells and may contain florid intraductal hyperplasia or intraductal papillary proliferations (Table 5–1).

Infiltrating syringomatous adenoma of the nipple (ISA) microscopically resembles syringoma of the skin and also presents as a firm, raised mass.[6-8] The overlying skin may be hyperkeratotic, but it shows no evidence of the ulceration often associated with NDA (Table 5–2). Pain, tenderness, or discharge from the nipple are also uncommon.

Adenomyoepithelioma (AME) and myoepitheliosis originate from myoepithelial cells and can occur in the nipple as well as elsewhere in the breast.[1-3, 9-11] Although adenomyoepithelioma usually presents as a palpable, well-circumscribed mass, myoepitheliosis is often grossly undetected except for the induration of mammary tissue. Serous discharge has been reported in patients with adenomyoepithelioma of the nipple.

Pleomorphic adenoma (PA), also known as benign mixed tumor, is a rare lesion that can occur in the nipple and subareolar region of the breast.[1-3, 12, 13] It is usually well circumscribed and shows a mixture of epithelial and myoepithelial elements as well as cartilage and bone. It is recognized by some as a variant of intraductal papilloma.

Other salivary gland type lesions that may be encountered in the breast include adenoid cystic carcinoma (discussed in Chapter 11) and rarer malignant tumors such as acinic cell carcinoma.

Table 5–1

VARIANTS OF NIPPLE DUCT ADENOMA AND SUBAREOLAR PAPILLOMATOSIS

Adenosis pattern	Resembles sclerosing adenosis: consists of crowded ducts lined by a double cell layer with no significant intraductal hyperplasia
Proliferative pattern	Shows crowded ducts containing florid benign intraductal hyperplasia; sometimes central necrosis and occasional mitotic figures
Papillomatosis and sclerosing papillomatosis pattern	Shows distended ducts with prominent papillary proliferations: Reactive fibrosis of the surrounding stroma may cause entrapment and distortion of some ducts, and may create a worrisome pattern of pseudoinfiltration

Table 5–2

HISTOLOGIC DIFFERENCES BETWEEN NIPPLE
DUCT ADENOMA (NDA) AND INFILTRATING
SYRINGOMATOUS ADENOMA (ISA)

NDA	ISA
Vague circumscription	Diffusely infiltrating pattern
Involvement of collecting ducts	Infiltrates around collecting ducts without direct involvement
Absence of smooth muscle and perineural invasion	Perineural and smooth muscle invasion often present
Can cause ulceration of the skin	Skin often hyperkeratotic but not ulcerated

Leiomyoma of the nipple is uncommon and is usually associated with the erector muscle.[14, 15] It consists of ill-defined bundles of smooth muscle that blend irregularly with the surrounding collagen.

Although nipple duct adenoma, infiltrating syringomatous adenoma, adenomyoepithelioma, pleomorphic adenoma, and leiomyoma are benign, they may recur if excision is incomplete. Myoepithelial carcinomas are rare and malignant.

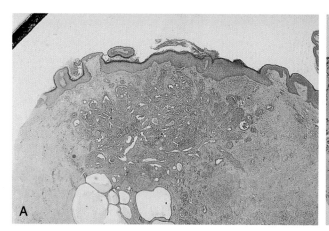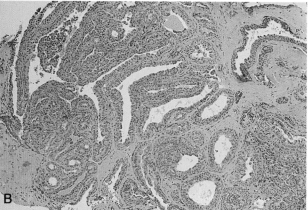

Figure 5–1. Nipple duct adenoma. *A,* The low-power view shows a superficially located and vaguely circumscribed nodular complex arrangement of ducts of different sizes and shapes.[1–5] *B,* Some ducts are small and compressed, and others have open lumens and may contain benign intraductal hyperplasia or papillary proliferations. (See Table 5–1 and Figures 5–2 to 5–5 for other specific patterns.)

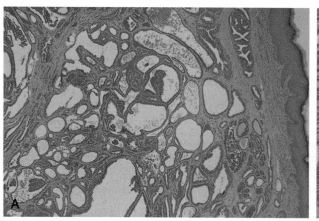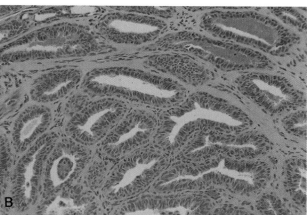

Figure 5–2. Nipple duct adenoma, adenosis type. *A,* The low-power view shows multiple ducts forming a rounded superficial nodule. There is no significant intraductal hyperplasia or papillary proliferation. *B,* Each duct is lined by an epithelial and myoepithelial cell layer.

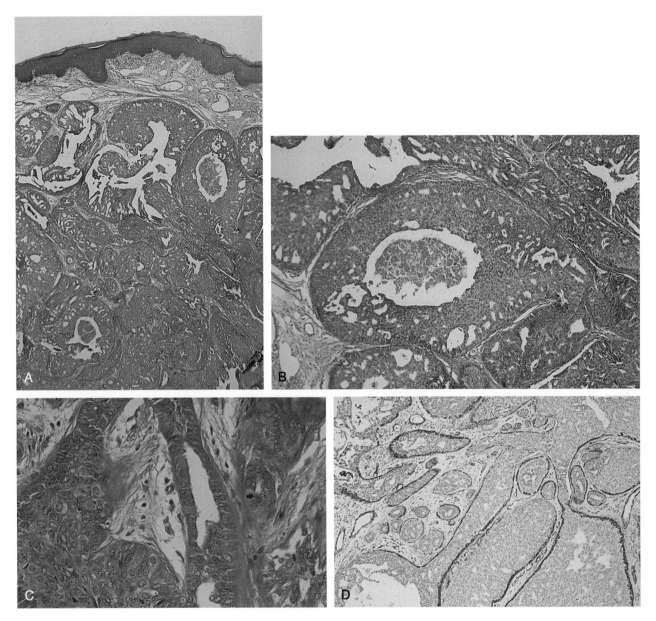

Figure 5–3. Nipple duct adenoma, proliferative type. *A,* The superficial arrangement of crowded and distended ducts shows florid benign intraductal hyperplasia. *B,* Some ducts reveal comedo-type necrosis and focal atypia. *C,* Scattered mitotic figures can also be identified. *D,* Immunostaining for smooth muscle actin highlights the presence of myoepithelial cells around the individual ducts and supports a benign interpretation for this lesion.

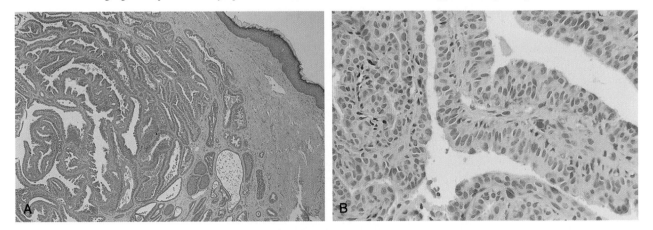

Figure 5–4. Nipple duct adenoma, papillomatosis type. *A,* Dilated ducts in the center of this lesion show multiple papillary structures projecting into the lumens. *B,* The double cell layer is easily identified within the papillary proliferations.

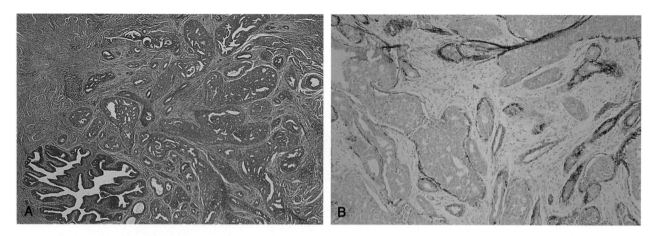

Figure 5–5. Nipple duct adenoma (NDA), sclerosing papillomatosis type. *A,* Reactive fibrosis and chronic inflammation within an NDA can cause distortion of ducts and may create a worrisome pattern mimicking infiltrating duct carcinoma. *B,* Immunostaining for smooth muscle actin helps to identify the double cell layer and to confirm the benign nature of this lesion.[16]

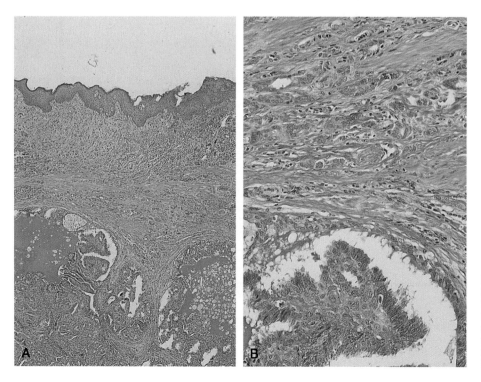

Figure 5–6. Nipple duct adenoma (NDA) associated with infiltrating duct carcinoma. *A, B,* The simultaneous occurrence of NDA and carcinoma is rare.[17] The figure shows small clusters and nests of atypical cells infiltrating fibrous stroma between the NDA and the epidermis.

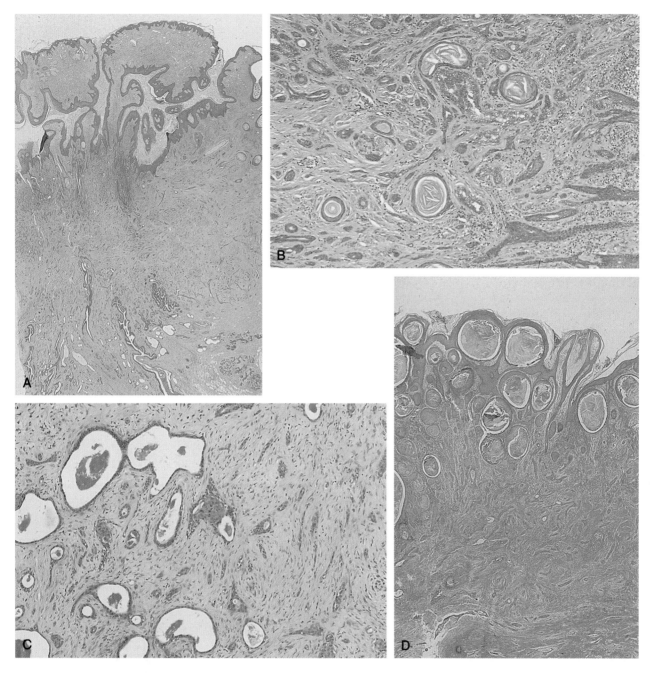

Figure 5–7. Infiltrating syringomatous adenoma (ISA). *A,* Despite the clinical presentation as a discrete nipple mass, microscopic examination of this ISA shows a diffusely infiltrating lesion (see Table 5–2).[1–3, 6–8] *B,* The haphazardly arranged ducts, cords, and keratin-filled cysts involve the skin and proliferate around collecting ducts. The presence of both an epithelial and myoepithelial layer and the superficial location help to differentiate this lesion from tubular carcinoma. *C,* The ducts in ISA are of variable size. Some are dilated and contain eosinophilic amorphous debris, others are compressed and have comma-like tails. Scattered around are single strands of ductal epithelium. The stroma is pale, cellular, and reactive. *D,* The overlying skin in ISA is often hyperkeratotic and shows prominent keratin-filled cysts.

Illustration continued on following page

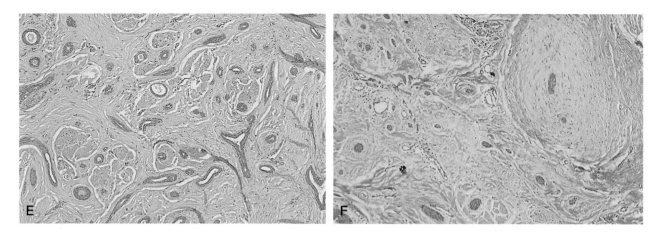

Figure 5–7. *Continued. E,* ISA often infiltrates smooth muscle (erector muscle) of the nipple. *F,* Perineural invasion may also be found within ISA.

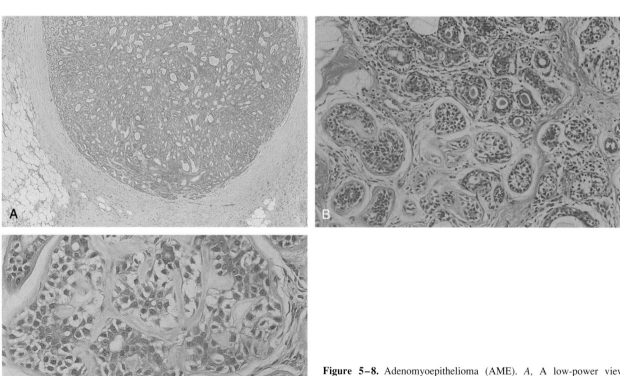

Figure 5–8. Adenomyoepithelioma (AME). *A,* A low-power view shows a well-circumscribed nodule surrounded by a rim of fibrous tissue.[1–3, 9–12] *B,* Another example of adenomyoepithelioma showing a mixture of tubular structures and solid aggregates of myoepithelial cells. *C,* High-power view shows small tubules in AME lined by an inner layer of deeply eosinophilic epithelial cells and an outer layer of prominent myoepithelial cells with abundant clear cytoplasm.

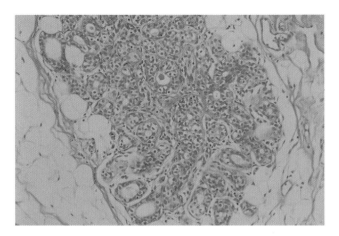

Figure 5–9. Myoepitheliosis. The diffuse myoepithelial proliferation typically involves a terminal ductal-lobular unit. Prominent myoepithelial cells in this figure are present around and in between the ductules.

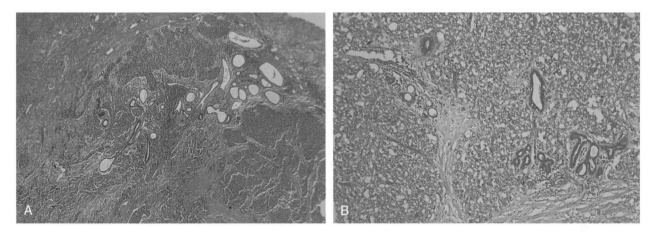

Figure 5–10. Myoepithelial carcinoma. *A,* A low-power photomicrograph shows small nests and large sheets of infiltrating tumor. *B,* At high power some ducts are preserved, while others are overgrown by the proliferation of atypical myoepithelial cells.

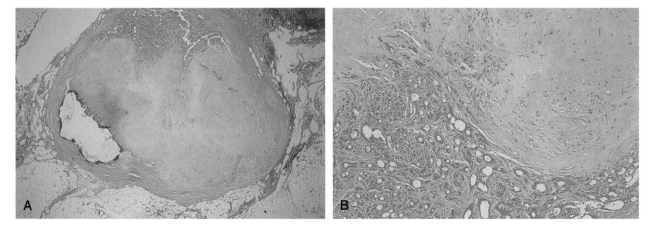

Figure 5–11. Pleomorphic adenoma. *A,* A low-power view shows a well-circumscribed margin, lobulated architecture, and a mixture of osseous, cartilaginous, epithelial, and myoepithelial elements.[1–3, 12, 13] *B,* Chondroid matrix and scattered epithelial and myoepithelial elements are commonly seen within the pleomorphic adenoma.

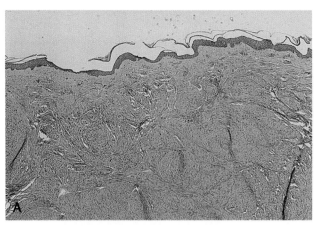
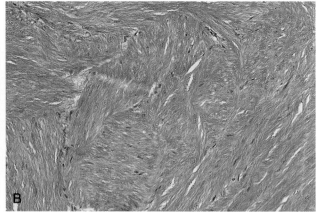

Figure 5–12. *A,* Leiomyoma of the nipple typically consists of irregularly arranged bundles of smooth muscle that form an ill-defined nodule.[14, 15] *B,* Smooth muscle proliferation shows no evidence of nuclear atypia or mitotic activity.

References

1. Tavassoli FA: Pathology of the Breast, Second Edition. Stamford, CT, Appleton & Lange, 1999.
2. Rosen PP: Rosen's Breast Pathology. New York, Lippincott-Raven, 1997.
3. Rosen PP, Oberman HA: Tumors of the mammary gland. In Atlas of Tumor Pathology, Series 3, Fascicle 7. Washington DC, Armed Forces Institute of Pathology, 1993.
4. Rosen PP, Caicco JA: Florid papillomatosis of the nipple. A study of 51 patients, including nine with mammary carcinoma. Am J Surg Pathol 10:87–101, 1986.
5. Lammie GA, Mills RR: Ductal adenoma of the breast. A review of fifteen cases. Hum Pathol 20:903–908, 1989.
6. Rosen PP: Syringomatous adenoma of the nipple. Am J Surg Pathol 7:739–745, 1983.
7. Ward BE, Cooper PH, Subramony C: Syringomatous tumor of the nipple. Am J Clin Pathol 92:692–696, 1989.
8. Jones MW, Norris HJ, Snyder RC: Infiltrating syringomatous adenoma of the nipple. A clinical and pathological study of 11 cases. Am J Surg Pathol 13:197–291, 1989.
9. Loose JH, Patchefsky AS, Hollander IJ, et al: Adenomyoepithelioma of the breast. A spectrum of biologic behavior. Am J Surg Pathol 16:868–876, 1992.
10. Rosen PP: Adenomyoepithelioma of the breast. Hum Pathol 18:1232–1237, 1987.
11. Tavassoli FA: Myoepithelial lesions of the breast. Myoepitheliosis, adenomyoepithelioma, and myoepithelial carcinoma. Am J Surg Pathol 15:554–568, 1991.
12. Chen KTK: Pleomorphic adenoma of the breast. Am J Clin Pathol 93:792–794, 1990.
13. Diaz NM, McDivitt RW, Wick MR: Pleomorphic adenoma of the breast: A clinicopathologic and immunohistochemical study of 10 cases. Hum Pathol 22:1206–1214, 1991.
14. Nascimento AG, Karas M, Rosen PP, et al: Leiomyoma of the nipple. Am J Surg Pathol 3:151–154, 1979.
15. Jones MW, Norris HJ, Wargotz ES: Smooth muscle and nerve sheath tumors of the breast. A clinicopathologic study of 45 cases. Int J Surg Pathol 2:85–92, 1994.
16. Diaz NM, Palmer JO, Wick MR: Erosive adenomatosis of the nipple: Histology, immunohistology and differential diagnosis. Mod Pathol 5:179–184, 1992.
17. Jones MW, Tavassoli FA: Coexistence of nipple duct adenoma and breast carcinoma: A clinicopathologic study of five cases and review of the literature. Mod Pathol 8:633–636, 1995.

CHAPTER 6

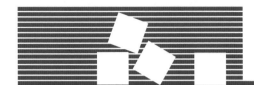

Nonproliferative and Benign Proliferative Epithelial Lesions

Arthur S. Patchefsky

INTRODUCTION

This chapter illustrates many of the microscopic abnormalities carried under the broad designation of fibrocystic disease or fibrocystic change. To what extent these represent an abnormal disease state is debatable, since it has long been observed that the vast majority of adult women and those who have borne children demonstrate one or more combinations of these histologic changes. Nevertheless, knowledge of the histology of the benign breast is necessary for the microscopist to evaluate the wide range of benign proliferative changes and to separate them from atypical hyperplasia and noninvasive carcinoma. This has been shown to be of paramount importance since the classic studies of Page and Dupont demonstrated that an increased risk of breast cancer can be directly related to epithelial hyperplasia and to the presence and degree of epithelial atypia in breast biopsy material.[1]

The terminology of both benign and malignant breast diseases has changed very little in decades. It is still referred to in terms of ductal or lobular abnormalities even though it is now clear, due largely to the subserial dissection studies of Wellings and coworkers, that the overwhelming majority of benign and malignant changes in the breast actually occur in the lobule or terminal duct lobular unit (TDLU).[2] The TDLU comprises portions of the terminal duct outside and within the intralobular stroma along with the florette-like branches, the individual acini or ductules. The wide variety of microscopic conditions commonly referred to as ductal hyperplasia, apocrine metaplasia, epithelial cysts, and others, are actually formed as the result of what has been termed "unfolding" or columnar cell change of the lobules which enlarge and expand and eventually evolve into the larger-diameter structures commonly referred to as "ducts."[2, 3]

Whether the following illustrations and captions conform to one's own ideas will depend on the relative balance between the criteria of the author compared with those of the reader. Suffice it to say that individual variation remains basic to the human condition. Some major differences notwithstanding, many nuances of the diagnostic process do not readily translate into written language, and it is hoped that the photomicrographs are sufficiently illustrative without having to rely on overly detailed microscopic descriptions. I apologize if examples of certain entities have been repeated too often, but this was done in order to emphasize their wide morphologic spectrum.

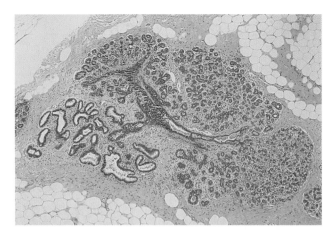

Figure 6–1. Unfolded lobule. Breast lobule shows partial unfolding *(lower left)*.

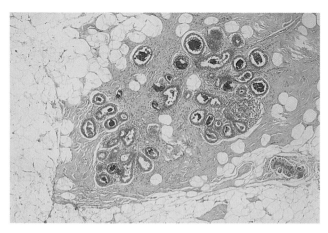

Figure 6–4. Unfolded lobule. Microcalcifications are often present in the acini of unfolded lobules.

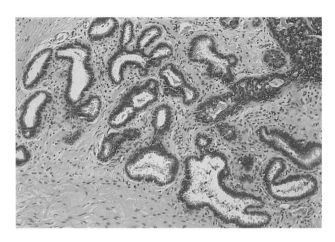

Figure 6–2. Unfolded lobule. Higher magnification of Figure 6–1 shows unfolded portion of lobule. Individual acini are dilated, and the area appears expanded. The epithelium shows no proliferation.

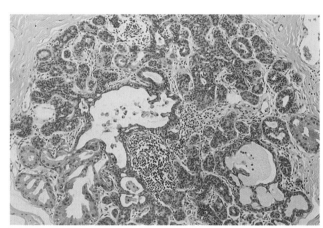

Figure 6–5. Unfolded lobule. Partially unfolded lobule shows focal apocrine metaplasia.

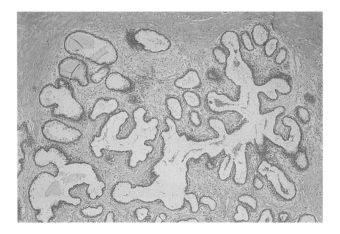

Figure 6–3. Unfolded lobule. Totally unfolded lobule shows dilated terminal ducts and acini that are transformed into a simplified and expanded structure that still retains the basic shape of the lobule and contains loose intralobular stroma.

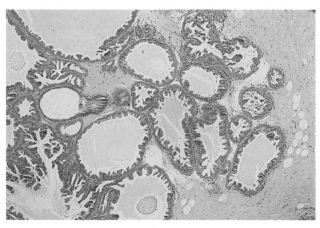

Figure 6–6. Unfolded lobule. More prominent lobular unfolding is seen with dilatation of individual acini and apocrine metaplasia.

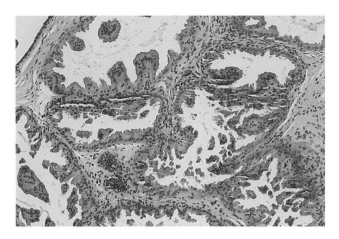

Figure 6–7. Unfolded lobule. Higher magnification of an area from the same case as Figure 6–6 shows acini lined with bland apocrine cells with micropapillary architecture.

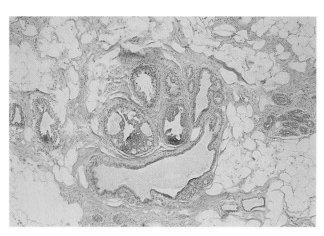

Figure 6–10. Unfolded lobule. This unfolded lobule is composed of a dilated terminal duct and expanded acini. The acini approach the diameter of the terminal duct and show fenestrated epithelial proliferation.

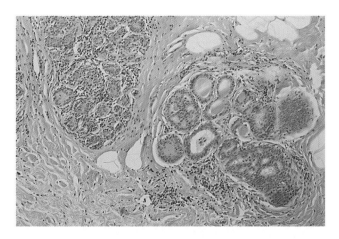

Figure 6–8. Unfolded lobule. Some unfolded lobules may show proliferation of epithelium resulting in cellular expansion of acini and terminal ducts.

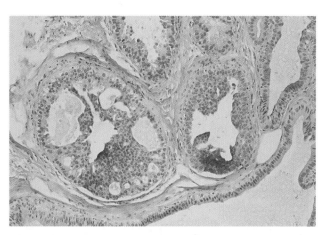

Figure 6–11. Unfolded lobule. This is a higher magnification view of Figure 6–10. The enlarged acini have a cribriform architecture with irregular lumens and rigid cohesive epithelial bridges. Although this process actually arises within an expanded or unfolded lobule, it is commonly referred to as "ductal hyperplasia," in everyday usage.

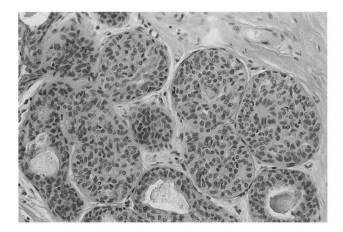

Figure 6–9. Unfolded lobule. Variation of cell types is evident with dark and light cells, variably shaped nuclei, incipient fenestrations, and irregular lumens. Acini are surrounded by a prominent layer of myoepithelial cells. This figure illustrates the origin of the majority of lesions commonly referred to as "ductal" as actually originating within the lobule.

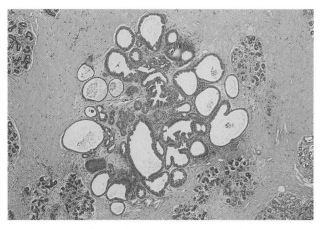

Figure 6–12. Unfolded lobule. Evolution of epithelial cysts from unfolded lobules is illustrated in the next two figures. Low power shows dilated acini with apocrine metaplasia. Compare this unfolded lobule to normal lobules adjacent to the lesion. The overall contour of the process conforms with the architecture and outline of the adjacent normal lobules. Distinction between acini and terminal duct cannot be appreciated.

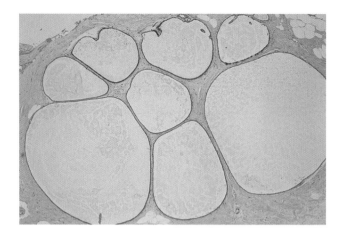

Figure 6–13. Unfolded lobule. Epithelial cysts still maintain a clustered lobulated appearance that signify their origin in expanded or unfolded lobule. The vast majority of gross and microscopic cysts develop in this way.

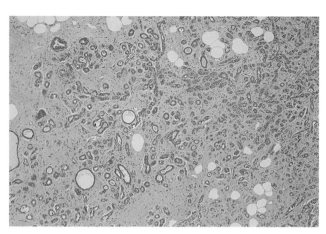

Figure 6–16. Sclerosing adenosis. More diffuse acinar proliferation tends to spread into sclerotic stroma. There is a vaguely lobular or symmetrical appearance, however, unlike the haphazard infiltration of invasive carcinoma.

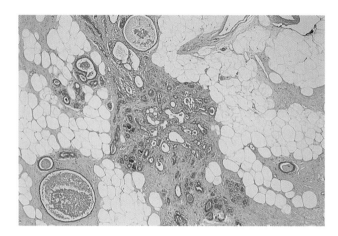

Figure 6–14. Sclerosing adenosis. Early, more exuberant phase of sclerosing adenosis shows dilatation of some acini and proliferation of others. The lesion is well circumscribed.

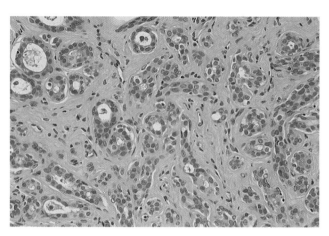

Figure 6–17. Sclerosing adenosis. Higher magnification view of Figure 6–16 shows benign acini being compressed and distorted by dense collagen. Occasional spindled myoepithelial cells are seen in individual acini. Myoepithelial cells may be difficult to discern in some examples, however.

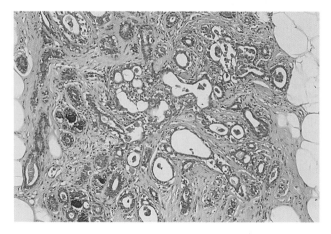

Figure 6–15. Sclerosing adenosis. Higher magnification view of Figure 6–14 shows the relationship of glands to stroma in which benign-appearing epithelial structures are molded by dense sclerotic collagen. There is no inflammatory reaction or loose reactive collagen, as is usually the case with invasive carcinoma.

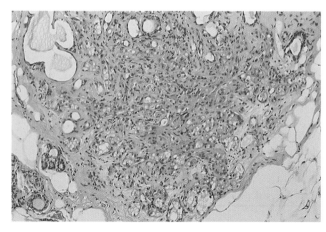

Figure 6–18. Sclerosing adenosis. Clearly lobular architecture of the process is apparent. Cellular variants such as this may be termed "florid adenosis."

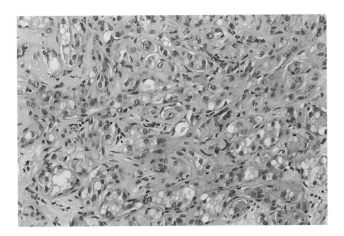

Figure 6–19. Sclerosing adenosis. Higher magnification view of Figure 6–18 shows more solid epithelial proliferation with few glandular lumens. There is a mixture of cell types varying from clearly cuboidal epithelium to spindle myoepithelial cells that are interspersed throughout the lesion.

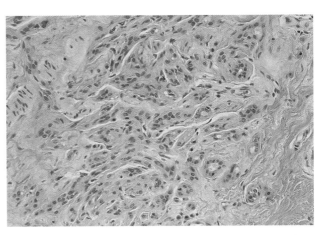

Figure 6–22. Sclerosing adenosis. Higher magnification view of Figure 6–21 shows that the dense stroma is increased and compresses the acini causing them to appear atrophic. A collarette of dense collagen and a spindle cell component to the lesion ensure that this is sclerosing adenosis.

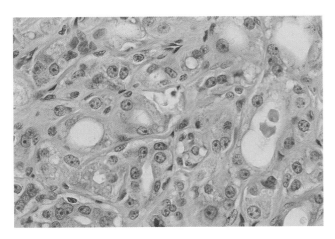

Figure 6–20. Sclerosing adenosis. Higher magnification view of Figure 6–19 shows pink apocrine nature of the epithelial cells that are arranged in compact glands and surrounded by an eosinophilic basement membrane. Spindled myoepithelial cells with dark nuclei are prominent. Apocrine metaplasia is not uncommon in sclerosing adenosis.

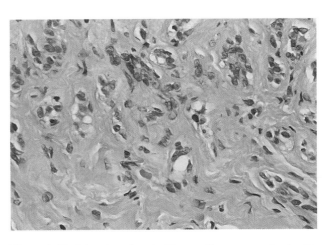

Figure 6–23. Sclerosing adenosis. Dense collagen surrounds atrophic acini containing spindle cells. Acini appear to be compressed and distorted by the stroma.

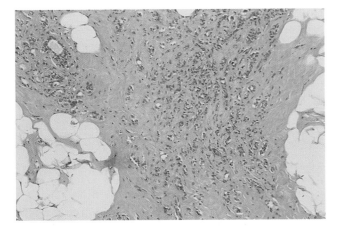

Figure 6–21. Sclerosing adenosis. More fibrous example of sclerosing adenosis illustrates the sclerosing phase. Note that while the overall contour of this focus appears to mimic invasive carcinoma, there is no inflammatory or stromal response, which is a clue that the process is benign.

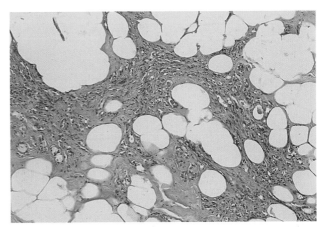

Figure 6–24. Sclerosing adenosis in fat. This example shows a lobular, whorled configuration to the process on low-power magnification.

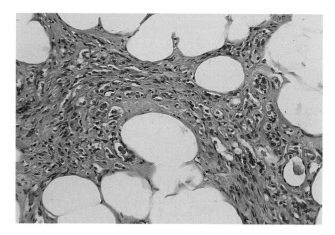

Figure 6–25. Sclerosing adenosis. Higher magnification view of Figure 6–24 shows predominant spindle myoepithelial cell population. The stroma is sclerotic, and the acini are compressed and atrophic.

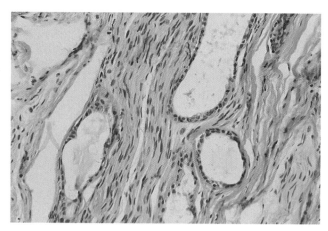

Figure 6–28. Sclerosing adenosis. Higher magnification view of Figure 6–27 shows the benign nature of the epithelial structures infiltrating the nerve sheath and the absence of inflammation or stromal reaction.

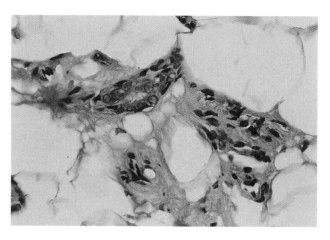

Figure 6–26. Sclerosing adenosis. Higher magnification view of Figure 6–25 shows atrophic acini containing dark-staining spindled myoepithelial cells adjacent to dense collagen. Absence of inflammation and stromal reaction, and the presence of spindle cells is consistent with sclerosing adenosis and not invasive carcinoma.

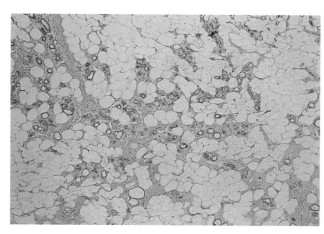

Figure 6–29. Microglandular adenosis.[5–7] Low-magnification view shows diffuse pattern of tissue involvement. Small acini seemingly infiltrate fat. The lobular architecture that characterizes sclerosing adenosis is inapparent. A similar pattern of acini may be seen in a background of fibrous tissue.

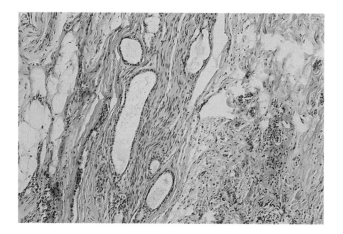

Figure 6–27. Sclerosing adenosis. Benign acini infiltrate nerve sheath. This is a rare feature of some examples of sclerosing adenosis.[4]

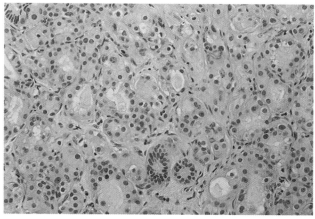

Figure 6–30. Microglandular adenosis. Rounded, closely packed acini with eosinophilic cells and intraluminal secretions are individually surrounded by a delicate basement membrane. Acini infiltrate around normal breast structures.

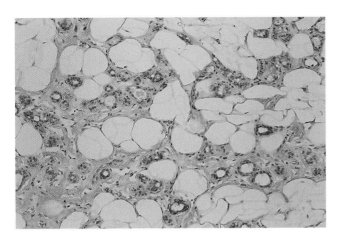

Figure 6–31. Microglandular adenosis. Dense stroma surrounds individual acini. These acini tend to be rounded and of more or less uniform size throughout the lesion.

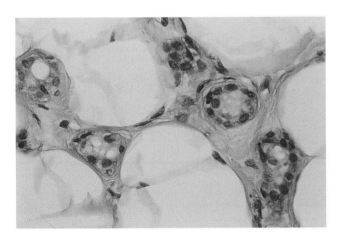

Figure 6–32. Microglandular adenosis. Small cytologically bland acini are surrounded by dense, undisturbed collagen. Cytoplasm is clear to amphophilic. Most acini of microglandular adenosis seemingly lack basal cells both immunohistochemically and ultrastructurally.[7] This may lead to confusion with invasive low-grade tubular carcinoma. Microglandular adenosis, however, lacks the angularly shaped glands and apocrine snouts common to tubular carcinoma. Atypical examples of microglandular adenosis have been described, and both in situ and invasive carcinoma have been observed.[8]

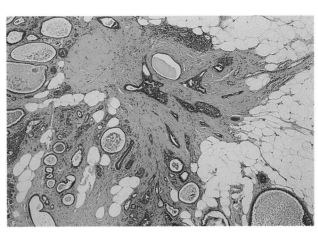

Figure 6–33. Radial scar. Low-magnification view shows stellate epithelial proliferation that is accompanied by dense collagen fibrosis. The center of the lesion has a "puckered" appearance as if the epithelial structures were being drawn into contracting stroma. Lesions are usually smaller than 1 cm and therefore are most commonly detected by mammography.[9]

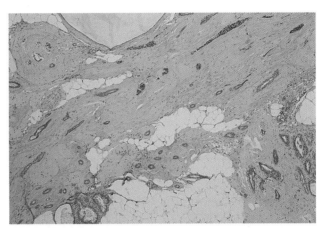

Figure 6–34. Radial scar. More peripheral, less cellular portion of the lesion shows elongated tubular epithelial structures within dense collagen. The stroma usually contains increased elastic tissue.[10]

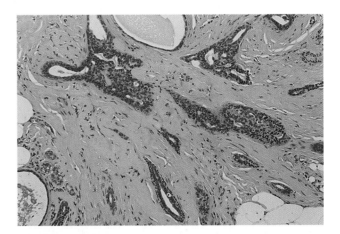

Figure 6–35. Radial scar. Higher magnification view of the central area of Figure 6–33 reveals irregularly shaped tubular ductal structures. There is seeming distortion of their shapes by sclerotic stroma. Irregular fenestrations and mild epithelial hyperplasia are characteristic features in the epithelium of radial scar. In situ carcinoma has been observed in rare instances.[11]

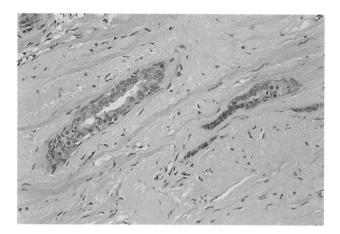

Figure 6–36. Radial scar. Elongated epithelial structures are seen with a prominent outer myoepithelial layer. Note the condensed rim of collagen around these structures and the absence of inflammation, both of which are characteristic of a benign process.

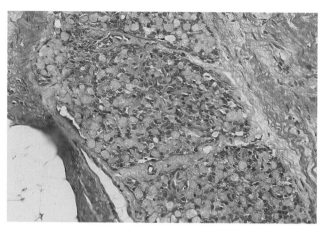

Figure 6–39. Collagenous spherulosis. Low-magnification view shows well-defined epithelial structure with closely apposed rings of cells. There is a prominent cylindromatous appearance to the lesion (trichrome stain).

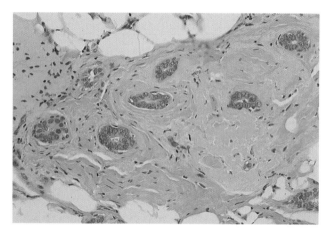

Figure 6–37. Radial scar. Small acini at the periphery of the lesion composed of bland epithelium and spindled myoepithelial cells are surrounded by laminated dense collagen. This appearance enables the separation of radial scar from invasive carcinoma.

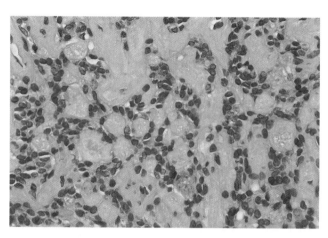

Figure 6–40. Collagenous spherulosis. Cylindromatous appearance is caused by a pronounced increase in extracellular matrix which forms small nodules that distort and compress the epithelium. The matrix has been shown to contain elastin, polysaccharides, and basement membrane material.[13, 14]

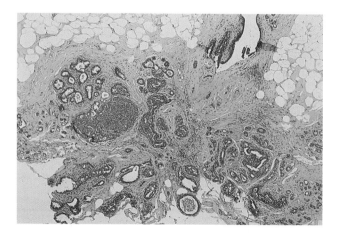

Figure 6–38. Radial scar. Another example of the lesion shows more exuberant proliferative changes. The central sclerosis appears to draw in the epithelium and results in the stellate architecture characteristic of radial scar. The premalignant nature of these lesions is controversial. A recent case-control study suggests increased risk.[12]

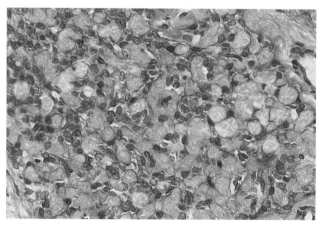

Figure 6–41. Collagenous spherulosis. Trichrome stain shows the connective tissue nature of the cylindromatous formations. Myoepithelial cells may surround the collagenous nodules. This is unlike adenoid cystic carcinoma, in which the lumens contain mucin and are unrelated to myoepithelium.

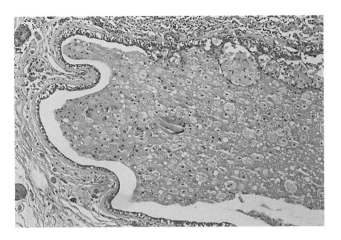

Figure 6–42. Duct ectasia. Dilated terminal duct shows pink granular intraluminal material that contains cellular debris. There is mild periductal chronic inflammation. Clinically, the patient presents with discharge from the nipple.

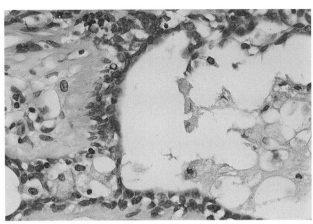

Figure 6–43. Duct ectasia. Foam cells and lymphocytes infiltrate the epithelium. Squamous metaplasia may be seen in some cases.

References

1. Page DL, VanderZwaag R, Rogers LW, et al: Relation between component parts of fibrocystic disease complex and breast cancer. J Natl Cancer Inst 61:1055–1063, 1978.
2. Wellings SR, Jensen HM, Marcum RG: An atlas of subgross pathology of the breast with special reference to possible precancerous lesions. J Natl Cancer Inst 55:231–273, 1975.
3. Page DL, Anderson TJ: Columnar alteration of lobules. In Diagnostic Histopathology of the Breast. New York, Churchill Livingstone, 1988, pp 86–88.
4. Taylor HB, Norris HJ: Epithelial invasion of nerves in benign diseases of the breast. Cancer 20:2245–2249, 1967.
5. Clement PB, Azzopardi JG: Microglandular adenosis of the breast. A lesion simulating tubular carcinoma. Histopathology 7:169–180, 1983.
6. Rosen PP: Microglandular adenosis. Am J Surg Pathol 7:137–144, 1983.
7. Tavasolli FA, Norris HJ: Microglandular adenosis of the breast. Am J Surg Pathol 7:731–737, 1983.
8. James BA, Cranor ML, Rosen PP: Carcinoma of the breast arising in microglandular adenosis. Am J Clin Pathol 100:507–513, 1993.
9. Adler DD, Helvie MA, Oberman HA, et al: Radial sclerosing lesion of the breast: Mammographic features. Radiology 176:737–740, 1990.
10. Anderson JA, Carter D, Linell F: A symposium of sclerosing duct lesions of the breast. Pathol Annu 21(2):145–179, 1986.
11. Mitnick JS, Vazquez MF, Roses DF et al: Stereotactic localization for fine needle aspiration breast biopsy: Initial experience with 300 patients. Arch Surg 126:1137–1140, 1991.
12. Jacobs TW, Byrne C, Colditz G, et al: Radial scars in benign breast-biopsy specimens and the risk of breast cancer. N Engl J Med 340:430–436, 1999.
13. Clement PB, Young RH, Azzopardi JG: Collagenous spherulosis of the breast. Am J Surg Pathol 11:414–417, 1987.
14. Grignon DJ, Ro JY, MacKay BN et al: Collagenous spherulosis of the breast. Immunohistochemical and ultrastructural studies. Am J Clin Pathol 91:386–392, 1989.

CHAPTER 7

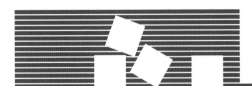

Intraductal Papillary Lesions

Ira J. Bleiweiss

INTRODUCTION

Papillary lesions of the breast are commonly encountered in routine surgical pathology practice either as distinct entities or as part of the spectrum of histology seen in fibrocystic changes. They may be solitary or multiple, with multiple lesions tending to be peripheral and somewhat more common in premenopausal patients.[1] Central lesions or those developing in larger or main lactiferous ducts may present clinically with a nipple discharge that is frequently bloody.[2] Although the premalignant potential of intraductal papillomas has long been a subject of debate, peripheral and multiple lesions have some increased associated risk.[3] The relative risk probably depends on the degree of epithelial hyperplasia contained in the papilloma and is akin to that ascribed respectively to florid duct hyperplasia and atypical duct hyperplasia without associated papilloma.

Solitary intraductal papillomas are usually nonpalpable lesions that may correspond mammographically to well-circumscribed radiodensities. Ultrasonography typically reveals mixed solid and cystic structures, often with associated dilated ducts. In some cases a soft, tan polypoid structure within a cyst may be seen grossly, often with associated hemorrhage. Frozen section analysis of such lesions is notoriously difficult, and attempts thereof are ill-advised, because the resultant artifact often makes the distinction from intracystic papillary carcinoma an even more arduous task.

The typical intraductal papilloma is easily recognized as composed of two types of cells (epithelial and myoepithelial) lining branching papillary structures with thick, often hyalinizing, fibrovascular cores within a cystically dilated duct. The cyst lining may similarly exhibit two cell layers, but it frequently has only an attenuated epithelium. Frequently the adjacent ducts are dilated, and fresh hemorrhage may be seen within the cystic spaces, as well as resorbing hemorrhage (hemosiderin-laden cells) both in the papilloma and cyst wall. Few benign lesions

of the breast exhibit as much histologic variation as intraductal papillomas, largely due to the degree of epithelial hyperplasia, sclerosis, and combinations of the two that may be seen, often creating immense difficulty distinguishing such lesions from both intraductal and invasive carcinoma. Apocrine metaplasia,[1] microcalcifications, and collagenous spherulosis[4] may also be seen within such lesions, as may occasional infarction.[1] Some authors (including the present) consider radial scars (or radial sclerosing lesions) variants of sclerosing intraductal papilloma in which the fibrosing component is dominant and produces the peculiar stellate configuration (see also Chapter 6). Although the nomenclature and pathogenesis of these lesions are a source of controversy, there is universal agreement that clinically, radiologically, and pathologically they may be difficult to distinguish from invasive carcinoma, especially the tubular type.[5]

The classic intracystic papillary carcinoma is typically composed of a single columnar type of epithelial cell lining thinner papillae containing a delicate capillary network.[6] The term *papillary carcinoma* has also been applied (incorrectly, in this author's view) to examples of other intraductal carcinoma patterns secondarily involving intraductal papillomas; such lesions are most often of cribriform and/or micropapillary pattern and of low to intermediate nuclear grade, although occasional cases of high-grade intraductal carcinoma may be encountered. A diagnosis of invasive carcinoma in the presence of a sclerosing papillary lesion must be made with great care and trepidation; it should be based on the presence of infiltration of breast tissue clearly beyond the lesion's fibrous capsule and not on examination of its sclerotic center.[1]

The current era of ultrasonography-guided and stereotactic core biopsy has introduced new difficulty in the differential diagnosis of papillary lesions. Such specimens are best interpreted with knowledge of the lesions' imaging characteristics, both to ensure diagnostic accuracy from the pathologist's point of view and to assure the radiologist that the targeted lesion was adequately sampled. Communication with the radiologist is extremely helpful, and, often in the case of intracystic papillary lesions, he or she will relate the partial or complete disappearance of the lesion during the sampling procedure. Sclerosing papillomas and radial scars may be particularly difficult diagnoses on core biopsies, and such cases deserve formal excision to rule out invasive carcinoma.[7]

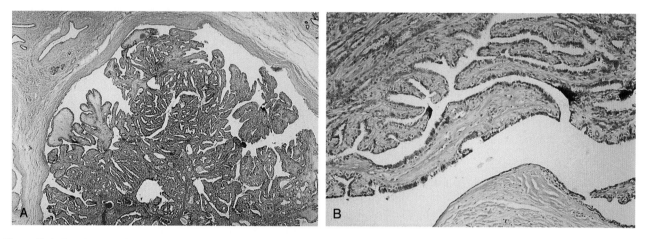

Figure 7–1. Intraductal papilloma. *A,* The prototypical intraductal papilloma shows branching papillary fronds with thick fibrovascular cores within a cystically dilated duct. *B,* High-power examination of papillary fronds reveals a two-cell-layer lining. Myoepithelial cells are prominent in this field, but they may be inapparent or discontinuous in other areas of the same lesion.

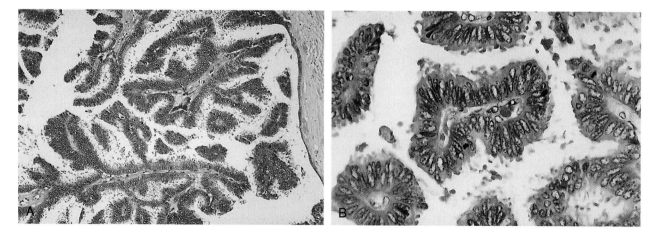

Figure 7–2. Intracystic papillary carcinoma (differential diagnosis). *A,* Intraductal papillomas must be differentiated from intraductal carcinoma. True papillary carcinoma is an uncommon lesion that constitutes a mass within a cystically dilated duct. The fronds contain a delicate vascular stroma and are lined by columnar epithelial cells with eosinophilic cytoplasm. Myoepithelial cells are absent. *B,* Higher-power magnification reveals rather uniform nuclei retaining a columnar polarity. Mitoses are evident but are not necessary for a malignant diagnosis.

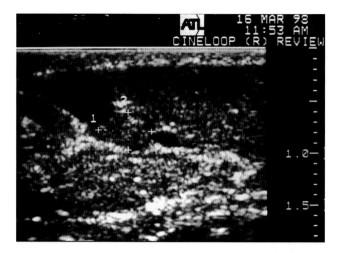

Figure 7–3. Intraductal papillary lesions—ultrasonographic appearance. In the subareolar region ultrasonography demonstrates a dilated duct containing a 5-mm by 3-mm echogenic (solid) mass outlined by the + marks. The imaging findings do not distinguish intraductal papilloma from papillary carcinoma. (Photo courtesy of Miriam Levy, MD.)

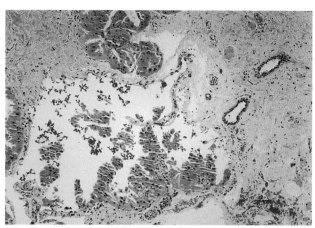

Figure 7–5. Papillary apocrine metaplasia. Apocrine metaplasia itself can exhibit papillary features. The cells in this field have classic apocrine cytology with abundant granular hypereosinophilic cytoplasm and thin, delicate fronds. This appearance is typically encountered as a solid proliferation in an apocrine metaplasia–lined cyst. Myoepithelial cells may be absent or not readily apparent.

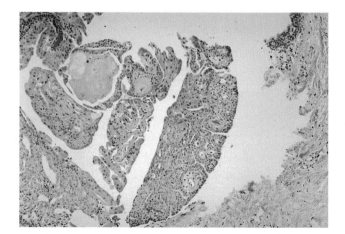

Figure 7–4. Papilloma with apocrine metaplasia. Apocrine metaplasia is a common histologic change within intraductal papillomas. As in this field, it is usually found in small foci admixed with the more typical epithelial- and myoepithelial-lined fronds or within duct hyperplasia associated with papilloma. Focal apocrine metaplasia in papillary lesions is nearly always associated with benign behavior, and its presence may therefore be quite helpful in difficult cases.

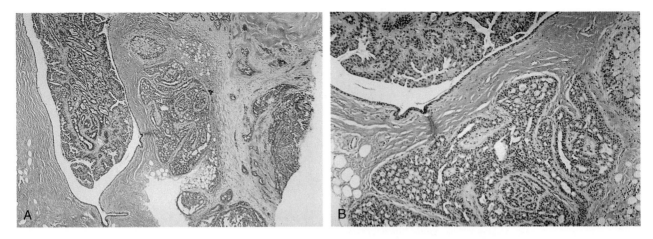

Figure 7–6. Collagenous spherulosis in intraductal papilloma. *A,* A low-power scan of this intraductal papilloma might generate concern over the seemingly uniform cribriform areas best seen at the center of the field. *B,* Closer examination reveals the pseudocribriform areas to actually contain glassy, lightly eosinophilic material typical of collagenous spherulosis. This secretion of basement membrane material and its resulting pattern must be distinguished from other forms of ductal hyperplasia, from atypical ductal hyperplasia, and, most importantly, from adenoid cystic carcinoma. Its occurrence within an intraductal papilloma is not uncommon, but it may add difficulty to the interpretation of hyperplastic areas.

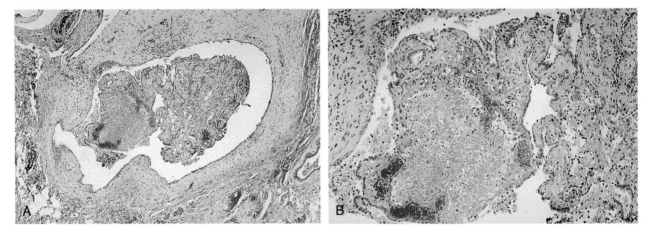

Figure 7–7. Infarction within intraductal papilloma. Intraductal papillomas can undergo partial or, rarely, complete infarction perhaps due to twisting of the stalk and secondary ischemia. Many papillomas show evidence of recent or ongoing hemorrhage and trauma, and infarcted areas may be spontaneous or associated with prior needle aspiration or biopsy. *A,* Approximately 40% of this small, solitary papilloma has undergone infarction. Note the slight chronic inflammatory reaction surrounding the duct, typical of such a lesion. *B,* At higher power a sharp demarcation is revealed between the infarcted area and the uninvolved papilloma. Such lesions are not indicative of rapid growth and must not be mistaken for evidence of malignancy.

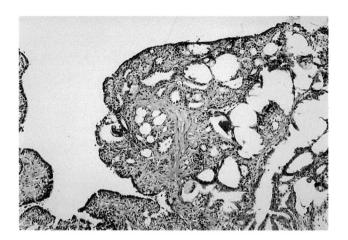

Figure 7–8. Calcifications in intraductal papilloma. Microcalcifications are an uncommon finding within a papilloma. They are more frequently encountered, in the author's experience, in areas of sclerosing adenosis or apocrine metaplasia (as in this figure) contained within the papilloma.

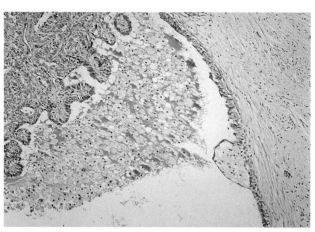

Figure 7–9. Degenerative changes in papilloma. Degenerative changes are an extremely common histologic feature of intraductal papilloma. As in this example, they may consist of intraductal and periductal histiocytes and periductal chronic inflammation or, more commonly, hemosiderin-laden macrophages and extensive fibrosis both within and surrounding the lesion.

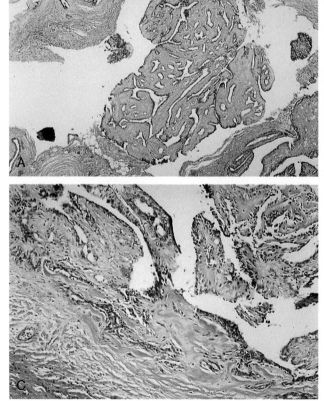

Figure 7–10. Sclerosing duct papilloma. *A,* Hyalinization within the fronds of a papilloma is typical and generally presents no diagnostic difficulty. *B,* Extensive sclerosis, however, both within and at the periphery of such lesions may entrap the epithelial component, often making the distinction from invasive carcinoma quite challenging. *C,* Entrapped glands such as these may or may not contain myoepithelial cells, and invasive carcinoma should be diagnosed only with clear-cut infiltration of the fibroadipose tissue beyond the confines of the papilloma.

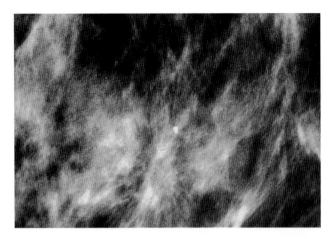

Figure 7–11. Radial scar—mammographic appearance. Mammography demonstrates an area of architectural distortion with radiating thin spiculations. There is no associated central radiodensity. (Photo courtesy of Barbara Braffman, MD.)

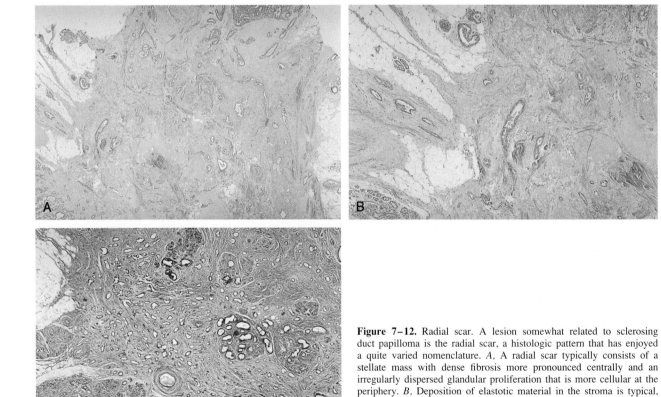

Figure 7–12. Radial scar. A lesion somewhat related to sclerosing duct papilloma is the radial scar, a histologic pattern that has enjoyed a quite varied nomenclature. *A,* A radial scar typically consists of a stellate mass with dense fibrosis more pronounced centrally and an irregularly dispersed glandular proliferation that is more cellular at the periphery. *B,* Deposition of elastotic material in the stroma is typical, and the glands, composed of two cell layers, do not directly invade the surrounding adipose tissue. *C,* In contrast, tubular carcinoma shows an even distribution of glands across the lesion with occasional angulated shapes and focal infiltration of adipose tissue.

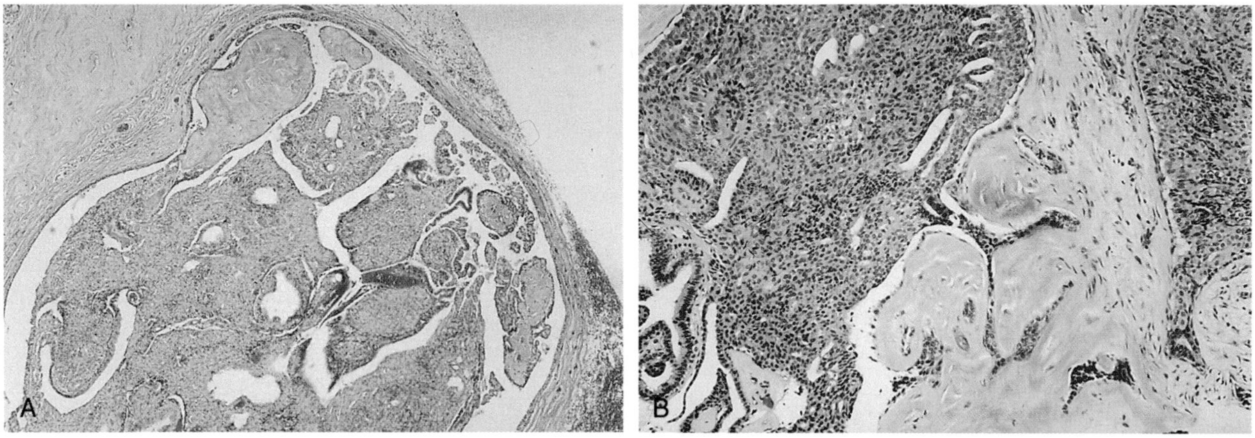

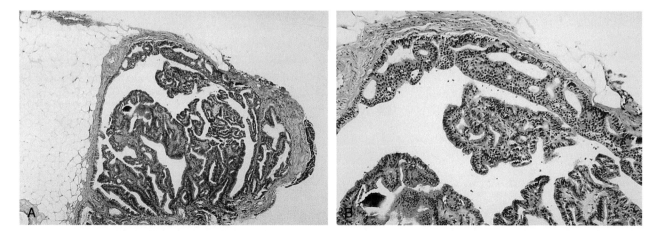

Figure 7–13. Intraductal papilloma with florid duct hyperplasia. The degree of epithelial hyperplasia in intraductal papilloma can be striking and among the most challenging aspects of breast pathology. The same rules of pattern recognition and cytology apply here as in nonpapillary proliferations. *A,* In this papilloma the ductal proliferation still contains a streaming pattern, and myoepithelial cells are still apparent. *B,* A higher-power view of a different area reveals a peripheral irregular cribriform pattern with curved (fishmouth) shapes. A streaming epithelial pattern is present centrally in the duct.

Figure 7–14. Intraductal papilloma with atypical ductal hyperplasia. The disagreements in interpretation inherent in atypical ductal hyperplasia are often compounded when the lesion occurs in the context of a papilloma. *A,* In this field atypical ductal hyperplasia is best seen at the edge of the duct *(top). B,* Although the cribriform pattern is rigid, and the epithelial proliferation is somewhat monotonous, it is only focal, not meeting minimal criteria for intraductal carcinoma.

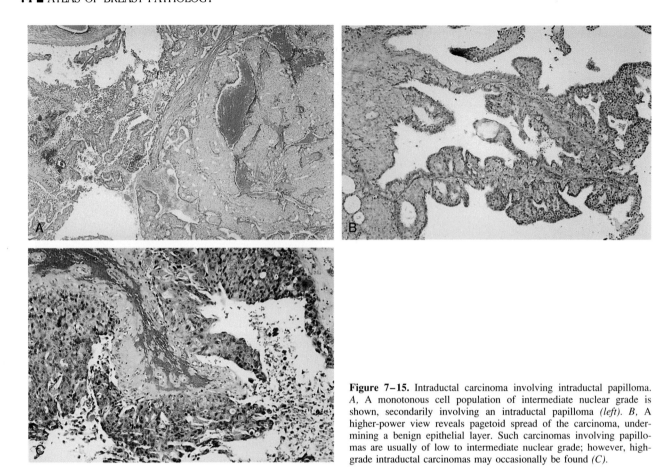

Figure 7–15. Intraductal carcinoma involving intraductal papilloma. *A,* A monotonous cell population of intermediate nuclear grade is shown, secondarily involving an intraductal papilloma *(left)*. *B,* A higher-power view reveals pagetoid spread of the carcinoma, undermining a benign epithelial layer. Such carcinomas involving papillomas are usually of low to intermediate nuclear grade; however, high-grade intraductal carcinomas may occasionally be found *(C).*

Figure 7–16. In situ lobular carcinoma involving intraductal papilloma. *A,* A uniform small cell population dilates and fills acini peripheral to this tiny intraductal papilloma. Pagetoid extension of the cells is seen within the papilloma, creating a difficult pattern to interpret. *B,* The lobular neoplasia cells have occasional signet ring features and are best seen at the lower part of this field.

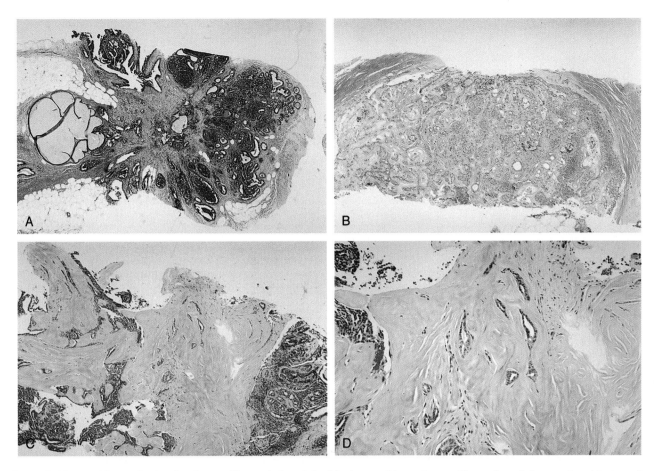

Figure 7–17. Core biopsy of sclerosing duct papilloma. *A,* Rare indeed is the core biopsy that provides a view of the overall architecture of a sclerosing papilloma. In this field typical papillary areas and duct hyperplasia are seen at the periphery of the fibrotic center. *B,* More difficult to interpret is this core biopsy, which some authors might classify as ductal adenoma. Combining a bland ductal proliferation with fibrosis, the lesion's circumscribed nature is evident even in the core biopsy. *C,* Even more difficult to interpret is this core biopsy in which extensive hyalinization has accentuated the entrapment phenomenon. *D,* Isolated foci at high-power magnification, if interpreted out of context, would be impossible to differentiate from invasive carcinoma. Such lesions should be correlated with imaging studies and probably deserve formal excision.

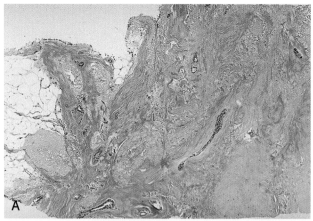

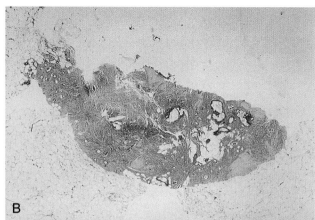

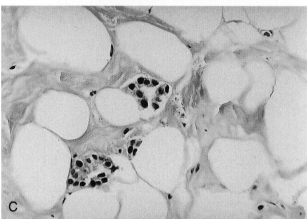

Figure 7–18. Core biopsy of radial scar versus tubular carcinoma. *A,* This core biopsy of a somewhat stellate mammographic area showed extensive fibrosis and elastosis with a minimal glandular component limited to the fibrous lesion. Excision of the area was performed, yielding identical histology. *B,* This core biopsy also emanated from a stellate radiodensity; however, the glandular proliferation is spread evenly across the core, consistent with tubular carcinoma. Elastosis is also present and is thus not pathognomonic for radial scar. *C,* Careful high-power examination reveals single cell layer glands directly invading adipose tissue at the lesion's periphery. This lesion was also excised and proved to be a tubular carcinoma. In general, even when core biopsy is highly suggestive of radial scar, surgical excision provides the only certain way to distinguish it from tubular carcinoma.

References

1. Rosen PP: Benign papillary tumors. In Rosen's Breast Pathology. Philadelphia, Lippincott-Raven, 1997, pp 67–104.
2. Cardenosa G, Eklund GW: Benign papillary neoplasms of the breast: Mammographic findings. Radiology 181:751–755, 1991.
3. Estabrook A: Are patients with solitary or multiple intraductal papillomas at higher risk of developing breast cancer? Surg Oncol Clin North Am 2:45–56, 1993.
4. Guarino M, Tricomi P, Cristofori E: Collagenous spherulosis of the breast with atypical epithelial hyperplasia. Pathologica 85:123–127, 1993.
5. Adler DD, Helvie MA, Oberman HA, et al: Radial sclerosing lesions of the breast: Mammographic features. Radiology 176:737–740, 1990.
6. Lefkowitz M, Lefkowitz W, Wargotz ES: Intraductal (intracystic) papillary carcinoma of the breast and its variants: A clinicopathological study of 77 cases. Hum Pathol 25:802–809, 1994.
7. Bassett L, Winchester DP, Caplan RB, et al: Stereotactic core-needle biopsy of the breast: A report of the joint task force of the American College of Radiology, American College of Surgeons, and College of American Pathologists. CA Cancer J Clin 47:171–190, 1997.

CHAPTER 8

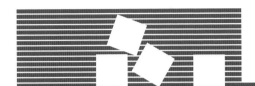

Ductal Carcinoma in Situ and Atypical Ductal Hyperplasia

Olga B. Ioffe
Steven G. Silverberg

INTRODUCTION

Ductal carcinoma in situ (DCIS) is a noninvasive neoplastic process that is relatively unifocal and is associated with a significantly increased risk of development of invasive cancer; it is also established as a direct precursor of invasive ductal carcinoma of the breast. The diagnosis of DCIS has increased dramatically since the 1980s with the advent of screening mammography.[1] This phenomenon is most certainly explained by the fact that most DCIS lesions are not palpable; they represent up to a third of nonpalpable cancers detected mammographically.[2] DCIS is a heterogeneous disease, ranging from high-grade lesions forming a mass, sometimes producing nipple discharge (Paget's disease of the nipple) and progressing to invasive carcinoma in most cases, to multifocal low-grade lesions, only a third of which become invasive with long-term follow-up. Quantitatively, DCIS ranges from extensive multicentric disease that is difficult to eradicate surgically to minimal forms bordering on atypical ductal hyperplasia (ADH).

Mammographic estimates of the size and extent of DCIS are usually based on the extent of microcalcifications; however, underestimation is common,[3] especially in low-grade DCIS of cribriform and micropapillary types.[4] Although the size of DCIS is one of the most important factors influencing the risk of recurrent and/or residual disease, it is often difficult to measure accurately. Although high-grade, especially comedo, DCIS typically forms a discrete, often palpable mass that can be measured clinically, mammographically, and grossly at pathologic examination, most in situ tumors are multifocal and/or multicentric, rendering even microscopic measurements highly inaccurate.

Multicentric distribution, by one definition, is that in which the tumor involves two or more remote areas separated by at least 3 to 4 mm of benign breast tissue[5]; another group defines multicentric DCIS as involving separate quadrants.[6] Because of varying definitions, the reported rates of multicentricity vary from 0% to 80%. Whole-organ studies have demonstrated that DCIS is not a multicentric disease, because it is confined to one "segment" of the breast.[3, 7] Unicentric tumor is confined to a single area and may be *multifocal,* involving multiple scattered ducts in several microscopic sections. Studies of Faverly and coworkers[8] showed that up to a half of all cases of DCIS show discontinuous, or multifocal, growth within the duct system.

Most in situ carcinomas in the male breast are intracystic papillary carcinomas and are usually of low nuclear grade; patients are usually older than women with DCIS.[9]

ADH is defined as a ductal proliferative process that possesses some, but not all, morphologic features of low-grade DCIS. Hence, the distinction between ADH and low-grade DCIS can be very difficult and subjective, with varying interobserver agreement.[10–13] However, even though the management of ADH and low-grade DCIS is quite different, they really represent a continuum[10, 14]; this concept received further development in the proposal of ductal intraepithelial neoplasia.[15] This continuum includes usual ductal epithelial hyperplasia, ADH, and low-grade DCIS, and it corresponds to increasing risk of developing breast cancer.[16–18]

In this chapter, we illustrate the architectural types and grading of DCIS and discuss its differential diagnosis with ADH, lobular lesions, and invasive carcinoma.

INTRADUCTAL CARCINOMA

Diagnostic Criteria for DCIS and Differential Diagnosis with ADH and IDH

Feature	IDH	ADH	Low-Grade DCIS
Extent/Size	Usually extensive, multifocal	Most very small, focal, rarely extensive. Two variants: only one duct profile completely diagnostic of DCIS, or one or more ducts not completely diagnostic of DCIS	Most cases >2 mm, may be extensive; has to involve at least two entire duct profiles
Architecture	Solid with fenestrations or micropapillary	Cribriforming or micropapillary structures not involving entire profile	Well developed cribriform, micropapillary, solid with rosettes or "mosaic" pattern, or cores with stratified columnar cells
Lumens/fenestrations	Irregular, slitlike, larger at periphery of duct	Mixture of punched out and irregular; may have some "Roman" bridges in part of lumen	Regular, "punched out"; round "Roman" bridges
Cell orientation	Streaming, swirling, parallel to axis in bridges; uneven cell spacing, overlapping	Focally even and regular but not in the entire space	Regular cell spacing; perpendicular to axis in bridges
Cellular population	Admixture of spindle and rounded cells, sometimes of apocrine cells	Focally monotonous; mixed population in the rest of the space	Monotonous uniform cells (single population)
Cell borders	Indistinct	May be distinct	Usually distinct
Nucleoli	Small	Small	Small
Mitoses	Rare	Rare	Rare
Necrosis	Rare	Rare	Rare
Keratin 34βE12 (see Fig. 8–37)	Positive	Focally positive	Negative

Figure 8–1. Definition and diagnostic criteria for ductal carcinoma in situ (DCIS) and differential diagnosis with atypical ductal hyperplasia (ADH) and usual intraductal hyperplasia (IDH). There are two most widely used minimal definitions of DCIS (this applies mostly to small amounts of low-grade DCIS, which can be difficult to distinguish from ADH). One definition, used by most authors, requires the presence of two duct epithelial profiles completely involved by changes typical of DCIS.[20] The other definition uses the size of 2 mm as the cutoff for the diagnosis of DCIS[16]; this cutoff is used for low-grade lesions only, while proliferations with high-grade cytology do not require a minimum measurement.[21]

Page and coworkers[17, 18, 22] and Lagios[4] developed a set of morphologic criteria for the diagnosis of DCIS and distinguished it from ADH and IDH, as summarized in the figure.

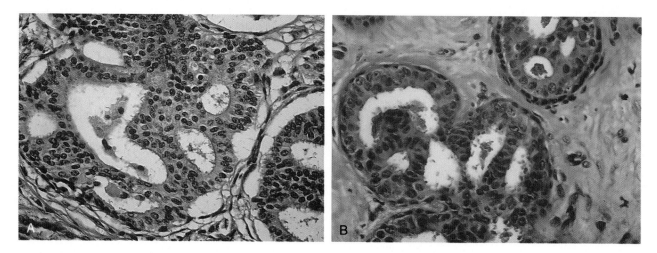

Figure 8–2. Microscopic features of ductal carcinoma in situ (DCIS). In this example of cribriform DCIS (low nuclear grade in A and intermediate nuclear grade in B), one can see many of the diagnostic features of DCIS listed in Figure 8–1: monotonous, uniform cells that are evenly spaced and perpendicularly oriented (B) to the axis of stiff bridges and arches, or to the lumen of the secondary space. Only one cell type is seen within the involved profile, without the admixture of myoepithelial cells.

Most Commonly Used Grading Schemes for DCIS

Scheme	Grade	Description
Nuclear grade (European Breast Screening Groups)	Low nuclear grade	Monomorphic, evenly spaced cells with inconspicuous nucleoli; few mitoses
	Intermediate nuclear grade	Mild to moderate nuclear pleomorphism, one or two nucleoli, high N/C ratio; occasional mitoses
	High nuclear grade	Marked pleomorphism, irregular spacing, loss of polarity, irregular nuclear contour, coarse chromatin and multiple nucleoli; frequent mitoses, may be abnormal forms
Lagios[23]	Low grade	Nuclear diameter equal to 1–1.5 red blood cells, diffuse chromatin, inconspicuous nucleoli; no necrosis
	Intermediate grade	Nuclear diameter equal to 1.5–2 red blood cells; coarse chromatin, rare nucleoli; mitoses; focal necrosis
	High grade	Nuclear diameter >2.5 red blood cells; vesicular chromatin, one or more prominent nucleoli, frequent mitoses; extensive necrosis
Van Nuys scheme[24]	Low grade/group 1	Low or intermediate nuclear grade without necrosis
	Intermediate grade/group 2	Low or intermediate nuclear grade with necrosis*
	High grade/group 3	High nuclear grade with or without necrosis
Tavassoli[25]	High grade	Cytologic atypia and necrosis
	Moderate grade	No atypia with necrosis; or cytologic atypia without necrosis
	Low grade	No atypia or necrosis

Figure 8–3. Grading of ductal carcinoma in situ (DCIS). Nuclear grade has been claimed to be the most prognostically powerful indicator of biologic behavior of DCIS, as it directly correlates with recurrence rate, tumor size, c-erbB-2 expression, cell proliferation fraction, and estrogen receptor/progesterone receptor expression.[26–31] The usefulness of the grading system based on nuclear grade rather than architectural type is also supported by the evidence that DCIS of mixed architectural type is much more common than DCIS of mixed nuclear grade—62% versus 16%,[32] leading to a greater consistency in classification using nuclear rather than architectural features. We generally prefer a system based on nuclear grade alone, because of studies of one of us[33] indicating that necrosis was the least important of three factors (grade, necrosis, and solid growth patterns) distinguishing pure DCIS from DCIS accompanying (and presumably progressed to) infiltrating carcinoma.

It should be noted that an effort must be made at avoiding the diagnosis of intermediate nuclear grade, as most studies showed a statistically significant difference in the outcome only between high-grade (grade 3) and non–high (low and intermediate)–grade DCIS.[34] This concept is confirmed by studies of biologic marker expression that showed separation only between high- and non–high-grade DCIS.[30]

* Determination of necrosis is based on a substantial amount of necrotic tumor cells; occasional desquamated or apoptotic cells do not qualify.

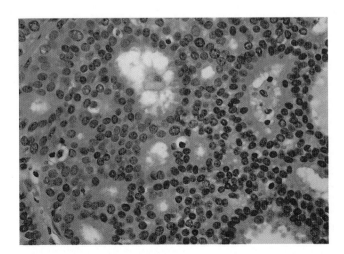

Figure 8–4. Low nuclear grade ductal carcinoma in situ (DCIS). This cribriform DCIS is classified as low nuclear grade. Note rather small, monomorphic, evenly spaced cells with inconspicuous nucleoli. Mitotic figures are not seen here, but a few mitoses may be present. Numerous or easily identifiable mitoses are usually not a feature of low-grade DCIS.

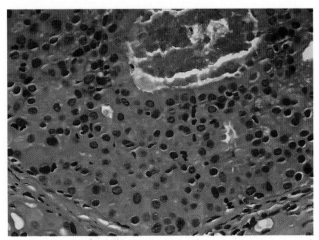

Figure 8–5. Intermediate nuclear grade ductal carcinoma in situ (DCIS). This solid DCIS with central necrosis displays nuclear features that are best characterized as intermediate grade. There is moderate nuclear pleomorphism and single rather small nucleoli. The nuclei are slightly larger than the ones seen in Figure 8–4.

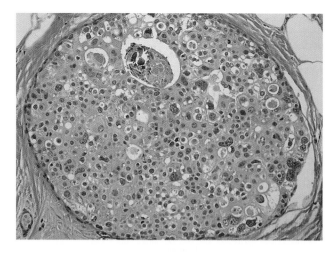

Figure 8–6. High nuclear grade ductal carcinoma in situ (DCIS). This solid type DCIS exhibits marked nuclear pleomorphism, with frequent large bizarre cells and multiple prominent nucleoli. Minimal central necrosis is present.

TYPES OF DUCTAL CARCINOMA IN SITU

Although the architectural patterns of DCIS are less important clinically than the nuclear grade, they are worth emphasizing because a presumed DCIS that lacks the classic appearance of at least one of these patterns has probably been overdiagnosed. In a case showing an admixture of several architectural patterns, all patterns should be listed in the diagnosis in the order of their relative amount.

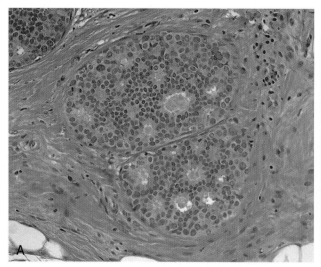
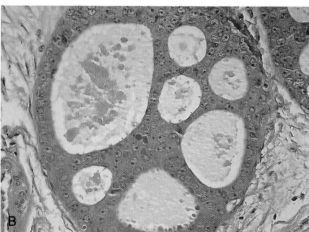

Figure 8–7. Cribriform ductal carcinoma in situ (DCIS). Among the several described architectural types of DCIS the cribriform pattern is the most common one, seen either in isolation or combined with other patterns; the cribriform pattern is the prototypical DCIS described by the set of diagnostic criteria used by most surgical pathologists.[4, 18, 22] The examples shown here (and in Fig. 8–2) illustrate these characteristics: round, uniform, "punched-out" spaces; the cells occupying the lumen of these profiles are uniform and evenly spaced without streaming or swirling. On the contrary, these cells are oriented perpendicularly to the axis of the arch, bridge, or the lumen of the secondary space. This type of DCIS is usually of low nuclear grade (A); the example shown in B is unusual in that it is of intermediate nuclear grade.

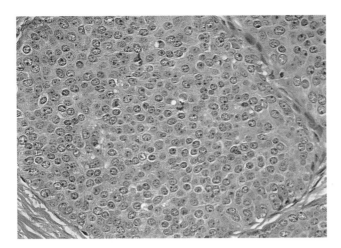

Figure 8–8. Solid ductal carcinoma in situ (DCIS). In this type of DCIS, the lumen is completely filled by uniform, monotonous cells that are evenly spaced. The nuclei of this DCIS qualify it as intermediate nuclear grade. No streaming or swirling is seen in this case; these latter findings, along with irregular slitlike secondary spaces, would make one diagnose florid ductal hyperplasia of usual type rather than DCIS.

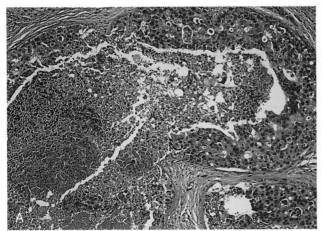 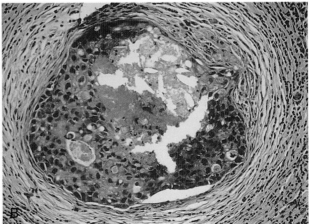

Figure 8–9. Comedocarcinoma. Comedocarcinoma, by definition, is solid high-grade ductal carcinoma in situ (DCIS) that exhibits central necrosis. Note the highly pleomorphic nuclei and abundant apoptotic bodies *(A, B)*. Frequent mitotic (and sometimes atypical mitotic) figures are often seen. Another feature commonly seen in comedocarcinoma is periductal stromal desmoplasia and inflammation *(B)*. This type of DCIS is worth separating from others because of its specific clinicopathologic features. Comedocarcinoma is more likely to present as a palpable mass, have a large size and positive resection margins, and recur locally. Most cases of comedocarcinoma progress (if they have not done so already) to invasive carcinoma (in contrast, only about 30% of low-grade DCIS becomes invasive with long-term follow-up.[35])

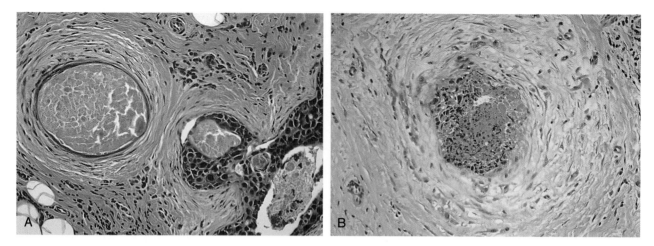

Figure 8–10. "Regressing" high-grade ductal carcinoma in situ (DCIS). *A,* The duct profile shown on the left is undergoing complete necrosis of epithelial cells and has only a thin layer of residual flattened epithelial cells with surrounding marked stromal desmoplastic reaction. Note the necrotic debris in the lumen. *B,* In this field, the duct outline is completely obliterated, and there are almost no residual epithelial cells.

This phenomenon is not uncommon in high-grade DCIS, and if it is the only finding (i.e., in a core needle biopsy), it may lead to significant diagnostic difficulty. High suspicion for a full-blown high-grade DCIS should be expressed in the diagnosis (especially if this is seen in a core needle biopsy).

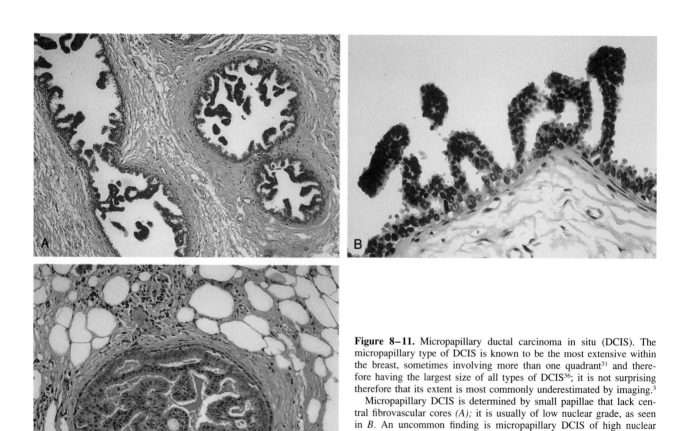

Figure 8–11. Micropapillary ductal carcinoma in situ (DCIS). The micropapillary type of DCIS is known to be the most extensive within the breast, sometimes involving more than one quadrant[31] and therefore having the largest size of all types of DCIS[36]; it is not surprising therefore that its extent is most commonly underestimated by imaging.[3]

Micropapillary DCIS is determined by small papillae that lack central fibrovascular cores *(A);* it is usually of low nuclear grade, as seen in *B.* An uncommon finding is micropapillary DCIS of high nuclear grade; however, nuclear grade has no bearing on the extent of micropapillary DCIS within the breast.[31] Occasionally, the papillae of this type of DCIS become very complex within the duct profile and the lesion acquires features of both micropapillary and cribriform DCIS *(C).*

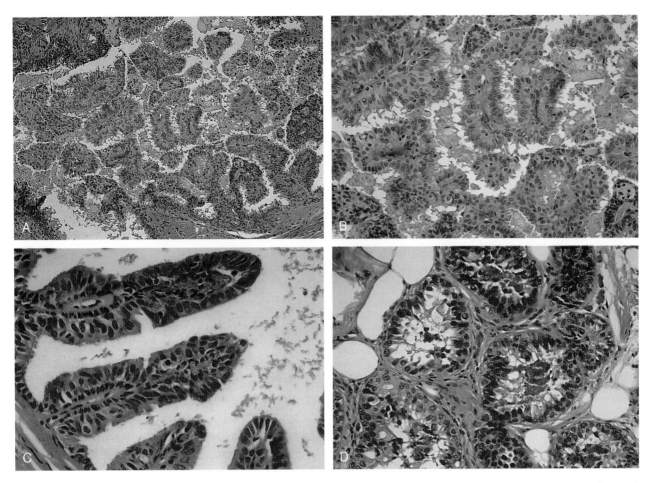

Figure 8–12. Stratified spindle cell papillary ductal carcinoma in situ (DCIS). In this less common type of DCIS, there are true papillae of larger size than those of the micropapillary type, usually filling a dilated duct *(A)*, and with fibrovascular cores that are lined by columnar cells exhibiting strikng nuclear stratification *(B)* (hence the designation). Note the nuclear hyperchromasia; occasional mitoses can be seen but are not necessary for the diagnosis *(C)*. Cancerization of lobules by this type of DCIS may present diagnostic difficulty because the acini are not filled but lined by malignant cells, in a clinging carcinoma pattern *(D)*.

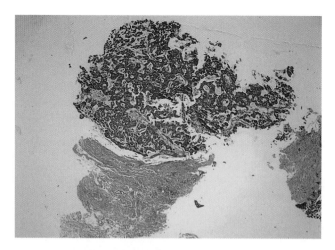

Figure 8–13. Intracystic papillary ductal carcinoma in situ (DCIS). (see also Chapter 7). Shown here is a core needle biopsy of an intracystic papillary DCIS. Note the thick fibrous wall outlining a space filled by a cribriform epithelial proliferation lacking fibrovascular cores. Most of these lesions occur in older patients and are of low or intermediate nuclear grade without necrosis, with strong estrogen receptor/progesterone receptor expression and no amplification of c-erbB-2.[37] This can be easily displaced from the cystic lumen during processing, leaving an empty space. The differential diagnosis from intraductal papilloma is helped by the predominance of epithelium over fibrovascular cores, unlike the prominent cores of a papilloma, and the presence of monotonous cells showing stratification, cribriforming, or solid growth pattern; myoepithelial cells are absent on hematoxylin-eosin and immunohistochemical stains. Necrosis is uncommon. In some cases, residual thick fibrous cores probably representing a preexisting intraductal papilloma may be present. The presence of DCIS involving small ducts surrounding the cyst ("tributary" ducts) is a common occurrence.

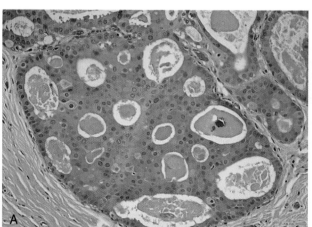

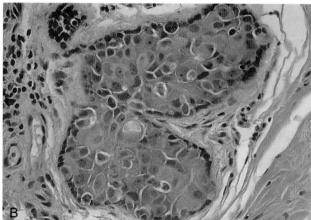

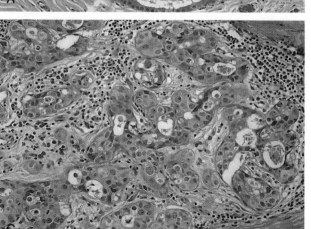

Figure 8–14. Apocrine ductal carcinoma in situ (DCIS). Apocrine DCIS is composed of cells demonstrating apocrine differentiation, but it is diagnosed by applying architectural criteria for the diagnosis of DCIS.[38] This is an important concept because even benign apocrine proliferations can exhibit significant nuclear atypia; therefore, only architectural findings typical of DCIS should be grounds for the diagnosis of apocrine carcinoma in situ. One important caveat is that the micropapillary pattern is not diagnostic of apocrine DCIS, as papillary tufts are a common feature of usual apocrine metaplasia. Although most cases of apocrine DCIS are of high or intermediate nuclear grade, some cases exhibit low-grade nuclear morphology.[39] Apocrine DCIS has a peculiar immunohistochemical profile in that it expresses androgen receptor and is negative for estrogen and progesterone receptors.[39] This case shows a cribriform architectural pattern of DCIS composed of modestly pleomorphic cells with abundant granular eosinophilic cytoplasm, the same cell type as seen in benign apocrine metaplasia *(A)*. Note distinct cell borders and prominent nucleoli in another case *(B)*. In the case of lobular cancerization by this type of DCIS *(C)*, stromal response may be prominent; this should not be overdiagnosed as evidence of invasive carcinoma.

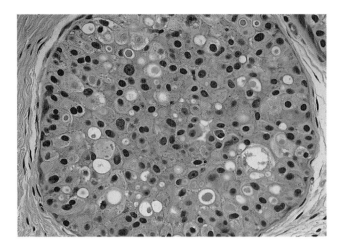

Figure 8–15. Ductal carcinoma in situ (DCIS) with intracytoplasmic lumens. Although the presence of intracytoplasmic lumina is the hallmark of lobular carcinoma (in situ and invasive), it is not uncommonly seen in ductal lesions, and therefore cannot be used as a pathognomonic feature of lobular lesions.

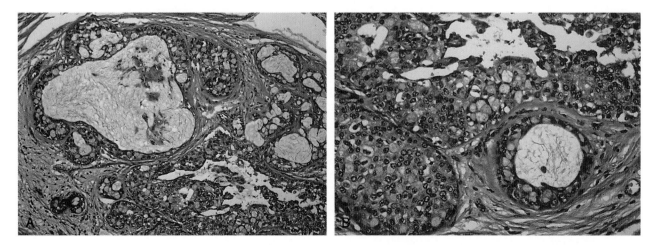

Figure 8–16. Mucinous ductal carcinoma in situ (DCIS) with prominent signet ring cells. This rare type of DCIS is most often seen adjacent to infiltrating mucinous carcinoma, and very seldom as a pure intraductal lesion. The characteristic feature of this type is the presence of intracytoplasmic mucin globules and extravasated mucin; the latter sometimes may present difficulties in distinguishing this from microinvasive mucinous carcinoma (see Fig. 8–17). The nuclear grade may vary but is usually low. Up to a third of mucinous DCIS may exhibit neuroendocrine differentiation. Prominent signet ring cells may raise a possibility of lobular carcinoma in situ; however, signet ring cells are not uncommon in ductal in situ and invasive lesions.

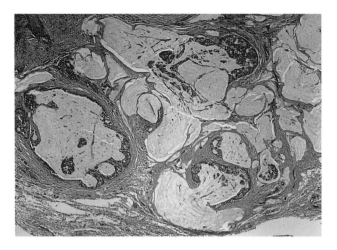

Figure 8–17. Mucocele-like lesion with intraductal carcinoma. Mucocele-like lesions have in common the presence of extravasated stromal mucin lakes, and they encompass a spectrum of disease from benign mucocele-like lesions, in which the epithelium lining the cysts is benign, to mucocele-like lesions with atypical ductal hyperplasia, to mucocele-like lesions with intraductal carcinoma, as shown in this figure.[40] Note that parts of the ruptured cystic spaces are filled with micropapillary and cribriform epithelium, diagnostic of DCIS. The most important differential diagnosis of mucocele-like lesions is mucinous carcinoma, in which malignant epithelial clusters are found floating within the mucin lakes.

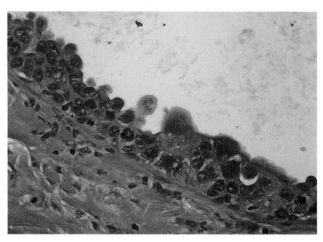

Figure 8–18. Clinging carcinoma pattern. This is an extremely difficult and controversial lesion that is characterized by ducts lined by a few layers of highly pleomorphic cells but no architectural features of ductal carcinoma in situ (DCIS).[41] Because not enough evidence exists regarding the behavior and significance of this rare pattern, we prefer to classify it as a form of atypical ductal hyperplasia (ADH). Recently, however, loss of heterozygosity identical to that seen in more overt types of DCIS was found in the majority of clinging carcinoma cases.[42]

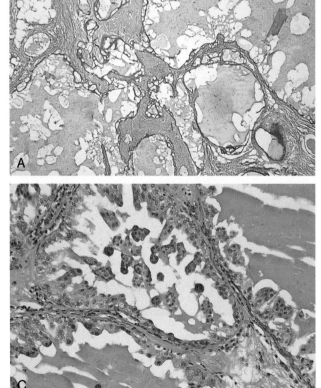

Figure 8–19. Cystic hypersecretory ductal carcinoma in situ (DCIS). Cystic hypersecretory DCIS is characterized by the presence of cystic spaces filled with colloid-like bright eosinophilic secretions. The cyst contents often show scalloped edges, retraction, and small round holes *(A)* or cracks *(B)*, similar to colloid. The epithelium in cystic hypersecretory lesions may range from flat and bland (cystic hypersecretory hyperplasia) to cytologically atypical or crowded with focal micropapillary formations (cystic hypersecretory hyperplasia with atypia), to fully developed intraductal carcinoma, usually of micropapillary architecture *(C)*.[40]

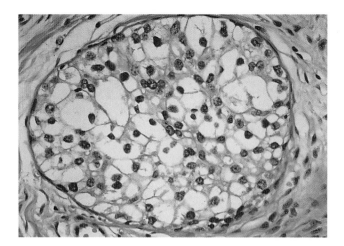

Figure 8–20. Clear cell ductal carcinoma in situ (DCIS). This is a very rare type of DCIS characterized by intraductal proliferation of usually relatively uniform cells with abundant clear cytoplasm, representing glycogen accumulation. Note the distinct cell borders, imparting a "mosaic"-like appearance. These lesions are thought to be precursors of glycogen-rich carcinoma. Some examples may represent a form of apocrine DCIS.

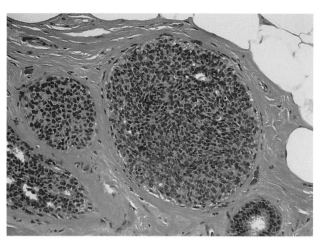

Figure 8–22. Spindle-cell ductal carcinoma in situ (DCIS). This type of DCIS is very uncommon but is worth mentioning because it can cause difficulty in differentiating it from florid ductal hyperplasia of the usual type. The spindle cell DCIS in this figure shows swirling and streaming of cells, which are usually attributed to usual ductal hyperplasia. The distinguishing feature diagnostic of DCIS is the presence of a single cell population.

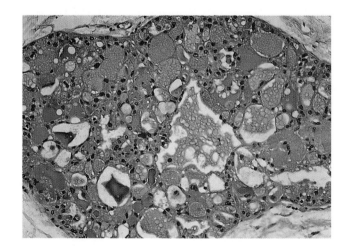

Figure 8–21. Secretory ductal carcinoma in situ (DCIS). Shown here is the intraductal component of secretory carcinoma, a rare type of invasive carcinoma that has been reported in older women as well as in children.[43] The secretory DCIS is usually cribriform (as in this figure) or micropapillary; rarely, it can display a solid pattern. Note the bland cytology and abundant vacuolated ("bubbly") luminal and intracytoplasmic amphophilic secretions.

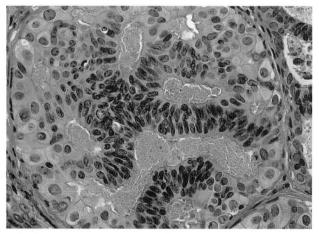

Figure 8–23. Dimorphic ductal carcinoma in situ (DCIS). Dimorphic variants of DCIS are unusual and contradict one of the main diagnostic concepts of DCIS, which requires the presence of a monotonous, single cell population. This intraductal carcinoma consists of two distinct cell populations: larger cells with more abundant cytoplasm at the periphery and smaller hyperchromatic cells in the center.

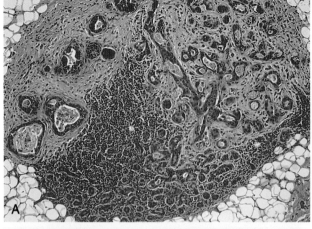

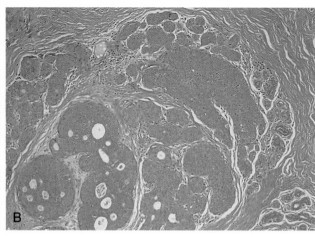

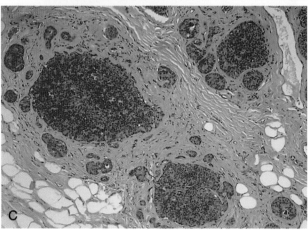

Figure 8–24. Cancerization of lobules. A lobule partially involved by intraductal carcinoma is shown in *A*. Note the associated stromal reaction and inflammation. An extensive lobular cancerization may mimic lobular carcinoma in situ *(B)*; in difficult cases, E-cadherin immunostain may be helpful (see Fig. 8–36). In some cases, such as seen in *C*, lobular cancerization may mimic invasive carcinoma and cause significant difficulties in diagnosis, especially when associated with pronounced desmoplastic stromal reaction, common in high-grade DCIS. Features that help rule out invasion include retention of low-power lobular architecture, albeit exaggerated and expanded by DCIS, in which one can mentally recreate a preexisting benign lobule with a terminal duct. In especially difficult cases the pathologist can resort to an immunohistochemical stain for smooth muscle actin, which helps confirm the presence of myoepithelial cells at the periphery of the suspicious cell nests. The presence of lobular cancerization, especially close to the surgical resection margins, has recently been claimed to be associated with increased risk of local recurrence.[44]

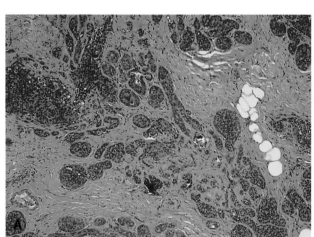

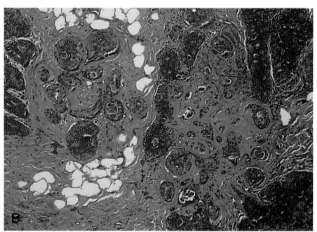

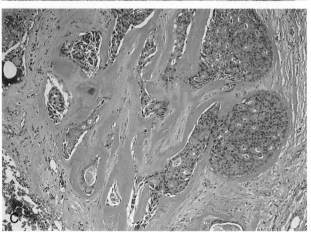

Figure 8–25. Involvement of sclerosing adenosis/complex sclerosing lesion by intraductal carcinoma. The question of invasion can arise when ductal carcinoma in situ (DCIS) involves a sclerosing lesion such as radial scar, sclerosing adenosis, sclerosing papilloma, or a combination thereof, the so-called complex sclerosing lesion. As in the case of lobular cancerization, the low-power architecture of the lesion is most helpful in ruling out invasive carcinoma. In *A*, the low-power picture is that of sclerosing adenosis, with compression of the epithelial profiles in the center and open spaces at the periphery; if one were to examine this area only at high power, invasive carcinoma would be difficult to rule out. Another diagnostic feature helpful to rule out invasion, seen usually in sclerosing lesions such as radial scar/complex sclerosing lesion, is the presence of stromal hyalinization/elastosis in the center of the lesion *(B, C)*, unlike the desmoplastic stromal reaction to invasive carcinoma. An important exception is tubular carcinoma, which is also frequently accompanied by stromal hyalinization. Actin immunostain can be of use in difficult cases to help demonstrate the presence of myoepithelial cells.

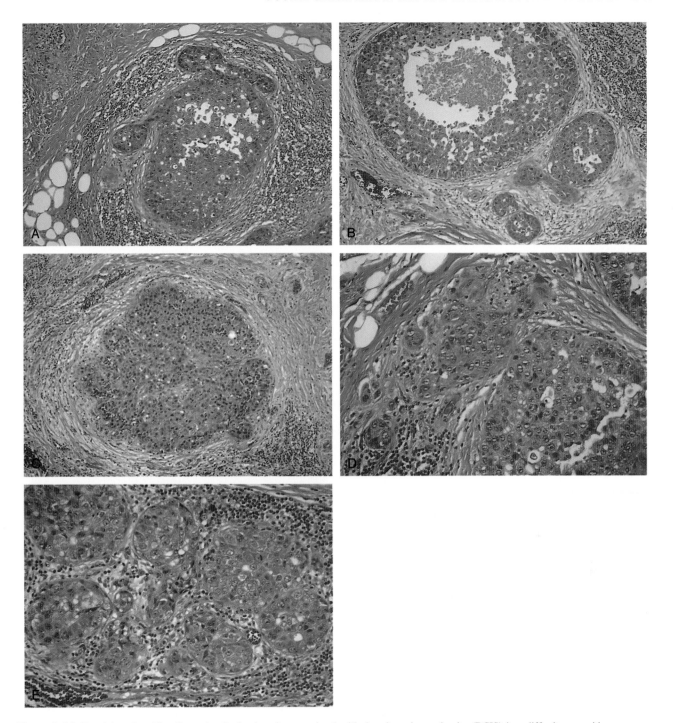

Figure 8–26. Pseudoinvasion. The diagnosis of microinvasion associated with ductal carcinoma in situ (DCIS) is a difficult one, with many more mimickers than true instances of invasion. In the several examples shown here, branching of a large duct *(A–C)* or cancerization of lobules *(D, E)*, especially in cases of high-grade DCIS associated with desmoplastic stromal reaction, may simulate invasion. Again, low-power architecture showing the epithelial nests in question confined within the duct/lobular outlines helps rule out invasive carcinoma. Actin stain, as discussed previously (see Figs. 8–24 and 8–25), may be used in case of doubt. It is important to use a conservative approach in these instances and diagnose only unequivocal invasion.

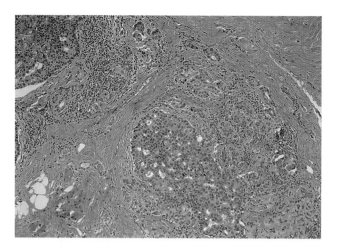

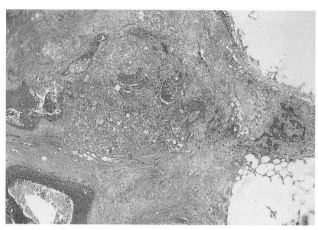

Figure 8–27. Microinvasion is defined as an area of invasive carcinoma measuring up to 1 mm in greatest dimension (see also Chapter 10). In the case shown here, two terminal duct/lobular units are involved by intraductal carcinoma; however, the focus of invasion seen between the two lobules clearly surpasses their confines and is thus diagnosed as invasive carcinoma. Compare this process with examples of lobular cancerization shown previously (see Figs. 8–24 and 8–26), in which the malignant process is limited by the confines of the terminal duct/lobular unit.

Figure 8–28. Epithelial displacement in intraductal carcinoma after core needle biopsy. This rare phenomenon may be seen after any needling procedure (fine-needle aspiration or core biopsy) and can lead to misdiagnosis of invasive carcinoma.[45, 46] Not only ductal carcinoma in situ (DCIS) but even benign epithelium may become displaced and mimic stromal or vascular space invasion. In this microphotograph, detached fragments of intraductal carcinoma are seen within organizing hemorrhage and show a clear linear distribution characteristic of needling artifact.

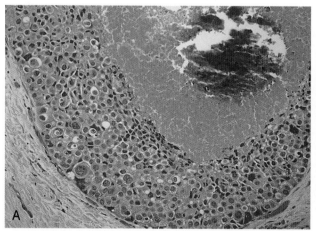

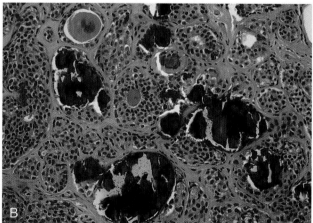

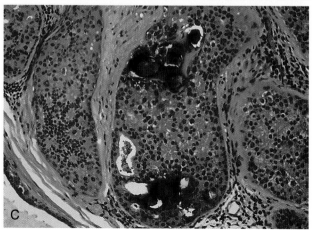

Figure 8–29. Microcalcifications. Microcalcifications are found in >70% of ductal carcinomas in situ (DCIS).[2] Other characteristic radiologic findings in DCIS include asymmetric density, with or without microcalcifications. Microcalcifications, if associated with DCIS, make for a better preoperative assessment of the extent of disease. Absence of microcalcifications was the only feature on multivariate analysis that was associated with recurrence in the study of Goldstein and coworkers.[47]

Microcalcifications seen in DCIS vary from early amorphous as seen here in comedocarcinoma *(A)* to laminated, shown in low-grade solid DCIS involving a sclerosing lesion *(B),* to psammoma-like *(C),* seen here in low-grade cribriform DCIS.

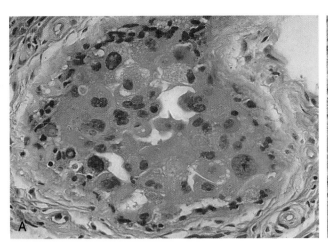
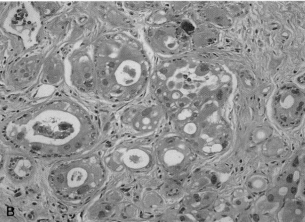

Figure 8–30. Ductal carcinoma in situ (DCIS) with treatment effect. In these microphotographs, DCIS with treatment effect is shown in a duct *(A)* and involving sclerosing adenosis *(B)*. Note marked cytomegaly with severe nuclear pleomorphism and abundant vacuolated cytoplasm. The nuclear grade cannot be assessed in these cases.

Margin Status at Excision of DCIS and Incidence of Recurrent or Residual Disease

Margin Status	Recurrence Rate/ Residual Disease	References
At least 1 mm	43%	48
<1 mm	76%	48
<1 mm	37.9%	49
<2 mm	31%	50
>2 mm	17%	50
≤5 mm	38%	51
>5 mm	6%	51
>10 mm	4.5%	49

Figure 8–31. Margin status. Using stereomicroscopic three-dimensional analysis, Faverly and colleagues showed that high-grade ductal carcinoma in situ (DCIS) grows continuously within the duct system, whereas the majority of low-grade DCIS showed discontinuous spread, with most gaps <10 mm long.[8] This has resulted in the recommendation by some institutions for a distance of at least 10 mm to be considered as a negative resection margin.

AXILLARY LYMPH NODE METASTASES

Examination of axillary lymph nodes in patients with DCIS is not a routine procedure but, when performed, identifies metastatic disease in up to 6% of patients, most of whom have high-grade/comedocarcinoma or, less frequently, very large low-grade DCIS.[19] The overwhelming majority of these metastases are micrometastases, most of which are detected only by cytokeratin immunostain.[19] We assume that foci of stromal invasion were present but missed in most (if not all) of the primary tumors in these cases.

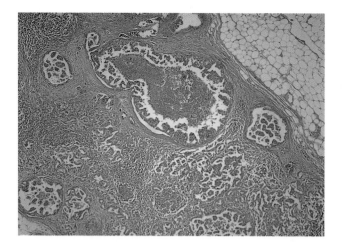

Figure 8–32. Revertant, or ductal carcinoma in situ (DCIS)–like, lymph node metastasis of invasive mammary carcinoma. Some metastases of invasive mammary carcinoma show the so-called revertant DCIS, or DCIS-like pattern.[52] This does not represent true DCIS, however, as no myoepithelial cells can be demonstrated in these cases. Interestingly, these DCIS-like areas exhibit a complete concordance with the primary intraductal component present elsewhere in the breast. This fascinating lesion is more common in cases with extensive axillary lymph node involvement, as seen in this figure.

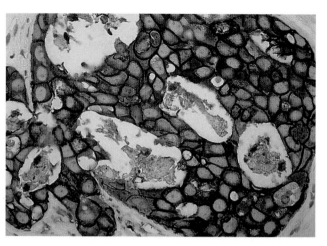

Figure 8–34. Strong c-erbB-2 immunostaining in comedocarcinoma. Amplification of c-erbB-2 is found by immunohistochemistry in a third of all ductal carcinomas in situ (DCIS) but is much more common in high-grade, especially comedo DCIS than in low-grade lesions.[54] c-erbB-2 positivity is associated with higher risk of local recurrence[34] and larger tumor size; overall it is seen in DCIS more commonly than in an associated invasive component of the same case, a paradox that awaits explanation.[55]

MOLECULAR/ IMMUNOHISTOCHEMICAL MARKERS

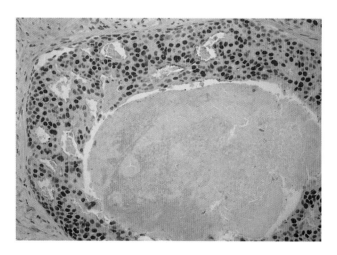

Figure 8–33. Estrogen receptor (ER) expression in ductal carcinoma in situ (DCIS). This microphotograph illustrates positive nuclear staining for ER in a low-grade cribriform DCIS. ER and progesterone receptor (PR) expression is observed in up to a third of intraductal carcinomas and is associated with low nuclear grade, and absence of c-erbB-2 overexpression.[53] Most low-grade DCIS cases express ER and PR, while only rare high-grade cases do so. This separation has served as a basis for recommendation for using steroid receptor status as a helpful discriminating feature in difficult cases.[30]

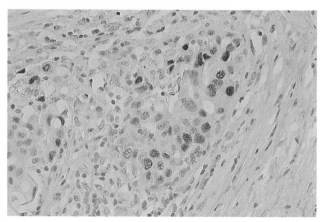

Figure 8–35. Positive nuclear immunoreactivity for p53 antigen in high-grade ductal carcinoma in situ (DCIS). Positive immunostaining is almost exclusively seen in high-grade DCIS[56]; this finding is supported by the finding of p53 mutations in microdissected DCIS in 41% of high-grade and 4% of intermediate-grade DCIS and none of low-grade DCIS.[57]

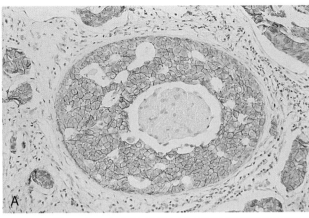

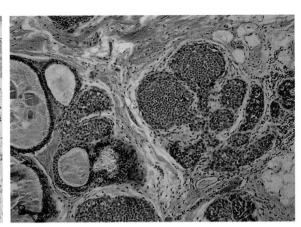

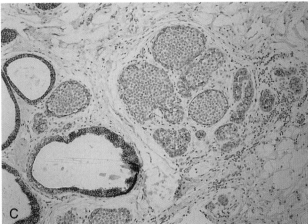

Figure 8–36. E-cadherin in the differential diagnosis of ductal carcinoma in situ (DCIS) and lobular carcinoma in situ (LCIS). Although in most cases, this distinction is easily made on hematoxylin and eosin stain, some cases of solid low-grade proliferations are difficult to classify accurately. One example of diagnostic problems is solid low-grade DCIS versus a lobular proliferation involving a terminal duct. In some cases, if the lesion occupies a lobule, the differential diagnosis is lobular cancerization by low-grade DCIS versus LCIS. In these instances, E-cadherin immunostaining becomes very useful and helps differentiate between ductal (E-cadherin–positive) and lobular (E-cadherin–negative) lesions.[58–60] *A,* Intraductal carcinoma shows characteristic strong membranous positivity for E-cadherin. *B,* In this case, a uniform cell population fills this terminal duct/lobular unit. *C,* E-cadherin immunostain is negative in this lesion, which is classified as LCIS. Note the positive internal control in benign ducts and lobules.

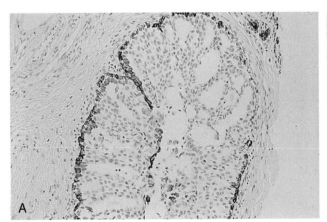

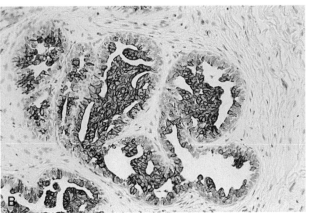

Figure 8–37. Use of keratin 34βE12 expression in the differential diagnosis of ductal hyperplasia and ductal carcinoma in situ (DCIS). Moinfar and associates[61] recently showed that keratin 34βE12 expression was lost in most cases of DCIS and atypical ductal hyperplasia (ADH) (90% of DCIS and 80% of ADH cases are negative), in contrast to usual intraductal hyperplasia (IDH), which showed heterogeneous but intense positivity in all cases. Immunostain for 34βE12 is negative in this case of DCIS *(A)* and is strongly positive in a profile involved by florid ductal hyperplasia *(B)*.

Recommendations for the Reporting of Breast Carcinoma with Respect to in situ Carcinoma

Gross Description

1. How the specimen was received—fresh, in formalin, intact, cut, margins inked or not.
2. How the specimen was identified and procedure—labeled with (name, number), designated as breast, right or left, and procedure: needle localization for calcifications, core biopsy, incisional biopsy, (excisional biopsy [lumpectomy], reexcision, quadrantectomy, simple mastectomy, modified mastectomy, other).
3. Size—the overall size of the excised specimen should be measured in three dimensions
4. Tumor description
   a. Presence or absence of a mass(es)
   b. Margins of the masses(es) (circumscribed, infiltrative)
   c. Distance of the mass(es) from nearest surgical margins (measured and recorded)
   d. Location of the mass(es) (e.g., quadrant if the specimen is a mastectomy)
   e. Size of the mass(es) (at least greatest diameter should be recorded, three dimensions are preferable)
   f. Texture of the masses(es) (e.g., soft, fleshy, hard, gritty)
5. Description of the prior biopsy site if present
6. Description of the remainder of the tissue (breast)
7. Number and appearance of lymph nodes if received
8. It is recommended that fresh tissue should not be submitted for special investigation because the most important information is the presence or absence of invasion. Blocks may be sectioned for special investigation if that information is desirable in an individual case
9. Whether a diagnostic frozen section was performed and the diagnosis that was made.

Diagnostic Information

1. Laterality of the breast and procedure
2. Histologic type—the Association recognizes that different terms are sometimes used for microscopically identified lesions (e.g., the term "lobular neoplasia" includes cases of atypical lobular hyperplasia). Moreover, ADASP recognizes that although the majority of cases of in situ carcinoma are readily categorized, there are borderline lesions. The criteria for diagnosing small borderline lesions as to either lobular carcinoma in situ (LCIS) or ductal carcinoma in situ (DCIS) vary. Different authors use different qualitative and quantitative criteria in arriving at the diagnosis of LCIS or DCIS in these circumstances.

   The Association realizes that the classification system for DCIS (intraductal carcinoma) is in a state of flux; because of this, it is recommended that the lesion be graded using the traditional system based primarily on architectural pattern as well as assigning a specific nuclear grade.

3. Architectural type
   a. Ductal carcinoma in situ (intraductal carcinoma) specify subtype—cribriform, micropapillary, solid (microacinar), papillary (includes most cases of intracystic), comedo (requires high grade nuclei; necrosis present)
   b. Lobular carcinoma in situ
4. Nuclear grade—because the architectural pattern may vary from area to area in the individual case and because nuclear grade may be important in regard to the potential for recurrence, the Association recommends that the ductal carcinoma in situ be divided into high, low, or intermediate nuclear grade in addition to providing type. Lobular carcinoma in situ is not routinely graded.
5. For ductal carcinoma in situ lesions only: margins of resection—the Association recognizes that at the present time, the clinical relevance of a positive margin is not clear, and further recognizes that there is no standard definition of what constitutes a positive or negative margin. However, margin involvement is used by many clinicians in forming therapeutic recommendations. In reporting the margins of resection state (a) whether sections of the margins have been taken parallel (shaved) or perpendicular to the surgical margin and (b) whether tumor is at margin (grossly or microscopically). If tumor is not present at a shaved margin or at an inked margin, the distance from the margin should be specified. Assessment of margins for lobular carcinoma in situ is not recommended.
6. For ductal carcinoma in situ lesions only: size—if a mass is present, obtain this from the gross; if not, several methods can be used to measure the size of an in situ process: (a) sectioning the biopsy from one end of the specimen to the other at 3–4-mm intervals and submitting the sections in sequence, thus allowing for an estimate of the size of the lesion based on the sections in which the lesion is present; or, (b) in small lesions, a measurement of size of the lesion may be obtained directly from the slide.
7. Microcalcifications—if the specimen was removed because of mammographic identification of microcalcifications, these should be identified in the tissue sections and the fact that they are found should be reported. A correlation with the location of the microcalcifications in the mammogram should be reported. It should be stated in which lesion the calcifications were identified (i.e., DCIS, adenosis). If they are not found or if the microcalcifications in the sections are not in the location indicated by the mammogram, this should be reported.
8. Other significant disease—atypical hyperplasias, papillomas, Paget's disease of the nipple, biopsy site changes.
9. If information required for prognosis or therapy is not available or cannot be adequately assessed (margins not assessable because specimen was cut before inking), this should be stated specifically in the report.

Figure 8–38. Recommendations for reporting of ductal carcinoma in situ (DCIS) by the Association of Directors of Anatomic and Surgical Pathology (ADASP). (From Association of Directors of Anatomic and Surgical Pathology: Recommendations for the reporting of breast carcinoma. Pathol Case Rev 3:241–247, 1998.)

ATYPICAL DUCTAL HYPERPLASIA

Clinical Significance of ADH in Various Clinical Settings

Setting	Significance	References
ADH in excisional biopsy and no other worse findings	Increased risk of developing breast cancer at long-term follow-up: 4 to 5-fold relative risk, or 8%–10% absolute risk at 10–15 years follow-up. No other surgery is needed; patients may benefit from chemoprevention therapy	16, 17
ADH at margin in excision with DCIS	Increased risk of local recurrence	44
ADH on core needle biopsy	Indication for excision, as incidence of malignancy at excision is 13%–66% (average 36.5%), including invasive carcinoma in up to 36% of cases	62–68

Figure 8–39. Clinical significance of atypical ductal hyperplasia (ADH). The finding of ADH in an excision is an indication of an increased risk of subsequent development of carcinoma in up to 10% of patients with follow-up of 2 decades or more.[16, 17, 69] Although this still applies to ADH found on core needle biopsy, malignancy can be seen in up to 66% on excision after the diagnosis of ADH in these patients, justifying a mandatory excision.

Although the management implications are drastically different among usual hyperplasia, ADH, and ductal carcinoma in situ (DCIS), in reality they belong to a continuum of proliferative breast disease with gradually increasing risk of breast cancer,[10, 14, 15] and the distinction can be very difficult in borderline cases. Some cases of ADH may be direct precursors of low-grade DCIS: ADH is aneuploid in 33%[70] and monoclonal in over 50% of cases.[71]

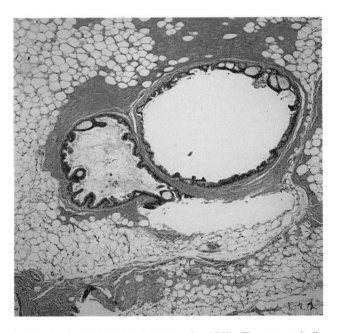

Figure 8–40. Atypical ductal hyperplasia (ADH). The two cystically dilated ducts seen in this figure are partially involved by epithelial proliferation with features of ductal carcinoma in situ (DCIS) (cribriform and micropapillary formations). The proliferation does not involve either profile completely, and the diagnosis of intraductal carcinoma cannot be made.

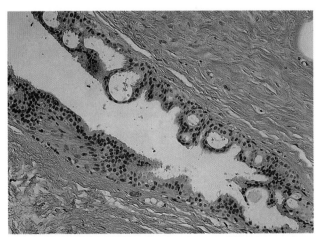

Figure 8–41. Atypical ductal hyperplasia (ADH). A proliferation similar to the one shown in Figure 8–40 is seen, with micropapillary and cribriform features. Note the presence of streaming in the arches, with nuclear axes oriented parallel to the arch.

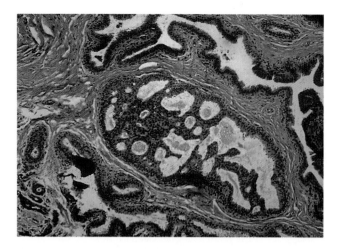

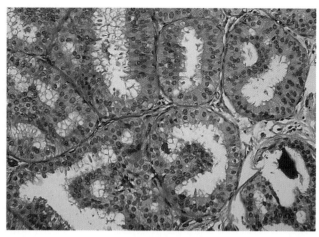

Figure 8–42. Atypical ductal hyperplasia (ADH). One duct profile in this case shows focal architectural changes resembling ductal carcinoma in situ (DCIS): there is cribriforming with some rounded, "punched-out" spaces; still other spaces show compression in the center with focal streaming. The epithelium of the uninvolved portion of this duct shows normal cuboidal lining. The diagnosis of ADH in this case is made because the changes have some features of DCIS but are admixed with areas more typical of usual ductal hyperplasia; in addition, these changes do not involve two complete duct profiles.

Figure 8–44. Atypical ductal hyperplasia (ADH) in pregnancy-like hyperplasia. In this lobule, the epithelium appears columnar with abundant cytoplasm and secretions. Focal micropapillary formations and round "Roman" arches are present, but these changes do not involve any given duct completely.

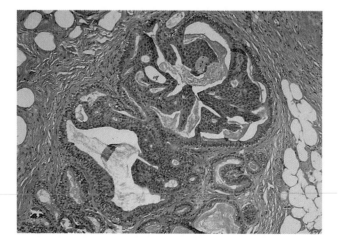

Figure 8–43. Atypical ductal hyperplasia (ADH), columnar cell type. In this case, there is micropapillary/cribriform proliferation of columnar cells approaching ductal carcinoma in situ (DCIS) in the profile on the top. The proliferation in the profile below does not involve it completely, and shows uneven spaces and streaming. The diagnosis of ADH is made here because the changes characteristic of DCIS do not involve two complete epithelial profiles.

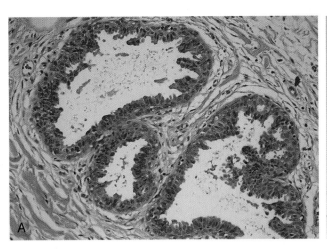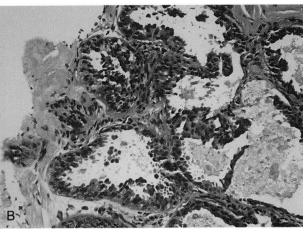

Figure 8–45. Atypical ductal hyperplasia (ADH) with micropapillary features. *A,* In this example, the architectural atypia is minimal, and this lesion may be considered borderline between micropapillary hyperplasia and ADH. Note that, unlike in micropapillary ductal carcinoma in situ (DCIS) (see Fig. 8–11), there is a dimorphic cell population, with a preserved layer of residual cuboidal duct lining in parts of these profiles. Some micropapillae have tapered ends, a feature of usual micropapillary hyperplasia, while occasional ones have a bulbous rounded shape, similar to micropapillary DCIS. *B,* This case shows much more pronounced architectural and cytologic atypia than seen in *A;* cellular crowding, hyperchromasia, and micropapillae with tufting approach DCIS. However, these changes do not involve any of the profiles completely.

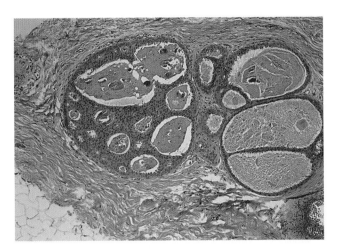

Figure 8–46. Atypical ductal hyperplasia (ADH). This lesion would be diagnostic of low-grade cribriform ductal carcinoma in situ (DCIS); however, it only involves a single duct in this case. Thus, this proliferation does not fulfill the quantitative requirement for the diagnosis of DCIS. It is important to remember, however, that in the case of overt cytologic atypia (equivalent to high- or intermediate-grade DCIS) this quantitative criterion does not have to be fulfilled.[21]

References

1. Ernster VL, Barclay J, Kerlikowske K, et al: Incidence of and treatment for ductal carcinoma in situ of the breast. JAMA 275: 913–918, 1996.
2. Dershaw DD, Abramson A, Kinne DW: Ductal carcinoma in situ: Mammographic findings and clinical implications. Radiology 172: 235–241, 1989.
3. Holland R, Hendriks JH, Vebeek AL, et al: Extent, distribution, and mammographic/histological correlations of breast ductal carcinoma in situ. Lancet 335:519–522, 1990.
4. Lagios MD: Duct carcinoma in situ: Pathology and treatment. Surg Clin North Am 70:853–871, 1990.
5. Fisher ER, Leeming R, Anderson S, et al: Conservative management of intraductal carcinoma (DCIS) of the breast. Collaborating NSABP investigators. J Surg Oncol 47:139–147, 1991.

6. Simpson T, Thirlby RC, Dail DH: Surgical treatment of ductal carcinoma in situ of the breast: 10- to 20-year follow-up. Arch Surg 127:468–472, 1992.
7. Holland R, Hendricks JHCL: Microcalcifications associated with ductal carcinoma in situ: Mammographic-pathologic correlation. Semin Diagn Pathol 11:181–192, 1994.
8. Faverly DR, Burgers L, Bult P, Holland R: Three dimensional imaging of mammary ductal carcinoma in situ: Clinical implications. Semin Diagn Pathol 11:193–198, 1994.
9. Hittmair AP, Lininger RA, Tavassoli FA: Ductal carcinoma in situ (DCIS) in the male breast: A morphologic study of 84 cases of pure DCIS and 30 cases of DCIS associated with invasive carcinoma—a preliminary report. Cancer 83:2139–2149, 1998.
10. Rosai J: Borderline epithelial lesions of the breast. Am J Surg Pathol 15:209–221, 1991.
11. Schnitt SJ, Connolly JL, Tavassoli FA, et al: Interobserver reproducibility in the diagnosis of ductal proliferative breast lesions using standardized criteria. Am J Surg Pathol 16:1133–1143, 1992.
12. Elston CW, Sloane JP, Amendoeira I, et al: Causes of inconsistency in diagnosing and classifying intraductal proliferations of the breast. Eur J Cancer 36:1769–1772, 2000.
13. Sloane JP, Amendoeira I, Apostolikas N, et al: Consistency achieved by 23 European pathologists from 12 countries in diagnosing breast disease and reporting prognostic features of carcinomas. European Commission Working Group on Breast Screening Pathology. Virchows Arch 434:3–10, 1999.
14. Page DL, Jensen RA, Simpson JF: Premalignant and malignant disease of the breast: The roles of the pathologist. Mod Pathol 11:120–128, 1998.
15. Tavassoli FA: Ductal carcinoma in situ: Introduction of the concept of ductal intraepithelial neoplasia. Mod Pathol 11:140–154, 1998.
16. Tavassoli FA, Norris H: A comparison of the results of long-term follow-up for atypical intraductal hyperplasia and intraductal hyperplasia of the breast. Cancer 65:518–529, 1990.
17. Page DL, Dupont WD, Rogers LW, Rados MS; Atypical hyperplastic lesions of the female breast: A long-term follow-up study. Cancer 55:2698–2708, 1985.
18. Page DL, Dupont WD, Rogers LW, Landenberger M: Intraductal carcinoma of the breast: Follow-up after biopsy only. Cancer 49:751–758, 1982.
19. Pendas S, Dauway E, Giuliano R, et al: Sentinel node biopsy in ductal carcinoma in situ patients. Ann Surg Oncol 7:15–20, 2000.
20. Page DL, Rogers LW: Carcinoma in situ (CIS). In Page D, Anderson TJ (eds): Diagnostic Histopathology of the Breast. New York, Churchill Livingstone, 1987, pp 157–192.
21. Lininger RA, Tavassoli FA: Atypical intraductal hyperplasia of the breast. In Silverstein MJ (ed): Ductal Carcinoma in Situ of the Breast. Baltimore, Williams Wilkins, 1997, pp 195–222.
22. Page DL, Rogers LW: Combined histologic criteria for the diagnosis of mammary atypical ductal hyperplasia. Hum Pathol 23:1095–1097, 1992.
23. Scott MA, Lagios MD, Axelsson K, et al: Ductal carcinoma in situ of the breast: Reproducibility of histological subtype analysis. Hum Pathol 28:967–973, 1997.
24. Silverstein MJ, Poller DN, Waisman JR, et al: Prognostic classification of breast ductal carcinoma-in-situ. Lancet 345:1154–1157, 1995.
25. Tavassoli FA: Pathology of the breast, 2nd ed. Stamford, Conn., Appleton & Lange, 1999.
26. Badve S, A'Hern RP, Ward AM, et al: Prediction of local recurrence of ductal carcinoma in situ of the breast using five histological classifications: A comparative study with long follow-up. Hum Pathol 29:915–923, 1998.
27. Ottesen GL, Graversen HP, Blichert-Toft M, et al: Carcinoma in situ of the female breast: 10 year follow-up results of a prospective nationwide study. Breast Cancer Res Treat 62:197–210, 2000.
28. Claus EB, Chu P, Howe CL, et al: Pathobiologic findings in DCIS of the breast: Morphologic features, angiogenesis, her-2/neu and hormone receptors. Exp Mol Pathol 70:303–316, 2001.
29. Leong AS, Sormunen RT, Vinyuvat S, et al: Biologic markers in ductal carcinoma in situ and concurrent infiltrating carcinoma. A comparison of eight contemporary grading systems. Am J Clin Pathol 115:709–718, 2001.
30. Moreno A, Lloveras B, Figueras A, et al: Ductal carcinoma in situ

31. of the breast: Correlation between histologic classifications and biologic markers. Mod Pathol 10:1088–1092, 1997.
31. Bellamy CO, McDonald C, Salter DM, et al: Noninvasive ductal carcinoma of the breast: The relevance of the histologic categorization. Hum Pathol 24:16–23, 1993.
32. Quinn CM, Ostrowski JL: Cytological and architectural heterogeneity in ductal carcinoma in situ of the breast. J Clin Pathol 50:596–599, 1997.
33. Moriya T, Silverberg SG: Intraductal carcinoma (ductal carcinoma in situ) of the breast. A comparison of pure noninvasive tumors with those including different proportions of infiltrating carcinoma. Cancer 74:2972–2978, 1994.
34. Silverstein MJ: Predicting local recurrence in patients with ductal carcinoma in situ. In Silverstein MJ (ed): Ductal Carcinoma in Situ of the Breast. Baltimore, Williams & Wilkins, 1997, p 275.
35. Page DL, Dupont WD, Rogers LW, et al: Continued local recurrence of carcinoma 15–25 years after a diagnosis of low grade ductal carcinoma in situ of the breast treated only by biopsy. Cancer 76:1197–1200, 1995.
36. Mack L, Kerkvliet N, Doig G, O'Malley FP: Relationship of a new histological categorization of ductal carcinoma in situ of the breast with size and the immunohistochemical expression of p53, c-erbB-2, bcl-2, and Ki-67. Hum Pathol 28:974–979, 1997.
37. Leal C, Costa I, Fonseca D, et al: Intracystic (encysted) papillary carcinoma of the breast: A clinical, pathological, and immunohistochemical study. Hum Pathol 29:1097–1104, 1998.
38. Tavassoli FA, Norris HJ: Intraductal apocrine carcinoma: A clinico-pathologic study of 37 cases. Mod Pathol 7:813–818, 1994.
39. Leal C, Henrique R, Monteiro P, et al: Apocrine ductal carcinoma in situ of the breast: Histologic classification and expression of biologic markers. Hum Pathol 32:487–493, 2001.
40. Rosen PP: Breast Pathology. Diagnosis by Core Needle Biopsy. Philadelphia, Lippincott Williams & Wilkins, 1999.
41. Eusebi V, Foschini MP, Cook MG, et al: Long-term follow-up of in situ carcinoma of the breast with special emphasis on clinging carcinoma. Semin Diagn Pathol 6:165–173, 1989.
42. Moinfar F, Man YG, Bratthauer GL, et al: Genetic abnormalities in mammary ductal intraepithelial neoplasia–flat type ("clinging ductal carcinoma in situ"): A simulator of normal mammary epithelium. Cancer 88:2072–2081, 2000.
43. Rosen PP, Cranor ML: Secretory carcinoma of the breast. Arch Pathol Lab Med 115:141–144, 1991.
44. Goldstein NS, Lacerna M, Vicini F. Cancerization of lobules and atypical ductal hyperplasia adjacent to ductal carcinoma in situ of the breast. Am J Clin Pathol 110:357–367, 1998.
45. Youngson BJ, Cranor M, Rosen PP: Epithelial displacement in surgical breast specimens following needling procedures. Am J Surg Pathol 18:896–903, 1994.
46. Youngson BJ, Liberman L, Rosen PP: Displacement of carcinomatous epithelium in surgical breast specimens following stereotaxic core biopsy. Am J Clin Pathol 103:598–602, 1995.
47. Goldstein NS, Kestin L, Vicini F: Intraductal carcinoma of the breast. Pathologic features associated with local recurrence in patients treated with breast-conserving therapy. Am J Surg Pathol 24:1058–1067, 2000.
48. Silverstein MJ, Gierson ED, Colburn WJ, et al: Can intraductal breast carcinoma be excised completely by local excision? Clinical and pathologic predictors. Cancer 73:2985–2989, 1994.
49. Chan KC, Knox WF, Sinha G, et al: Extent of excision margin width required in breast conserving surgery for ductal carcinoma in situ. Cancer 91:9–16, 2001.
50. Ratanawichitrasin A, Rybicki LA, Steiger E, et al: Predicting the likelihood of residual disease in women treated for ductal carcinoma in situ. J Am Coll Surg 188:17–21, 1999.
51. Arnesson LG, Smeds S, Fagerberg G, Grontoft O: Follow-up of two treatment modalities for ductal cancer in situ of the breast. Br J Surg 76:672–675, 1989.
52. Barsky SH, Doberneck SA, Sternlicht MD, et al: "Revertant" DCIS in human axillary breast carcinoma metastases. J Pathol 183:188–194, 1997.
53. Poller DN, Snead DR, Roberts EC, et al: Oestrogen receptor expression in ductal carcinoma in situ of the breast: Relationship to flow cytometric analysis of DNA and expression of the c-erbB-2 oncoprotein. Br J Cancer 68:156–161, 1993.
54. Iwase H, Ando Y, Ichihara S, et al: Immunohistochemical analysis

on biological markers in ductal carcinoma in situ of the breast. Breast Cancer 8:98–104, 2001.

55. Wilbur DC, Barrows GH: Estrogen and progesterone receptor and c-erbB-2 oncoprotein analysis in pure in situ breast carcinoma: An immunohistochemical study. Mod Pathol 6:114–120, 1993.

56. Poller DN, Roberts EC, Bell JA, et al: p53 protein expression in mammary ductal carcinoma in situ: Relationship to immunohistochemical expression of estrogen receptor and c-erbB-2 protein. Hum Pathol 24:463–468, 1993.

57. Done SJ, Eskandarian S, Bull S, et al: p53 missense mutations in microdissected high-grade ductal carcinoma in situ of the breast. J Natl Cancer Inst 93:700–704, 2001.

58. Acs G, Lawton TJ, Rebbeck TR, et al: Differential expression of E-cadherin in lobular and ductal neoplasms of the breast and its biologic and diagnostic implications. Am J Clin Pathol 115:85–98, 2001.

59. Goldstein NS, Bassi D, Watts JC, et al: E-cadherin reactivity of 95 noninvasive ductal and lobular lesions of the breast. Implications for the interpretation of problematic lesions. Am J Clin Pathol 115: 534–542, 2001.

60. Lehr HA, Folpe A, Yaziji H, et al: Cytokeratin 8 immunostaining pattern and E-cadherin expression distinguish lobular from ductal breast carcinoma. Am J Clin Pathol 114:190–196, 2000.

61. Moinfar F, Man YG, Lininger RA, et al: Use of keratin 34βE12 as an adjunct in the diagnosis of mammary intraepithelial neoplasia-ductal type—benign and malignant ductal proliferations. Am J Surg Pathol 23:1048–1058, 1999.

62. Ioffe OB, Berg WA, Rucker C, Silverberg SG: Can we predict malignancy at excision of atypical ductal hyperplasia diagnosed on core needle biopsy of the breast? [abstract]. Mod Pathol 14:28A, 2001.

63. Burak WE, Owens KE, Tighe MB, et al: Vacuum-assisted stereotactic breast biopsy: Histologic underestimates of malignant lesions. Arch Surg 135:700–703, 2000.

64. Jackman RJ, Nowels KW, Rodriguez-Soto J, et al: Stereotactic, automated, large-core needle biopsy of nonpalpable breast lesions: False-negative and histologic underestimation rates after long-term follow-up. Radiology 210:799–805, 1999.

65. Darling ML, Smith DN, Lester SC, et al: Atypical ductal hyperplasia and ductal carcinoma in situ as revealed by large-core needle breast biopsy: Results of surgical excision. AJR Am J Roentgenol 175:1341–1346, 2000.

66. O'hea BJ, Tornos C: Mild ductal atypia after large-core needle biopsy of the breast: Is surgical excision always necessary? Surgery 128:738–743, 2000.

67. Lin PH, Clyde JC, Bates DM, et al: Accuracy of stereotactic core-needle breast biopsy in atypical ductal hyperplasia. Am J Surg 175: 380–382, 1998.

68. Philpotts LE, Shaheen NA, Carter D, et al: Comparison of rebiopsy rates after stereotactic core needle biopsy of the breast with 11-gauge vacuum suction probe versus 14-gauge needle and automatic gun. AJR Am J Roentgenol 172:683–687, 1999.

69. London S, Connolly J, Schnitt S, Colditz G: A prospective study of benign breast disease and the risk of breast cancer. JAMA 267: 941–944, 1992.

70. Schmitt FC, Leal C, Lopes C: p53 protein expression and nuclear DNA content in breast intraductal proliferations. J Pathol 176:233–241, 1995.

71. Lakhani SR, Collins N, Stratton MR, Sloane JP: Atypical ductal hyperplasia of the breast: Clonal proliferation with loss of heterozygosity on chromosomes 16q and 17p. J Clin Pathol 48:611–615, 1995.

CHAPTER 9

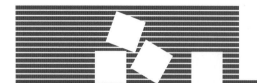

Atypical Lobular Hyperplasia, Lobular Carcinoma In Situ, and Infiltrating Lobular Carcinoma

Andra R. Frost

INTRODUCTION

Foote and Stewart[1, 2] were among the first to recognize infiltrating lobular carcinoma (ILC) as a specific histologic type of carcinoma identified by its linear pattern of infiltration and associated desmoplastic reaction. They were also aware of its frequent concurrence with a type of in situ carcinoma involving small ducts and lobules, which they named lobular carcinoma in situ (LCIS), and concluded that ILC arose from LCIS. They also recognized that LCIS is a multicentric process that is not detectable by physical examination or grossly in resected specimens, LCIS extends from involved lobules into adjacent ducts but rarely causes Paget's disease of the nipple, the cells of LCIS frequently have a mucin content, and LCIS is often associated with invasive carcinomas, including lobular and ductal types.[3, 4]

Subsequently, other observers have confirmed the findings of Foote and Stewart and have provided new information about the behavior and significance of ILC and LCIS. It has been determined that, in addition to being multicentric, LCIS has a higher incidence of bilaterality, with carcinoma involving both breasts synchronously or metachronously, than does DCIS. The frequent association of LCIS with invasive carcinoma, especially ILC, was confirmed by other authors who reported an increased likelihood of subsequent invasive carcinoma in patients with a diagnosis of LCIS. In addition, both the breast involved by LCIS and the opposite breast were at an increased risk for developing invasive carcinoma. This observed multicentricity, bilaterality, and increased risk for subsequent invasive carcinoma resulted in treating LCIS with mastectomy of the involved breast and either mastectomy or biopsy of the opposite breast.[3, 5]

As it gradually became apparent that less than half of patients with LCIS have bilateral disease, and the majority (approximately 80%) of patients with LCIS do not develop invasive carcinoma even after long-term follow-up, the necessity of bilateral mastectomy or mastectomy with biopsy of the opposite breast in every woman with LCIS came into question. In efforts to identify those cases of LCIS that were more likely to progress, the extent of lobular involvement appeared to be a prognostic indicator. Less extensive in situ lobular lesions (e.g., those with residual acinar lumens, acini lacking distention, or involvement of only one lobule) were termed atypical lobular hyperplasia (ALH), although definitions varied from author to author. Studies comparing the relative risk of patients with ALH and LCIS for developing subsequent carcinoma have demonstrated a lower relative risk for ALH (approximately 4.0) than for LCIS (approximately 9.0). ALH and LCIS are now considered to be markers for an increased risk of developing carcinoma rather than being obligate precursors of invasive carcinoma, and close clinical follow-up, rather than mastectomy, is now the more common treatment recommendation.[3, 5, 6] A study of loss of heterozygosity at chromosome 11q13 in LCIS, ALH, and ILC has shown that cases of LCIS with loss of heterozygosity at chromosome 11q13 were more likely to be associated with ILC, which demonstrated a similar loss of heterozygosity.[7] In addition, several examples of LCIS that have progressed to microinvasive disease have been reported.[8] These findings suggest an etiologic link between LCIS and ILC, as previously suggested by Foote and Stewart.

Patients with ILC have been demonstrated to have a higher frequency of bilateral carcinoma than patients with other types of invasive carcinoma, including infiltrating duct carcinoma (IDC). In addition, ILC has a tendency to be multifocal. ILC also differs from IDC in its distribution of metastatic sites, with a higher frequency of involvement of peritoneal surfaces, gastrointestinal tract, uterus, and ovaries.[9] Biomarker expression in ILC differs from that of IDC, with ILC being less likely to express c-erbB-2, P-cadherin, vascular endothelial growth factor, or E-cadherin than does IDC.[9–14] Additionally, the immunohistochemical pattern of expression of cytokeratin 8 differs in IDC, with a prominent peripheral or membrane staining pattern, and ILC, which has a perinuclear staining pattern.[12] In spite of these differences, most studies of survival in ILC have concluded that when compared stage for stage, overall survival is similar in ILC and IDC.[9] Consequently, standard treatment for ILC is similar to IDC. Breast conserving therapy, which has been demonstrated to be as effective as mastectomy in many patients with IDC, has also proven to be efficacious in treating ILC, despite its frequent multifocality.[15, 16]

As with all invasive breast cancers, the search continues to identify prognostic features of carcinomas that will allow us to more effectively treat patients. Because of apparent biologic differences between ILC and IDC, prognostic indicators applicable to IDC, such as histologic grade, may not be applicable to ILC. After the initial descriptions of classic ILC were reported, it was noted that some cases with the typical cytologic features of ILC infiltrated in solid sheets or nests of cells. These alternate patterns of infiltration became known as variant patterns. In the search for prognostic features of ILC, patients with the variant patterns have had a worse prognosis than patients with classic ILC in some studies, but not in others. Thus far, the most important prognostic determinants in ILC are tumor size and nodal status.[9, 17, 18] As we continue to identify prognostic indicators, assess alternate forms of treatment and develop strategies for the prevention of breast cancer, their applicability to this distinct histologic subtype of invasive breast carcinoma, ILC, should be evaluated.

Clinical Features of ALH and LCIS

Incidence	0.3%–3.8% of breast biopsies
Presentation	Discovered coincidentally
Average age at diagnosis	44 to 54
Bilaterality	35%–59% of cases
Multicentricity	60%–85% of cases
Gross pathology	Dependent on associated lesion

Figure 9–1. Clinical features of atypical lobular hyperplasia (ALH) and lobular carcinoma in situ (LCIS). Histologic definitions of ALH and LCIS vary among authors (see Fig. 9–2), and these entities are combined into a single designation of lobular neoplasia (LN) by some; consequently, the reported clinical features of ALH and LCIS overlap and are presented together. ALH and LCIS are usually incidental histologic findings in breast biopsies or mastectomies performed for a coexisting mass lesion or a mammographic abnormality; consequently, their true incidence is unknown. However, they have been reported to occur in up to 3.8% of breast biopsies, and they have been identified in women ranging in age from 15 to 80, but are most common in premenopausal women. The incidence of bilateral ALH and LCIS is not well documented in many reports because both breasts are not routinely examined by biopsy or mastectomy; however, involvement of both breasts is common. ALH and LCIS are often found in multiple foci in the same breast. These lesions are not detectable in gross specimens, but they are often present in tissue that is grossly abnormal as a result of another benign or malignant neoplasm.[3, 4, 19]

Histologic Definitions of ALH and LCIS

Cellular Characteristics (ALH and LCIS)	
Author	*Description*
Page	Cells lack regular cohesion or orientation, but are similar in appearance and placement with regard to each other
	Round to oval nuclei, usually without hyperchromasia; may have small nucleoli
	Cytoplasm tends to be clear; cytoplasmic vacuoles are frequently present
Rosen	Loss of cellular cohesion
	Typically small, round, cytologically bland nuclei that lack nucleoli, with scant cytoplasm
	May be larger, more pleomorphic nuclei that sometimes have nucleoli and more abundant cytoplasm
	Intracytoplasmic vacuoles containing mucin are usually present
Tavassoli	Classically, relatively uniform, loosely cohesive, often small and round cells with sparse cytoplasm and round nuclei
	May display minor variations in size and cytoplasmic changes (e.g., apocrine, secretory, signet ring cell)
	Intracytoplasmic lumens and mucous globules are common
	Rare to observe distinct cell margins

Extent of Lobular Involvement

	ALH	LCIS
Page	Less than 50% of the acini in a lobular unit are filled, distorted, and distended by characteristic cells	Characteristic cells must comprise the entire population of cells in a lobular unit
	Characteristic cells must be increased in number (>2 above basement membrane) over that normally present in acinus	Filling (no interspersed spaces between cells) of all acini is required
		Expansion and/or distortion of at least 50% of the acini in one lobular unit required
Rosen	Less than 75% of one lobular unit shows the features of LCIS	Characteristic cells replace the normal epithelium of at least 75% of acini and intralobular ductules in one lobular unit
	Borders of acini and intralobular ductules remain indistinct	Involved acini are clearly delineated
		Lobular distention is not an absolute criterion
		Complete absence of glandular lumens is not necessary

	LN1	LN2	LN3
Tavassoli	Partial or complete replacement or displacement of normal acinar cells within a lobule by characteristic cells	Characteristic cells fill and distend some or all acini	Characteristic cells distend the acini to the point that they appear almost confluent, *or*
	Lumens may be filled	Acinar outlines remain distinct and separate from one another with intervening stroma	Acini are distended by a solid, occlusive population of signet ring cells
	Acini are not distended when compared with adjacent uninvolved acini	Residual lumens may persist	Residual lumens are absent

Figure 9–2. Histologic definitions of atypical lobular hyperplasia (ALH) and lobular carcinoma in situ (LCIS). The definitions presented are those of three respected authorities on breast pathology and are the most widely used.[3–5, 19] The cytologic descriptions of the cells comprising ALH and LCIS are similar, although the degree of pleomorphism allowed may vary somewhat. There is agreement that lobular epithelium must be replaced or displaced by these cells, but there are significant differences in the extent of lobular involvement required for ALH and LCIS, with more extensive involvement being required to define LCIS in Page's criteria than in Rosen's. All three of these authorities require involvement of only one lobule, whereas other authors have demanded involvement of more than one lobule to qualify for a diagnosis of LCIS, as discussed by Rosen.[3] Rather than splitting the spectrum of lobular involvement into ALH and LCIS, Tavassoli has chosen to follow the lead of Haagensen[20] and use the designation of lobular neoplasia (LN) to encompass both entities. To convey the extent of lobular neoplasia present, the degree of involvement can be graded as LN1 to LN3. (Data from references 3–5, 19.)

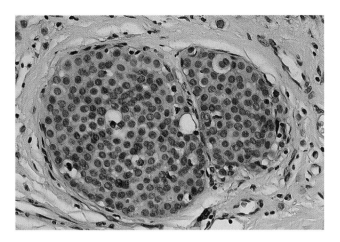

Figure 9–3. Cytologic features of lobular carcinoma in situ (LCIS) and atypical lobular hyperplasia (ALH). The cells of LCIS and ALH are usually relatively uniform, similar to one another, and without hyperchromasia. The cytoplasm is not abundant and is often vacuolated. Nucleoli may be present but are not prominent. Loss of cellular cohesion is also typical, but it may not be readily apparent when acini are completely filled and expanded.

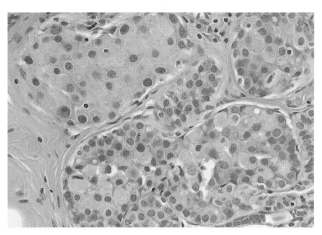

Figure 9–5. Apocrine metaplasia in lobular carcinoma in situ (LCIS). The cells of LCIS and atypical lobular hyperplasia (ALH) can undergo apocrine metaplasia, as depicted in this figure, as well as clear cell change and secretory change. The cells involved by apocrine metaplasia can be expected to have prominent nucleoli.

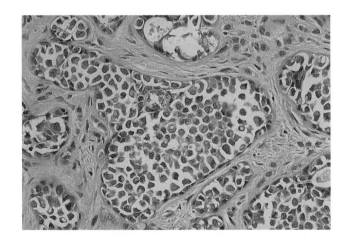

Figure 9–4. Cytologic features of lobular carcinoma in situ (LCIS) and atypical lobular hyperplasia (ALH). The cells of LCIS and ALH do not always exhibit the uniform "classic" appearance. The nuclei may be more pleomorphic, with greater variability in nuclear size and shape than presented in Figure 9–3. The cytoplasm may be abundant and eosinophilic. Nucleoli are often present. These more pleomorphic cells have been referred to as type B cells, and the classic, more uniform cells as type A cells.[3] In addition to the greater degree of pleomorphism demonstrated in this figure, prominent cytoplasmic vacuolization and lack of cellular cohesion are also present. Cytoplasmic vacuolization and/or the presence of intracytoplasmic lumens are characteristic of LCIS and ALH. These cytoplasmic structures often contain mucin, which can be demonstrated by a mucicarmine stain. As seen in the figure, cytoplasmic distention by vacuoles may result in signet ring cells, which can be numerous.

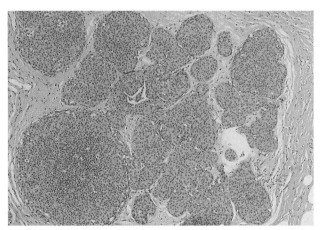

Figure 9–6. Lobular carcinoma in situ (LCIS). In this well developed example of LCIS, lobular acini are filled and >50% are distended or expanded by neoplastic cells with the characteristic cytologic features of LCIS and atypical lobular hyperplasia (ALH). There is marked distention of some acini. The degree of involvement of the lobule in this example meets the criteria of Rosen and possibly Page (although there is a residual lumen in a central intralobular duct) for LCIS and would likely be classified as lobular neoplasia grade 3 (LN3) by Tavassoli.

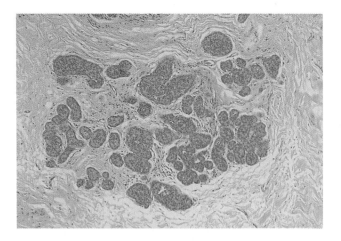

Figure 9–7. Lobular carcinoma in situ (LCIS). In this figure the extent of lobular involvement is less than is seen in Figure 9–6, although >50% of the acini appear expanded, and all are filled with no intercellular lumens or spaces present. The definition of acinar expansion or distortion is often not provided when criteria are presented; however, most authorities compare the size of involved acini with adjacent uninvolved acini, realizing that normal acinar size may vary from lobule to lobule.[3, 5] The degree of involvement of the lobule seen in this figure meets the criteria of both Page and Rosen for LCIS and would probably be classified as lobular neoplasia grade 2 (LN2) by Tavassoli.

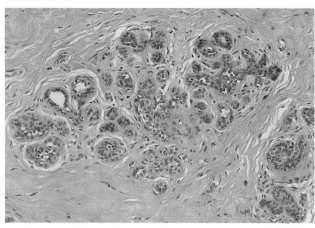

Figure 9–9. Atypical lobular hyperplasia (ALH). This is an example of minimal involvement of a lobule by ALH. Only a portion (<50%) of the acini in this lobular group is involved by the characteristic cells. There is an increased number of cells in involved acini, but only a few of the acini are distended when compared to adjacent uninvolved acini. This lesion would qualify as lobular neoplasia grade 1 (LN1) in Tavassoli's classification system.

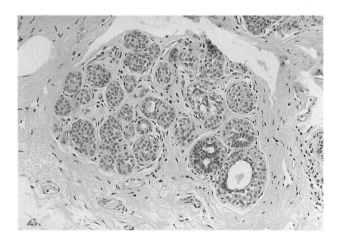

Figure 9–8. Atypical lobular hyperplasia (ALH). The diagnosis of ALH depends on the extent of involvement of the lobular unit by the characteristic cells. In this figure residual acinar lumens are present and slightly less than half of the acini appear distended; thus Page's criteria for a diagnosis of lobular carcinoma in situ (LCIS) are not met, resulting in a designation of ALH. Because complete filling and distention of acini are not absolute requirements in Rosen's definition of LCIS and the normal epithelium of acini and intralobular ductules is replaced in >75% of the lobular unit, this lobule meets Rosen's definition of LCIS. Applying the classification system of Tavassoli would result in a designation of lobular neoplasia grade 2 (LN2). Note the residual normal acinar or intralobular ductal epithelium with undermining lobular neoplasia in the lower right corner.

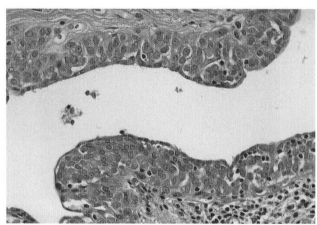

Figure 9–10. Extension of lobular carcinoma in situ (LCIS) into interlobular ducts. The cells of LCIS and atypical lobular hyperplasia (ALH) may extend from the involved lobular unit into interlobular ducts. In this figure, the proliferating cells have formed a thick layer between residual, attenuated normal ductal epithelium at the luminal surface and the basement membrane and residual myoepithelial cells at the duct periphery. This pattern of ductal involvement has been termed "pagetoid" because of its similarity to Paget's disease. LCIS involves the epithelium of ducts in 65% to 75% of patients. Both ALH and LCIS can involve ducts, but the distinction between the two requires examination of involved lobules.

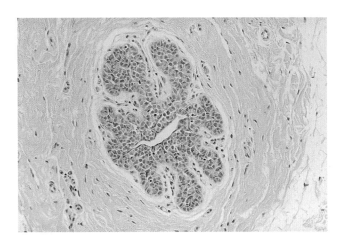

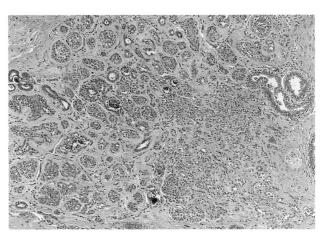

Figure 9–11. Lobular carcinoma in situ (LCIS). Here the lobular involvement by LCIS has resulted in acini pulling away from the intralobular terminal duct, located in the center of the lobule, creating a "cloverleaf" configuration. This process has been referred to as "unfolding" of a lobule, gradually transforming the lobule into a ductlike structure.[5] Some examples of this "cloverleaf" pattern have been interpreted as ductal involvement by LCIS or ALH by others.[3, 4]

Figure 9–13. Lobular carcinoma in situ (LCIS) involving sclerosing adenosis. LCIS may extend into areas of sclerosing adenosis or occasionally may be identified only in sclerosing adenosis. The diagnosis requires recognition of the characteristic cells replacing the native epithelium, as seen in this figure. Because the usual lobular configuration is sometimes markedly distorted in sclerosing adenosis, involvement by LCIS in such distorted foci can resemble invasive carcinoma, as is demonstrated in the right portion of the photomicrograph. On high-power examination, the presence of basement membrane and myoepithelial cells surrounding the clusters of neoplastic cells within the adenosis is usually evident and allows distinction from invasive carcinoma. Immunostains for actin can be used to highlight myoepithelial cells and for laminin and type IV collagen to mark basement membrane. In addition, the overall rounded configuration of the lesion on low-power examination is further evidence of its noninvasive nature. To qualify for invasion, carcinoma cells should be identified in stroma outside the boundary of the sclerosing lesion. In this example, calcifications are also present.

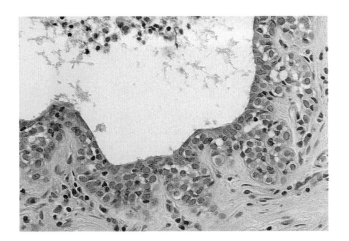

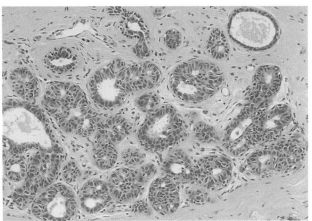

Figure 9–12. Lobular carcinoma in situ (LCIS). This "cloverleaf" structure is less involved by the characteristic cells of LCIS than the one shown in Figure 9–11. This structure could be interpreted as pagetoid extension of LCIS into a duct or as involvement of an unfolding lobule. Diagnostic LCIS was present in nearby lobules.

Figure 9–14. Ductal hyperplasia involving a lobular unit. Ductal hyperplasia and atypical ductal hyperplasia (ADH) can extend into lobular units and are entities in the differential diagnosis of atypical lobular hyperplasia (ALH) and lobular carcinoma in situ (LCIS). Ductal hyperplasia and ADH can usually be distinguished from ALH or LCIS by the presence of lumen formation and cytologic features not characteristic of LCIS or ALH. In this figure, there is lumen formation in intralobular ducts and acini by cells typical of ductal hyperplasia, which exhibit variability in nuclear size and shape and nuclear elongation. The same criteria used to distinguish ductal hyperplasia and ADH in ducts are applicable to these processes in lobular units.

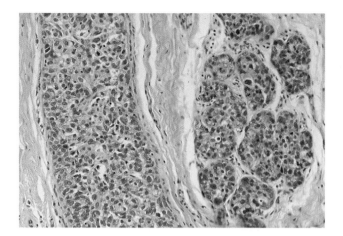

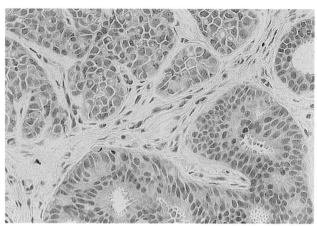

Figure 9–15. Ductal carcinoma in situ (DCIS) involving a lobule. DCIS can also extend into a lobular unit and enters into the differential diagnosis of lobular carcinoma in situ (LCIS) or atypical lobular hyperplasia (ALH). In this figure, the cells involving the lobule and adjacent duct are identical and exhibit a greater degree of pleomorphism than expected in LCIS or ALH. Distinguishing lobular involvement by DCIS with a low nuclear grade from LCIS or ALH can be difficult because the cytologic features of the cells are often similar. Formation of small secondary lumens and a rosetting arrangement of cells suggest ductal differentiation. The presence of distinct cell margins in foci of solid growth has also been identified as a ductal feature.[5] Cytoplasmic vacuolization, intracytoplasmic lumens and signet ring cells are more typical of LCIS or ALH, but they can be seen in DCIS. In some instances, the most helpful feature is finding architecturally diagnostic DCIS with similar cytology in adjacent ducts.

Figure 9–16. Coexisting lobular carcinoma in situ (LCIS) and ductal carcinoma in situ (DCIS). In this figure, there are two cytologically and architecturally different cell populations present. The lobule (*upper*) is expanded and filled by dyscohesive cells with cytologic features of LCIS; however, the adjacent duct (*lower*) contains a more cohesive and slightly less pleomorphic cell population with the cribriform growth pattern of DCIS. DCIS and LCIS can coexist within the same breast and even within the same duct. When this occurs the presence of both should be reported.

Relative Risk for Subsequent Carcinoma in Women with ALH and LCIS*

	Anderson[21]	Rosen et al[22]	Haagensenen et al[20]	Page et al[23]	Bodian et al[24]	Page et al[25]	Page et al[26]
ALH						4.2(126)	4.3(125)
ALH with DIALH							6.8(47)
LCIS	12.0(47)	9.0(99)		9.0(44)			
LN			7.2(211)		5.7(99)		

Figure 9–17. Relative risk for subsequent carcinoma in women with atypical lobular hyperplasia (ALH) and lobular carcinoma in situ (LCIS). Women with ALH and LCIS have an increased risk of developing (or having concurrently) invasive carcinoma in the ipsilateral or contralateral breast. Histologic definitions of ALH and LCIS have varied in studies evaluating the relative risk (RR) of developing subsequent carcinoma when compared to age-matched controls, but the results are consistent and indicate a higher RR for LCIS than ALH. When no distinction was made between ALH and LCIS (i.e., lobular neoplasia (LN) was used), the RR was intermediate between the two. When ALH coexists with a pagetoid extension of the process into interlobular ducts (ductal involvement by ALH, or DIALH), a RR intermediate between ALH and LCIS has resulted.[26] In addition, a family history of breast carcinoma in a mother, sister, or daughter of a woman with ALH will elevate the RR to 11.[5] It is interesting that the RR ascribed to LCIS by Rosen and coworkers and Page and colleagues is similar, despite the fact that their quantitative histologic criteria are significantly different. These results, in addition to the lack of a uniform definition of ALH and LCIS, put in doubt the prognostic significance of splitting the spectrum of lobular involvement into two groups, and have been used to support the use of the general term "lobular neoplasia."

* Relative risk is followed by the total number of cases in parentheses.

Histologic Type of Subsequent or Concurrent Invasive
Carcinoma

Histologic Type	% of Subsequent or Concurrent Invasive Carcinomas
Infiltrating lobular carcinoma	43–70
Infiltrating duct carcinoma	10–50
Tubular carcinoma	20

Figure 9–18. Histologic type of subsequent or concurrent invasive carcinoma. In follow-up studies of women who have not received mastectomy following a biopsy diagnosis of lobular carcinoma in situ (LCIS), 20% to 30% of these women developed invasive breast carcinoma within 15 to 20 years after initial biopsy. Approximately 50% of these invasive carcinomas develop in the contralateral breast.[4] Some series have indicated a preponderance of infiltrating duct carcinoma (IDC) in associated invasive carcinomas, and in others, infiltrating lobular carcinoma (ILC) predominated.[3, 23] The high frequency of bilaterality and multicentricity of atypical lobular hyperplasia (ALH) and LCIS, their prognostic implication of an increased risk for the development of subsequent invasive carcinoma in the ipsilateral or contralateral breast, and their association with infiltrating carcinomas of histologic types other than ILC, has led to the conclusion that they are markers for an increased risk of invasive carcinoma but are not necessarily precursors of invasive carcinoma.

Biomarker Expression and Chromosomal
Alterations in LCIS

	Percentage of Positive Cases
Estrogen receptor[5, 22]	67%–90%
Progesterone receptor[27]	36%
c-erbB-2[5, 28]	0%
Type IV collagen[5]	100%
B72.3[5]	7%
E-cadherin[10]	0%
LOH at 11q13[7]	33%
Chromosomal loss at	
16p[29]	55%
16q[29, 30]	30%, 45%
17p[29, 30]	8%, 29%
22q[29]	52%
Chromosomal gain at	
16q[29]	16%

Figure 9–19. Biomarker expression and chromosomal alterations in lobular carcinoma in situ (LCIS). Information on the expression of molecular markers, hormone receptors, and chromosomal changes in LCIS is limited and practically nonexistent for atypical lobular hyperplasia (ALH). A few studies have demonstrated that LCIS typically possesses estrogen receptors by immunohistochemistry, but it is less frequently positive for progesterone receptors.[5, 27] Type IV collagen can be consistently demonstrated by immunohistochemistry around acini containing the characteristic cells and corresponds to a persistent basal lamina.[5] Unlike ductal carcinoma in situ (DCIS), which frequently expresses c-erbB-2, LCIS does not exhibit immunohistochemical staining for this marker.[5, 28] Also unlike most ductal carcinomas and similar to the majority of infiltrating lobular carcinomas (ILC), LCIS does not express E-cadherin, a cell adhesion molecule that plays a role in cell-cell interactions.[10] Truncating mutations of the E-cadherin gene have been reported in LCIS.[31] Loss of E-cadherin expression may reflect the loss of cellular cohesion typical of LCIS. Nayar and coworkers[7] have demonstrated loss of heterozygosity (LOH) at chromosome 11q13 in approximately one third of informative cases of LCIS examined. In addition, LCIS with concurrent ILC more frequently exhibited LOH than did cases of LCIS without ILC. This suggests that LOH at chromosome 11q13 may play a role in the development of ILC. Such genetic changes in LCIS may indicate a lesion that is more likely to progress to invasive carcinoma than LCIS lacking these alterations. Microdissected samples of ALH and LCIS have been analyzed by comparative genomic hybridization for gains and losses of genetic material. Loss of chromosomal material from 16p, 16q, 17p, and 22q and gain of material from 6q was found at a similar frequency in ALH and LCIS, indicating a similar genetic stage of development for these histologic entities.[29, 30]

Clinical Management of ALH and LCIS

1941	LCIS is designated as "carcinoma" and mastectomy is recommended
1941–1970	Mastectomy with contralateral biopsy is favored over observation
1970	Introduction of mammographic screening and increased public awareness of breast cancer
1978	Rosen and colleagues reported that invasive carcinoma subsequent to LCIS was exceptional
1985	NSABP legitimized breast preservation as alternative to mastectomy
1986	Haagensen reports that the majority of patients with LCIS never develop invasive carcinoma
1996	Observation is favored over mastectomy with contralateral biopsy

Figure 9–20. Clinical management of atypical lobular hyperplasia (ALH) and lobular carcinoma in situ (LCIS). Currently, the recommended management for ALH and most LCIS is a lifetime of close clinical follow-up.[3] This was not always the case, however. Foote and Stewart were the first to designate LCIS as a carcinoma. They conceptualized LCIS and infiltrating lobular carcinoma (ILC) as a single entity and a rare form of breast carcinoma. Consequently, mastectomy was the recommended treatment. Soon the frequent bilaterality of LCIS became apparent, and biopsy of the contralateral breast in addition to mastectomy of the initially biopsied breast containing LCIS was standard therapy. At the same time, another approach to the management of LCIS was initiated by Haagensen, who recognized that all patients with LCIS did not progress to invasive carcinoma. He advised close surveillance of both breasts to allow early detection of carcinomas that might develop, rather than mastectomy. In the 1970s and 1980s, the introduction of mammographic screening and an increased public awareness of breast cancer spawned an increased number of breast biopsies. Consequently ALH and LCIS were detected more frequently, and our understanding of LCIS and ALH as markers of increased risk for invasive carcinoma developed. The 1985 report of the National Surgical Adjuvant Breast Project (NSABP) indicating that breast preservation was as effective as mastectomy in treating stage I and II invasive breast carcinoma resulted in women questioning the need for more aggressive treatment of a marker of increased risk for invasive cancer than for invasive cancer itself. Gradually, the preferred treatment of ALH and LCIS has shifted to long-term observation over mastectomy as indicated by a survey of members of the Society of Surgical Oncology and the American Society of Breast Disease in 1996, in which 85% of respondents favored observation.[6, 32] In a recent assessment of 137 patients with LCIS and associated invasive breast carcinoma (i.e., infiltrating duct carcinoma [IDC], ILC, and mixed ILC and IDC) treated with breast conserving surgery, neither the presence nor extent of LCIS affected the risk of developing recurrent cancer compared with 1044 similarly treated patients without LCIS.[33]

Clinical Features of ILC

Incidence	0.7%–14% of all invasive carcinogams
Presentation	Palpable mass with ill-defined margins
Median age at diagnosis	45–57 years
Bilaterality	6%–47% of cases
Multifocality	Tends to form multiple small nodules
Gross pathology	Firm to hard tumor with irregular borders that blend with surrounding breast parenchyma

Figure 9–21. Clinical features of infiltrating lobular carcinoma (ILC). The reported incidence of ILC varies with differences in histologic definitions between series. The inclusion of the more recently described variant histologic subtypes has resulted in a higher incidence in reports including these subtypes. ILC is relatively more common in women older than 75 years than in those 35 years or younger (11% versus 2%, respectively). Patients generally present with a palpable breast mass, which may be only a vague thickening, a fine diffuse nodularity or a large lesion, sometimes with skin fixation or nipple retraction. Paget's disease of the nipple is rare in ILC. Mammographically, ILC does not produce a single characteristic appearance, but presents in a variety of patterns. An asymmetric, ill defined density is the most common presentation. A disproportionate number of ILCs are missed mammographically when compared with other types of breast carcinoma. Women with ILC have a higher frequency of bilateral carcinomas than do women with other types of breast carcinoma. ILC varies from microscopic in size to involvement of the entire breast. Grossly, ILC forms a firm nodule, often with indistinct borders that may be clearly identifiable only by palpation. Alternatively, the carcinoma may not be visible grossly and detectable only by a slight firmness to palpation, or it may form numerous, tiny, hard nodules in the breast parenchyma.[9, 34]

Histology of ILC

Cytologic Features	
Classic	Similar to cells of LCIS
	Small uniform cells with round to ovoid nuclei and inconspicuous nucleoli
	Mucin-containing intracytoplasmic lumina or vacuoles are variably present; may impart a signet ring cell configuration if prominent
Pleomorphic	More pleomorphic nuclei, often with distinct nucleoli and eccentric placement
	Relatively abundant eosinophilic cytoplasm, often with apocrine differentiation
Histologic Patterns	
Classic	Cells exhibit a lack of cohesion by infiltrating singly or in linear strands one or two cells thick in at least 70%–85% of the tumor
	Diffuse infiltration of breast parenchyma with entrapment of normal structures
	Often assumes a concentric arrangement around ducts and lobules ("targetoid")
Variant Patterns	
Solid	Confluent or solid groups of cells with cytologic features of classic lobular carcinoma constitute the majority of the tumor
	Groups of cells are separated by delicate vascularized stroma
Alveolar	Rounded aggregates or, less commonly, irregularly shaped clumps of ≥20 cells with classic cytologic features of lobular carcinoma constitute the majority of the tumor
Mixed	An admixture of classic and/or variant patterns is present
	There may be a cell population that is more atypical than in classic lobular carcinoma

Figure 9–22. Histology of infiltrating lobular carcinoma (ILC). The initial description of ILC presented by Foote and Stewart in the 1940s was that of classic infiltrating lobular carcinoma, and most clinicopathologic studies published afterward followed their definition. In the 1970s, the variant histologic patterns were recognized, and subsequent series of ILC included these subtypes. A trabecular variant, consisting of classic lobular carcinoma cells infiltrating in trabeculae one or more cells in thickness, has also been described. This particular variant has not gained wide acceptance because of its significant morphologic overlap with the classic and mixed patterns.[9] Most ILCs are not composed completely of any one histologic pattern. The proportion of a single histologic pattern required for classification as a particular histologic subtype has varied from 70% to 80%.[9, 34] More recently, a pleomorphic variant of ILC has been described. This variant exhibits the classic pattern of infiltration, but it is composed of cells with pleomorphic nuclei and often relatively abundant eosinophilic cytoplasm. It has been demonstrated to behave more aggressively than classic ILC.[35–37] The reported incidence of variant subtypes has varied with the histologic criteria employed, but it ranges from 23% to 70%.[9, 38]

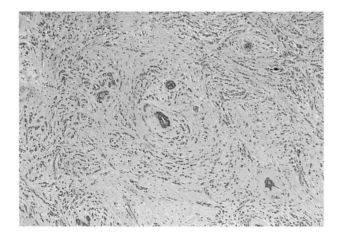

Figure 9–23. Classic infiltrating lobular carcinoma (ILC). This figure is an example of the classic pattern of ILC as initially described by Foote and Stewart. Malignant cells with characteristic cytologic features (see Fig. 9–26) infiltrate as single cells or as groups of cells in a linear arrangement one or two cells thick or as small clusters composed of only a few cells. The cells often infiltrate in a concentric fashion, referred to as "targetoid," around ducts and lobules, as in this figure. Classic ILC can have several patterns, but in general there is a lack of cohesion of the infiltrating cells and an absence of solid, papillary, or alveolar growth and gland formation.

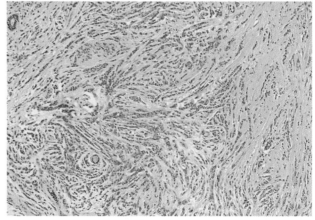

Figure 9–24. Classic infiltrating lobular carcinoma (ILC). In this classic example of ILC, the neoplastic cells have a tendency to form broader, linear aggregates, three to four cells in thickness. This pattern is sometimes referred to as trabecular, but it often occurs with the classic pattern or other variant patterns and, consequently, is usually designated as the classic or mixed histologic pattern.

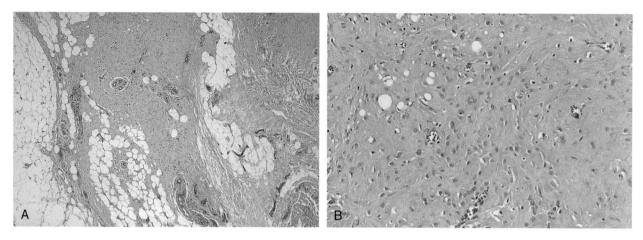

Figure 9–25. Classic infiltrating lobular carcinoma (ILC). *A,* Because of the dispersed pattern of infiltration and tendency to form multiple small nodules, classic ILC can be subtle microscopically, particularly at low power, as demonstrated in this figure. This presentation of ILC has been referred to as "occult." *B,* On higher power examination of the carcinoma seen in *A,* the single cell pattern of infiltration by small neoplastic epithelial cells with relatively uniform nuclei is apparent. This classic ILC has more single cells with fewer cell aggregates than the other examples. This pattern of infiltration can easily be confused with scattered inflammatory cells, particularly at low magnification.

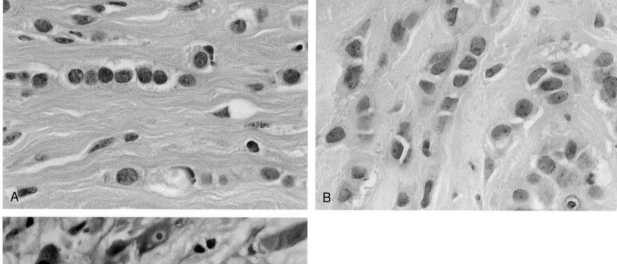

Figure 9–26. Cytology of infiltrating lobular carcinoma (ILC). *A,* The cells of classic ILC are usually small and uniform with round nuclei and small nucleoli, as demonstrated in this figure. *B,* In some examples of classic ILC, the cells, although small, may have notched nuclei and a greater degree of pleomorphism than depicted in *A.* *C,* Cytoplasmic vacuolization, intracytoplasmic lumens, and signet ring cells are present to a variable degree in ILC. Ultrastructurally, intracytoplasmic lumens are large vacuoles with microvilli protruding into the lumens.[39] In some, a central mucin droplet is present. Histologically, this luminal content is identifiable as a central dot. Signet ring cells result when the cytoplasmic vacuoles indent the nucleus. This photomicrograph displays two signet ring cells with intracytoplasmic lumens. One of the cells contains two intracytoplasmic lumens. Other signet ring cells are also present without the cytoplasmic dot.

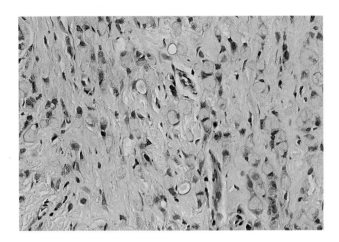

Figure 9–27. Signet ring cells in infiltrating lobular carcinoma (ILC). ILC is rarely composed almost entirely of signet ring cells, as seen in this figure. In nearly half of ILC, signet ring cells comprise ≥10% of the neoplastic cells present.[40] Carcinomas in which there is a preponderance of signet ring cells have been designated as signet ring cell carcinomas, but they are usually ILC. However, abundant signet ring cells can also be found in infiltrating duct carcinoma (IDC).

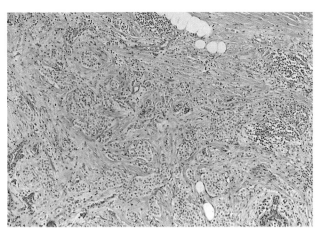

Figure 9–29. Alveolar variant of infiltrating lobular carcinoma (ILC). In the alveolar variant, cells typical of classic ILC are arranged in globular aggregates or clumps composed of ≥20 cells. This growth pattern can be mixed with classic and solid patterns, but it should constitute at least 70% of the tumor to be classified as alveolar.

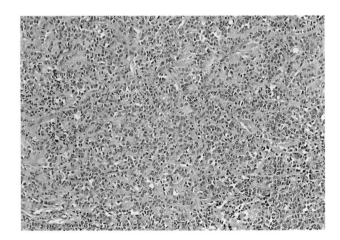

Figure 9–28. Solid variant of infiltrating lobular carcinoma (ILC). Infiltrating carcinomas with the typical cytologic features of classic lobular carcinoma, but without significant areas of the dispersed or linear invasive pattern of classic ILC have been classified as variant ILC. This figure is an example of the solid variant, consisting of confluent or solid groups of neoplastic cells. Often the classic or alveolar patterns are also present. To be classified as the solid variant, the solid pattern should constitute at least 70% of the tumor. The growth pattern of this variant could cause confusion with lymphoma; however, special stains for mucin or immunohistochemical stains for cytokeratin and lymphoid markers should be diagnostic.

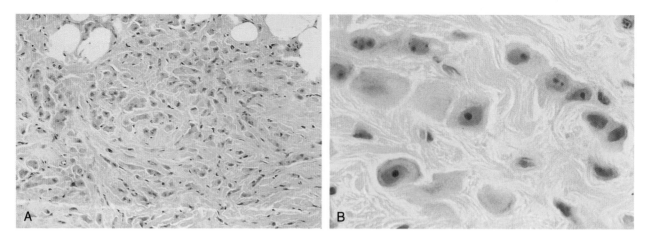

Figure 9–30. Pleomorphic infiltrating lobular carcinoma (ILC). *A,* In the pleomorphic variant of ILC, the growth pattern is that of classic ILC, but the nuclei are of a higher grade than is typical of ILC. *B,* The cells are pleomorphic, sometimes with prominent nucleoli, as in this figure. They have more abundant cytoplasm and often a plasmacytoid appearance. Eusebi and coworkers emphasized the apocrine differentiation which is often present and depicted in this figure.[35] These carcinomas have been reported to have a more aggressive behavior, with a greater likelihood of recurrence, than other forms of ILC.[35–37] Pleomorphic ILC exhibits more chromogranin and p53 protein expression and less estrogen receptor and progesterone receptor expression, as assessed by immunohistochemistry, than classic ILC.[41]

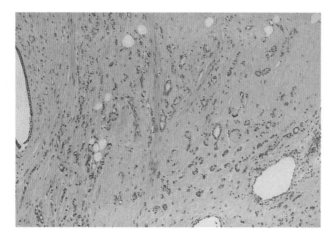

Figure 9–31. Tubulolobular carcinoma. Tubulolobular carcinomas have been considered to be a variant of infiltrating lobular carcinoma (ILC) by some authors. These carcinomas have relatively low-grade nuclei with an invasive pattern similar to classic ILC but with foci of tubule formation, as demonstrated in this figure. The histologic features and clinical behavior are intermediate between tubular carcinoma and ILC.[9, 42] Consequently, tubulolobular carcinoma should be regarded as a distinct tumor type.

Prognosis of Patients with ILC

Overall Survival			
Stratified by Stage			
Stage	% Survival	Follow-up (yr)	Study
I	86	8	Newman[43]
I	72	10	Richter et al[44]
I	74	10	Ashikari et al[45]
I	~85	10	DiCostanzo et al[38]
II	54	8	Newman[43]
II	9.3	10	Richter et al[44]
II (+ level I nodes)	80	10	DiCostanzo et al[38]
II (+ level II/III nodes)	~28	10	DiCostanzo et al[38]
Stratified by Subtype			
Probability of Survival		Study	
Classic > alveolar > mixed > solid		Dixon et al[46]	
Classic > mixed > solid		du Toit et al[47]	
Classic = variants		DiCostanzo et al[38]	
Classic = variants		Frost et al[17]	

Figure 9–32. Prognosis of patients with infiltrating lobular carcinoma (ILC). Although a number of studies including from 73 to 344 patients have evaluated the prognosis of patients with ILC, they have not demonstrated a consistent difference in survival compared to patients with infiltrating duct carcinoma (IDC) when stratified by stage of disease. Most patients with stage I ILC have a survival similar to those with stage I IDC.[38, 44, 45] In some studies, patients with stage II ILC have a poorer overall survival than stage-matched patients with IDC, whereas in others the survival has been similar to stage-matched patients with IDC.[38] In comparisons of the clinical behavior of histologic subtypes of ILC, some authors have shown a greater probability of survival with classic ILC than the variant forms,[46, 47] and others have found no statistically significant differences.[17, 38] When comparing only women with classic ILC with a group of women with IDC matched for age and stage, there was no difference in survival in stage II patients, but recurrence-free survival was significantly better for patients with stage I classic ILC.[38]

Biomarker Expression and Chromosomal
Alterations in ILC

Estrogen receptor	49%–92% positive cases
Progesterone receptor	63%–75% positive cases
c-erbB-2	0%–43% positive cases
p53	4.2%–9% positive cases
E-cadherin	0%–20% positive cases
P-cadherin	0% positive cases
Fibronectin	Decreased around tumor cells
Vascular endothelial growth factor	Less mRNA and protein than IDC
Ki-67/MIB1 (proliferation index)	Less than IDC
Chromosomal losses/imbalances	8p,16q frequent in ILC

Figure 9–33. Biomarker expression and chromosomal alterations in infiltrating lobular carcinoma (ILC). The presence of estrogen and progesterone receptors has been reported in classic and variant patterns, with reports that the alveolar variant is the one most commonly positive for estrogen receptors.[9, 17] c-erbB-2 expression demonstrated by immunohistochemistry has been reported to occur in ILC less often than or with a similar frequency as in infiltrating duct carcinoma (IDC).[11, 48] p53 expression detected by immunohistochemistry is typically lower in ILC than in IDC.[49, 50] E-cadherin, assessed by immunohistochemical staining, has been reported to be consistently absent or expressed much less frequently in ILC than in IDC.[10, 11, 14] Expression of P-cadherin, another cell adhesion protein, has also been reported to be absent in ILC.[14] The decreased expression of these cell adhesion molecules may contribute to the typical single cell and linear growth pattern in ILC. In addition, fibronectin, which is a glycoprotein associated with basement membrane that contributes to cell adhesiveness, has been observed to be decreased in the stroma adjacent to ILC tumor cells in comparison to IDC.[9] This decrease in fibronectin may also contribute to the infiltrative pattern of ILC. Vascular endothelial growth factor protein and messenger RNA (mRNA) have been shown to be expressed at a higher level in IDC compared with ILC, although no significant differences in vascular density were identified between the two histologic types.[13] It has been demonstrated that losses of chromosome arms 1p, 3q, 11q, and 18q are more prevalent in IDC than ILC, while losses or imbalances of 8p are more frequent in ILC.[51] Deletion of chromosome arm 16q is highly recurrent in ILC and may be related to the loss of expression of E-cadherin, the gene of which is located on 16q.[52] Mutations of the E-cadherin gene have been reported in 56% of ILC[53] and also detected in adjacent lobular carcinoma in situ (LCIS).[31] In addition, microsatellite instability has been observed in almost 40% of ILC, but in only 13% of IDC. Microsatellite instability has been linked to defects in a group of mismatch repair genes. Replication errors resulting from the defective mismatch repair genes are believed to cause genomic instability.[51] Cell proliferation, as assessed by immunohistochemical staining for Ki-67/MIB1, is significantly lower in ILC than IDC.[54] These differences in expression of a variety of biomarkers and chromosomal alterations suggest that ILC and IDC are distinct pathologic entities that may arise by different mechanisms of carcinogenesis.

Markers Indicating a Poor Prognosis in ILC

Consistently reported
  Stage of Disease
    Large tumor size
    Positive axillary lymph nodes
Inconsistently reported
  Variant histologic subyptes
  Nuclear grade other than 1 (low)
  Presence of ≥10% signet ring cells
  Diploid carcinomas with a high SPF

Figure 9–34. Markers indicating a poor prognosis in infiltrating lobular carcinoma (ILC). The majority of studies addressing this issue have found that the stage of disease, including tumor size and axillary lymph node status, is the most reliable indicator of prognosis. Other potential prognostic indicators have either not been widely assessed or have not provided consistent results. Some studies have demonstrated that classic ILC has a better prognosis than variant patterns, whereas other studies have shown no statistically significant differences between subtypes.[9] Nuclear grade has not been widely assessed, but patients with ILC having a nuclear grade of 1, rather than 2, were less likely to exhibit axillary nodal metastases in one study.[17] Breast carcinomas rich in signet ring cells are typically considered to be aggressive neoplasms. In one study of ILC, patients with stage I disease and tumors having ≥10% signet ring cells were more likely to have recurrences or metastases than patients with stage I tumors and <10% signet ring cells (25%).[40] Additional examination of the same group of patients revealed that ILC is usually diploid (80%) and that those patients with stage I diploid tumors having a high S-phase fraction were more likely to have disease recurrence than those with a low S-phase fraction.[55]

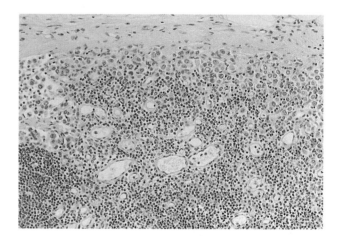

Figure 9–35. Axillary lymph node involved by metastatic infiltrating lobular carcinoma (ILC). Metastatic ILC to axillary lymph nodes is typically sinusoidal and spares the lymphoid areas. In this figure, lobular carcinoma occupies the nodal subcapsular sinus. This pattern can be mistaken for sinus histiocytosis, and the neoplastic cells, because of their small size and low degree of atypia, can resemble histiocytes. On the other hand, sinusoidal histiocytes may be vacuolated and resemble the signet ring cells of ILC. The content of these histocytes can be weakly mucicarminophilic; therefore, immunohistochemical stains should be relied on to distinguish these entities.[56]

Comparison of Metastatic Sites in ILC and IDC

Metastatic Sites More Common in ILC	Metastatic Sites More Common in IDC
Peritoneum	Lungs
Retroperitoneum	Pleura
Gastrointestinal tract	Brain parenchyma
Genitourinary tract	
Leptomeninges	

Figure 9–36. Comparison of metastatic sites in infiltrating lobular carcinoma (ILC) and infiltrating duct carcinoma (IDC). The metastatic patterns of ILC and IDC differ. ILC more commonly involves the peritoneum, retroperitoneum, intestines, ovaries, and uterus. Metastases of ILC to the central nervous system usually involve the meninges, whereas IDC is more commonly metastatic to brain parenchyma. Metastases of ILC to bone marrow are also common. ILC is sometimes difficult to detect, especially in the endometrium and bone marrow, because of the small cell size and diffuse pattern of infiltration.[3, 5]

References

1. Foote FW Jr, Stewart FW: A histologic classification of carcinoma in the breast. Surgery 19:74–99, 1946.
2. Foote FW Jr, Stewart FW: Lobular carcinoma in situ. A rare form of mammary cancer. Am J Pathol 7:491–496, 1941.
3. Rosen PP: Lobular carcinoma in situ and atypical lobular hyperplasia. In Rosen's Breast Pathology. Philadelphia, Lippincott-Raven, 1997, pp 507–544.
4. Page DL, Anderson TJ, Rogers LW: Carcinoma in situ (CIS). In Page DL, Anderson TJ (eds): Diagnostic Histopathology of the Breast. New York, Churchill Livingstone, 1987, pp 157–192.
5. Tavassoli FA: Lobular neoplasia (lobular carcinoma in situ). In Tavassoli FA (ed): Pathology of the Breast. 2nd ed. Norwalk, Conn., Appleton & Lange, 1999, pp 263–291.
6. Gump FE, Kinne D, Schwartz GF: Current treatment for lobular carcinoma in situ. Ann Surg Oncol 5(1):33–36, 1998.
7. Nayar R, Zhuang Z, Merino MJ, et al: Loss of heterozygosity on chromosome 11q13 in lobular lesions of the breast using tissue microdissection and polymerase chain reaction. Hum Pathol 28: 277–282, 1997.
8. Nemoto T, Castillo N, Tsukada Y, et al: Lobular carcinoma in situ with microinvasion. J Surg Oncol 67(1):41–46, 1998.
9. Rosen PP: Invasive lobular carcinoma. In Rosen's Breast Pathology. Philadelphia, Lippincott-Raven, 1997, pp 545–565.
10. Hashizume R, Koizumi H, Ihara A, et al: Expression of beta-catenin in normal breast tissue and breast carcinoma: A comparative study with epithelial cadherin and alpha-catenin. Histopathology 19:139–146, 1996.
11. Palacios J, Benito N, Pizarro A, et al: Relationship between erbB2 and e-cadherin expression in human breast cancer. Virchows Arch 427:259–263, 1995.
12. Lehr HA, Folpe A, Yaziji H, et al: Cytokeratin 8 immunostaining pattern and E-cadherin expression distinguish lobular from ductal breast carcinoma. Am J Clin Pathol 114:190–196, 2000.
13. Lee AH, Dublin EA, Bobrow LG, et al: Invasive lobular and invasive ductal carcinoma of the breast show distinct patterns of vascular endothelial growth factor expression and angiogenesis. J Pathol 185(4):394–401, 1998.
14. Peralta Soler A, Knudsen KA, Salazar H, et al: P-cadherin expression in breast carcinoma indicates poor survival. Cancer 86(7): 1263–1272, 1999.
15. White JR, Gustafson GS, Wimbish K, et al: Conservative surgery and radiation therapy for infiltrating lobular carcinomas of the breast: The role of preoperative mammograms in guiding treatment. Cancer 74:640–647, 1994.
16. Francis M, Cakir B, Bilous M, et al: Conservative surgery and radiation therapy for invasive lobular carcinoma of the breast. Austr N Z J Surg 69(6):450–454, 1999.
17. Frost AR, Terahata S, Yeh I, et al: An analysis of prognostic features of infiltrating lobular carcinoma of the breast. Mod Pathol 8:830–836, 1995.
18. Moreno-Elola A, Aguilar A, Roman JM, et al: Prognostic factors in invasive lobular carcinoma of the breast: A multivariate analysis. A multicentre study after seventeen years of follow-up. Ann Chir Gynaecol 88(4):252–258, 1999.
19. Page DL, Anderson TJ, Rogers LW: Epithelial hyperplasia. In Page DL, Anderson TJ (eds): Diagnostic Histopathology of the Breast. New York, Churchill Livingstone, 1987, pp 120–156.
20. Haagensen CD, Lane N, Lattes R, et al: Lobular neoplasia (so-called lobular carcinoma in situ) of the breast. Cancer 42:737–769, 1978.
21. Andersen J: Lobular carcinoma in situ: A long-term follow-up in 52 cases. Acta Pathol Microbiol Scand [Sect A] 82:519–533, 1974.
22. Rosen PP, Lieberman PH, Braun DW Jr, et al: Lobular carcinoma in situ of the breast. Detailed analysis of 99 patients with average follow-up of 24 years. Am J Surg Pathol 2:225–251, 1978.
23. Page DL, Kidd TE Jr, Dupont WD, et al: Lobular neoplasia of the breast: Higher risk for subsequent invasive cancer predicted by more extensive disease. Hum Pathol 22:1232–1239, 1991.
24. Bodian CA, Perzin KH, Lattes R, et al: Prognostic significance of benign proliferative breast disease. Cancer 71:3896–3907, 1993.
25. Page DL, Dupont WD, Rogers LW, et al: Atypical hyperplastic lesions of the female breast. A long-term follow-up study. Cancer 55:2698–2708, 1985.
26. Page DL, Dupont WD, Rogers LW: Ductal involvement by cells of atypical lobular hyperplasia in the breast: A long-term follow-up study of cancer risk. Hum Pathol 19:201–207, 1988.
27. Pallis L, Wilking N, Cedermark B, et al: Receptors for estrogen and progesterone in breast carcinoma in situ. Anticancer Res 12(6B): 2113–2115, 1992.
28. Ramachandra S, Machin L, Ashley S, et al: Immunohistochemical distribution of c-erbB-2 in in-situ breast carcinoma—a detailed morphologic analysis. J Pathol 161:7–14, 1990.
29. Lu YJ, Osin P, Lakhani SR, et al: Comparative genomic hybridization analysis of lobular carcinoma in situ and atypical lobular hyperplasia and potential roles for gains and losses of genetic material in breast neoplasia. Cancer Res 58(20):4721–4727, 1998.
30. Lishman SC, Lakhani SR: Atypical lobular hyperplasia and lobular carcinoma in situ: Surgical and molecular pathology. Histopathology 35:193–200, 1999.
31. Vos CB, Claton-Jonsen AM, Berx G, et al: E-cadherin inactivation

in lobular carcinoma in situ of the breast: An early event in tumorigenesis. Br J Cancer 76:1131–1133, 1997.

32. Gump FE: Implications and management of lobular carcinoma in situ of the breast (LCIS). The Breast J 3:196–199, 1997.

33. Abner AL, Connolly JL, Recht A et al: The relation between the presence and extent of lobular carcinoma in situ and the risk of local recurrence for patients with infiltrating carcinoma of the breast treated with conservative surgery and radiation therapy. Cancer 88(5):1072–1077, 2000.

34. Tavassoli FA: Infiltrating carcinomas, common and familiar special types. In Tavassoli FA (ed): Pathology of the Breast. Norwalk, Conn., Appleton & Lange, 1992, pp 293–333.

35. Eusebi V, Magalhaes F, Azzopardi JG: Pleomorphic lobular carcinoma of the breast: An aggressive tumor showing apocrine differentiation. Hum Pathol 23:655–662, 1992.

36. Weidner N, Semple JP: Pleomorphic variant of invasive lobular carcinoma of the breast. Hum Pathol 23:1167–1171, 1992.

37. Bentz JA, Yassa N, Clayton F: Pleomorphic lobular carcinoma of the breast: Clinicopathologic features of 12 cases. Mod Pathol 11:814–822, 1998.

38. DiCostanzo D, Rosen PP, Gareen I, et al: Prognosis in infiltrating lobular carcinoma. An analysis of "classical" and variant tumors. Am J Surg Pathol 14:12–23, 1990.

39. Ferguson DJP, Anderson TJ, Wells CA, et al: An ultrastructural study of mucoid carcinoma of the breast: Variability of cytoplasmic features. Histopathology 10:1219–1230, 1986.

40. Frost AR, Terahata S, Yeh I, et al: The significance of signet ring cells in infiltrating lobular carcinoma of the breast. Arch Pathol Lab Med 119:64–68, 1995.

41. Radhi JM: Immunohistochemical analysis of pleomorphic lobular carcinoma: Higher expression of p53 and chromogranin and lower expression of ER and PgR. Histopathology 36(2):156–160, 2000.

42. Page DL, Anderson TJ: Uncommon types of invasive carcinoma. In Page DL, Anderson TJ (eds): Diagnostic Histopathology of the Breast. New York, Churchill Livingstone, 1987, pp 244–246.

43. Newman W: Lobular carcinoma of the female breast. Report of 73 cases. Ann Surg 164:305–314, 1966.

44. Richter GO, Dockerty MB, Clagett OT: Diffuse infiltrating scirrhous carcinoma of the breast. Cancer 20:363–370, 1967.

45. Ashikari R, Huvos AG, Urban JA, et al: Infiltrating lobular carcinoma of the breast. Cancer 31:110–116, 1973.

46. Dixon JM, Anderson TJ, Page DL, et al: Infiltrating lobular carcinoma of the breast. Histopathology 6:149–161, 1982.

47. du Toit RS, Locker AP, Ellis IO, et al: Invasive lobular carcinomas of the breast—the prognosis of histopathologic subtypes. Br J Cancer 60:605–609, 1989.

48. Rosen PP, Lesser ML, Arroyo CD, et al: Immunohistochemical detection of HER2/neu in patients with axillary lymph node negative breast carcinoma. A study of epidemiologic risk factors, histologic features and prognosis. Cancer 75:1320–1326, 1995.

49. Martinazzi M, Crivelli F, Zampatti C, et al: Relationship between p53 expression and other prognostic factors in human breast carcinoma. An immunohistochemical study. Am J Clin Pathol 100:213–217, 1993.

50. Rosen PP, Lesser ML, Arroyo CD, et al: p53 in node-negative breast carcinoma: An immunohistochemical study of epidemiologic risk factors, histologic features and prognosis. J Clin Oncol 13:821–830, 1995.

51. Brenner AJ, Aldaz CM: The genetics of sporadic breast cancer. In Aldaz CM (ed): Etiology of Breast and Gynecological Cancers. New York, Wiley-Liss, 1997, pp 63–82.

52. Flagiello D, Gerbault-Seureau M, Sastre-Garau X, et al: Highly recurrent der(1;16)(q100) and other 16q arm alterations in lobular breast cancer. Genes Chromosomes Cancer 23(4):300–306, 1998.

53. Berx G, Cleton-Jansen AM, Strumane K, et al: E-cadherin is inactivated in a majority of invasive human lobular breast cancers by truncation mutations throughout its extracellular domain. Oncogene 13(9):1919–1925, 1996.

54. Kruger S, Fahrenkrog T, Muller H: Proliferative and apoptotic activity in lobular breast carcinoma. Int J Mol Med 4(2):171–174, 1999.

55. Frost AR, Karcher DS, Terahata S, et al: DNA analysis and S-phase fraction determination by flow cytometric analysis of infiltrating lobular carcinoma of the breast. Mod Pathol 9:930–937, 1996.

56. Frost AR, Shek YH, Lack EE: "Signet ring" sinus histiocytosis mimicking metastatic adenocarcinoma: Report of two cases with immunohistochemical and ultrastructural study. Mod Pathol 5:497–500, 1992.

CHAPTER 10

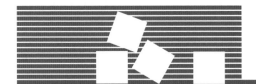

Infiltrating Carcinoma: Infiltrating Duct Carcinoma Not Otherwise Specified and Prognostic Factors Other Than Histologic Type

Olga B. Ioffe
Steven G. Silverberg

INTRODUCTION

With the increased spread of screening for breast cancer, more and more women present at an early stage of disease. Nevertheless, about 20% to 30% of node-negative breast cancer patients develop a relapse of some sort and eventually die of disease. This subset of patients benefits from adjuvant therapy, and the remaining 70% to 80% of early-stage breast cancer patients are essentially cured and should not need additional treatment. There is a need for prognostic markers that would stratify patients at the time of diagnosis for appropriate treatment decisions. In addition, we need tumor markers that can help in the selection of specific adjuvant therapy.

There are about 100 putative prognostic factors reported in the literature, including ones that are well known to help clinicians stratify patients into low- and high-risk groups as well as other candidate and experimental markers that are currently being investigated for clinical relevance. These markers range from those routinely used and required in the surgical pathology report (i.e., tumor size, nodal status, histologic type and grade) to the ones that are widely accepted and reported by most laboratories (i.e., S-phase, immunohistochemical assay for estrogen and progesterone receptors, c-erbB-2), to a host of potentially useful but not well studied markers that await clinical validation.

Infiltrating duct carcinoma (IDC) represents the largest group of malignant breast tumors, comprising 65% to 80% of infiltrating breast carcinomas.[1, p 275] IDC not otherwise specified (NOS) is conventionally defined by what it is not, that is, it is a carcinoma that is not classified as any special type of mammary carcinoma. This diagnostic category includes tumors that have minor foci of special types of breast carcinoma (e.g., tubular, medullary, colloid) but are not entirely or in very large part composed of those patterns; such features of special types are observed in approximately one third of breast carcinomas.[2] The prognostic differences characteristic of the special types of mammary carcinoma do not apply to these mixed tumors.

In this chapter, we review well established and putative prognostic markers as related to infiltrating duct carcinoma NOS; prognostic implications of special types of breast carcinoma are addressed in the chapters devoted to those special types.

INFILTRATING DUCT CARCINOMA, NOT OTHERWISE SPECIFIED

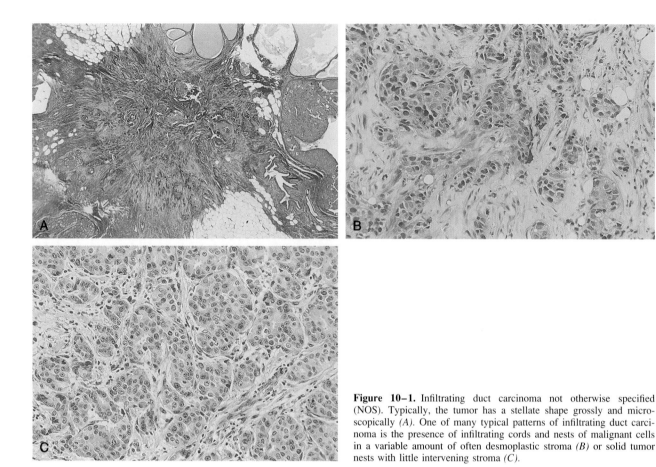

Figure 10–1. Infiltrating duct carcinoma not otherwise specified (NOS). Typically, the tumor has a stellate shape grossly and microscopically *(A)*. One of many typical patterns of infiltrating duct carcinoma is the presence of infiltrating cords and nests of malignant cells in a variable amount of often desmoplastic stroma *(B)* or solid tumor nests with little intervening stroma *(C)*.

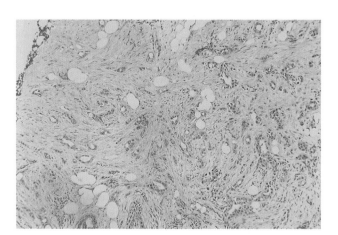

Figure 10–2. Infiltrating duct carcinoma with focal tubule and single cell cord formation, reminiscent of lobular and tubulolobular carcinoma. Only tumors with classic, very low-grade uniform nuclei and low cell density, in addition to the characteristic growth pattern, should be classified as classic lobular carcinoma. The tumor is termed mixed ductal and lobular if the ductal component comprises from 10% to 90% of the tumor mass. If there is <10% of the ductal component, the tumor should be classified as an infiltrating lobular carcinoma; the reverse is true for infiltrating carcinoma with <10% lobular morphology, which should be classified as ductal carcinoma not otherwise specified (NOS).[3, p 296]

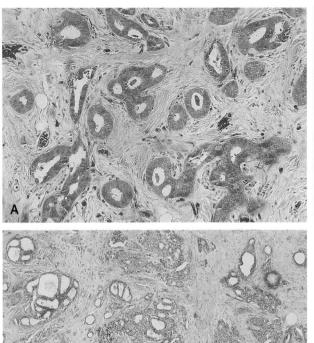

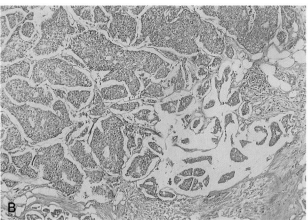

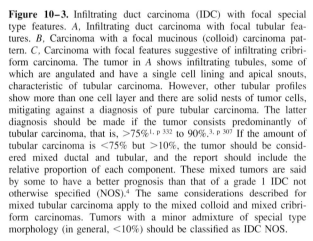

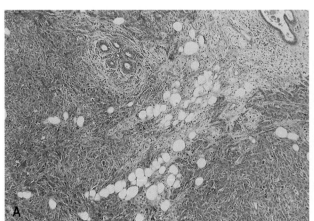

Figure 10–3. Infiltrating duct carcinoma (IDC) with focal special type features. *A,* Infiltrating duct carcinoma with focal tubular features. *B,* Carcinoma with a focal mucinous (colloid) carcinoma pattern. *C,* Carcinoma with focal features suggestive of infiltrating cribriform carcinoma. The tumor in *A* shows infiltrating tubules, some of which are angulated and have a single cell lining and apical snouts, characteristic of tubular carcinoma. However, other tubular profiles show more than one cell layer and there are solid nests of tumor cells, mitigating against a diagnosis of pure tubular carcinoma. The latter diagnosis should be made if the tumor consists predominantly of tubular carcinoma, that is, >75%[1, p 332] to 90%.[3, p 307] If the amount of tubular carcinoma is <75% but >10%, the tumor should be considered mixed ductal and tubular, and the report should include the relative proportion of each component. These mixed tumors are said by some to have a better prognosis than that of a grade 1 IDC not otherwise specified (NOS).[4] The same considerations described for mixed tubular carcinoma apply to the mixed colloid and mixed cribriform carcinomas. Tumors with a minor admixture of special type morphology (in general, <10%) should be classified as IDC NOS.

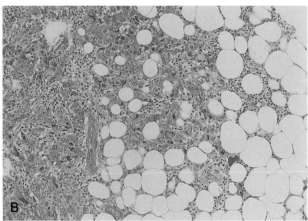

Figure 10–4. Infiltrating duct carcinoma (IDC) with features of medullary carcinoma (medullary-like carcinoma). When strict criteria for the diagnosis of medullary carcinoma are not met, but the tumor shows some of the features of medullary carcinoma, it should be classified as a medullary-like carcinoma. Any of the following features (poor circumscription, absence of high nuclear grade or syncytial growth pattern, absent or weak lymphocytic infiltrate), excludes the diagnosis of classic medullary carcinoma. *A,* This tumor has an overall good circumscription but focally engulfs benign lobules, thus ruling out a diagnosis of classic medullary carcinoma. *B,* Extensive infiltration of fat also precludes the diagnosis of medullary carcinoma.

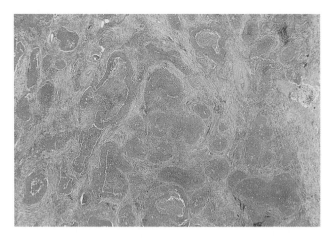

Figure 10-5. Differential diagnosis between ductal carcinoma in situ (DCIS) and infiltrating duct carcinoma (IDC). Some growth patterns of IDC make it difficult to distinguish from intraductal carcinoma. One example of this diagnostic problem is shown in the figure. This infiltrating tumor grows in a pattern mimicking comedo DCIS. The desmoplastic stromal reaction and irregular, bizarre shapes of the epithelial nests point toward an infiltrating carcinoma. In this case, as well as in cases of solid or cribriform invasive tumor nests mimicking solid or cribriform DCIS, it is a challenge to ascertain the relative amounts of intraductal and invasive components of the tumor.

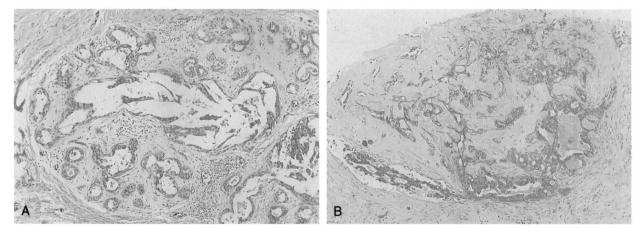

Figure 10-6. Pseudoinvasion. *A,* In cases of lobular cancerization with marked desmoplastic stromal reaction such as shown in this figure, a suspicion of invasion is sometimes raised. However, the preserved terminal duct/lobular architecture helps avoid overdiagnosis of invasive carcinoma. *B,* Another challenge is the differential diagnosis between true invasion and an intraductal carcinoma involving a sclerosing lesion. Usually, the low-power architecture consistent with, for example, sclerosing adenosis (with epithelial profiles compressed in the center and open at the periphery of the lesion) helps in making the distinction. The presence of a circumscribed outer border and of hyalinized stroma and the absence of desmoplastic stromal reaction are additional but not always reliable features suggesting the absence of invasion.

TUMOR SIZE

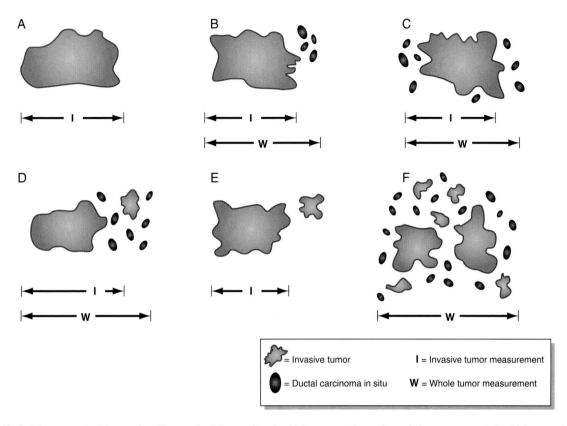

= Invasive tumor   **I** = Invasive tumor measurement

= Ductal carcinoma in situ   **W** = Whole tumor measurement

Figure 10–7. Measurement of tumor size. The maximal tumor size should be measured grossly, and the measurement should be repeated on the histologic sections, if the tumor size is such that its maximal diameter can be confined to a single slide. Alternatively, the tumor slice may be divided between two blocks and the two dimensions added; this, however, may lead to inaccuracies. The measurement on histologic sections may slightly underestimate the tumor size due to tissue shrinkage, but it is more accurate in several circumstances, for example, in tumors with an extensive intraductal component that accounts for a large portion of the tumor mass seen grossly, invasive lobular carcinoma, small invasive carcinomas that may not be appreciated grossly, and extensive desmoplastic or lymphoid stromal reaction around the tumor. Thus, in many cases, the microscopic measurement takes precedence and should be used in reporting. The measurement of the invasive component only should be used for accurate staging and prognostication.[5] One largest tumor dimension (after the tumor has been measured in at least two dimensions) should be included in the report. If more than one separate tumor is present, each is measured and reported separately. It also should be noted that adding the tumor size in the primary excision and at re-excision is highly inaccurate and should be discouraged. (Adapted from Elston CW, Ellis IO, Goulding H, Pinder SE: Role of pathology in the prognosis and management of breast cancer. In Elston CW, Ellis IO [eds]: The Breast. New York, Churchill Livingstone, 1998, p 387.)

A. Tumor Size and Relapse-Free Survival of Breast Cancer Patients

Tumor Size (mm)	Relapse-Free Survival
<10	88%
11–13	73%
14–16	65%
17–22	59%

B. Correlation of Tumor Size and Incidence of Axillary Lymph Node Metastases

Tumor Size (mm)	Roger et al	Silverstein et al
<5	3%	3%
6–10	10%	17%
11–15	21%	
16–20	35%	32%(11–20 mm)
21–50		44%
>51		60%

Figure 10–8. Impact of tumor size on prognosis. Tumor-node-metastasis (TNM) stage is the most important predictor of outcome in breast cancer patients. Tumor size is one of the most important prognostic factors *(A, B)*. It has been shown in many large studies that patients with smaller tumors have a significantly better long-term survival and lower incidence of nodal metastases.[6] Patients with *minimal mammary carcinoma* carry a very good prognosis[7]; however, the definition of minimal mammary carcinoma is not well defined. It initially was restricted to tumors <5 mm in diameter,[7] but this size limitation has been redefined as 9 mm,[8, 9] or up to and including 10 mm.[10] Tumors measuring ≤10 mm have an excellent prognosis, especially if their histologic grade is not high.[11, 12] (Data from Rosen PP, Groshen S: Factors influencing survival and prognosis in early breast carcinoma (T1N0M0–T1N1M0). Assessment of 664 patients with median follow-up of 19 years. Surg Clin North Am 70:937–962, 1990; Roger V, Beito G, Jolly PC: Factors affecting the incidence of lymph node metastases in small cancers of the breast. Am J Surg 157:501–502, 1989, Silverstein MJ, Gierson ED, Waisman JR, et al: Axillary lymph node dissection for T$_{1a}$ breast carcinoma. Cancer 73:664–667, 1994.)

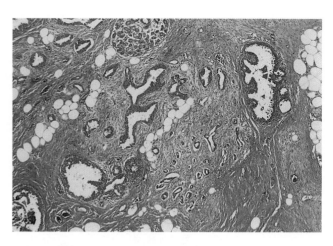

Figure 10–9. Microinvasive mammary carcinoma. Within the category of minimal mammary carcinoma a category of *microinvasive carcinoma* is recognized as having an excellent prognosis.[13, 14] Microinvasive carcinoma is defined as invasive tumor <1 mm in size.[1, p 289]

HISTOLOGIC GRADING

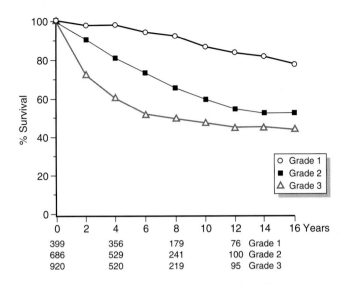

<table>
<tr><td colspan="2">A. Summary of Nottingham Histologic Grading Method</td></tr>
</table>

Feature	Score
Tubule formation	
Majority of tumor (>75%)	1
Moderate degree (10%–75%)	2
Little or none (<10%)	3
Nuclear pleomorphism	
Small, uniform nuclei	1
Moderate pleomorphism and increase in size	2
Marked variation	3
Mitotic counts per 10 high-power field	
Depend on microscopic field area (see Fig. 10–15)	1–3

B. The scores for each factor are added to result in a final score according to which the histologic grade is allocated

3–5 points: Nottingham grade 1
6–7 points: Nottingham grade 2
8–9 points: Nottingham grade 3

Figure 10–10. Correlation between histologic grade and long-term survival in 2005 patients with primary operable carcinoma of the breast. Histologic grade has been shown to be a powerful prognostic factor for women with infiltrating duct carcinoma.[15–21] The grade correlates well with other prognostic markers (e.g., proliferative rate, ploidy, c-erbB-2 expression, hormone receptor status). Numbers at bottom of the graph represent patients surviving at each time point. (From Elston CW, Ellis IO: Assessment of histological grade. In Elston CW, Ellis IO [eds]: The Breast. New York, Churchill Livingstone, 1998, p 378.)

Figure 10–11. Nottingham breast cancer grading scheme. The most precisely defined and most commonly used system of grading is a modification of the Scarff-Bloom-Richardson grading scheme[22] by Elston and Ellis[15] referred to as Nottingham grade. The method is summarized in *A* and *B*. (Adapted from Elston CW, Ellis IO: Assessment of histological grade. In Elston CW, Ellis IO [eds]: The Breast. New York, Churchill Livingstone, 1998, pp 369, 375.)

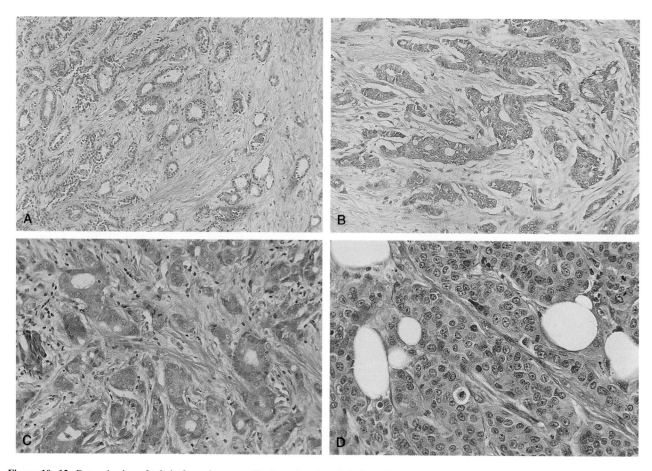

Figure 10–12. Determination of tubule formation score. To determine the tubule formation score, the entire tumor should be scanned at low power and the relative percent of tubule formation is estimated. *A,* At low power, this tumor shows tubule formation in almost all nests, and is given a score of 1 for tubule formation. *B,* In this carcinoma, the tubule formation was seen in <75% but >10% of all fields, and the tubule formation score is 2. Tubules must show clear central lumina *(C);* spaces created by shrinkage, necrosis, or apoptosis should not be mistaken for tubular structures; no tubule formation is seen in this field *(D).*

Assignment of Nuclear Pleomorphism Score

Nuclear Pleomorphism Score	Features
1	Nuclei not much larger than benign
	Minimal anisonucleosis (<2-fold)
	Smooth outline, regular shape, uniform chromatin
	Nucleoli absent or pinpoint
2	Nuclei larger than normal
	Moderate variation in size and shape (2- to 3-fold)
	Open, vesicular, or coarse chromatin
	Visible, usually single nucleolus
3	Very large, occasionally bizarre nuclei
	Marked anisonucleosis (>3-fold)
	Vesicular, coarse chromatin
	Prominent, often multiple nucleoli

Figure 10–13. Assignment of nuclear pleomorphism score. The entire tumor should be scanned, and the overall impression should be used to assess the nuclear pleomorphism score. Benign epithelial cells adjacent to the tumor should be used as a reference point to ascertain the size of the malignant cells. If no normal breast epithelium is present for comparison, lymphocytes can be used with the understanding that they are smaller than benign epithelial cells.

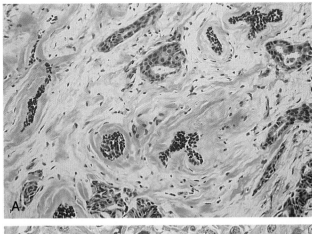

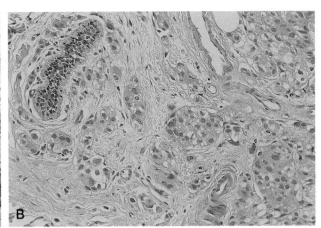

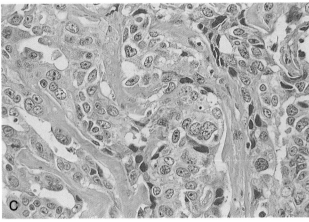

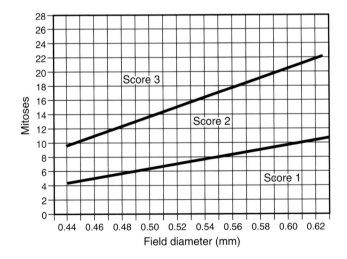

Figure 10–14. Nuclear pleomorphism score. *A,* score 1; *B,* score 2; *C,* score 3. Relatively small, uniform nuclei with regular outlines and inconspicuous nucleoli *(A)* qualify for a nuclear pleomorphism score of 1. Note that grade 1 nuclei are not significantly larger than nuclei in the adjacent and partially infiltrated benign lobule. Nuclei larger than in the adjacent benign duct *(B),* showing moderate variation in size and shape, coarse chromatin, and predominantly single nucleoli should be given a nuclear pleomorphism score of 2. *C,* Large, occasionally bizarre nuclei with multiple nucleoli; there is marked variation in nuclear size and shape. Nuclear pleomorphism score is 3.

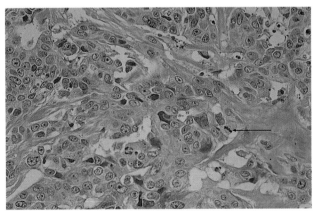

Figure 10–15. Microscope field diameter and number of mitoses. This graph shows correlation between the microscope field diameter and mitotic count. Mitotic count is allocated points according to the size of the high-power field by plotting the actual mitotic count against the field diameter. This calibration procedure needs to be performed only once for a given microscope and the resulting cutoffs can be used for score assignment. (From Elston CW, Ellis IO: Assessment of histological grade. In Elston CW, Ellis IO [eds]: The Breast. New York, Churchill Livingstone, 1998, p 376.)

Figure 10–16. Mitoses counting. The photomicrograph shows one unequivocal mitotic figure *(arrow);* crushed cells and apoptotic bodies should not be counted. Mitoses are counted at the tumor's advancing edge because that is the most mitotically active area. Some authors advocate screening the periphery of the tumor and starting the 10-field count in the most mitotically active area. Only unequivocal mitotic figures should be counted; apoptotic bodies, pyknotic nuclei, and crushed intratumoral lymphocytes should be ignored. Although proliferative activity as assessed by mitotic index is a very important part of histologic grade and is even claimed to be an independent prognostic factor,[23] mitosis counting has always been fraught with problems, and not only in breast pathology. The variables include difference in criteria and definition of mitotic figures, staining and section thickness variability, heterogeneity in distribution of mitotically active cells, amount of tumor examined, amount of stroma, and microscopic field area.

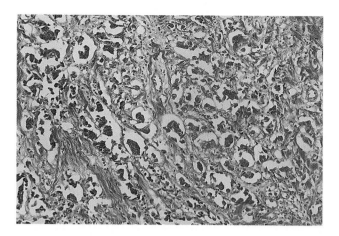

Figure 10–17. Importance of fixation. Fixation is of paramount importance in assessment of all components of the histologic grading of breast cancer. None of these components can be accurately gauged in the poorly fixed material shown in this figure. Formalin infiltrates tissues slowly; the effect of delay in fixation was studied in breast carcinoma and it has been shown that a delay of 6 hours decreased the number of mitoses by up to 76%, causing a reduction in histologic grade.[24]

LYMPH NODE STATUS

Five Year Overall Survival According to Number of Positive Axillary Lymph Nodes

No. of Positive Lymph Nodes	Overall 5-Year Survival (%)
0	82.8
1–3	73.0
4–12	45.7
>13	28.4

Figure 10–18. The lymph node stage is the single most important prognostic factor in breast cancer. Clinical assessment is inaccurate and the assignment of lymph node stage is based only on histologic examination of axillary lymph nodes. Patients with regional lymph node involvement have a significantly reduced long-term survival: 25% to 30% 10-year survival versus 75% in patients without lymph node involvement.[6] The number of lymph nodes involved is prognostically relevant; the survival data are often based on whether the number of lymph nodes involved is <4 versus ≥4. (Adapted from Osborne CK: Prognostic factors in breast cancer. Princ Pract Oncol 4: 1–11, 1990.)

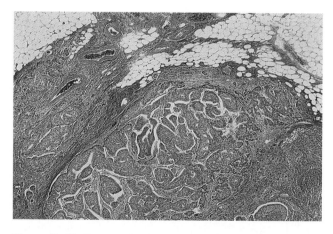

Figure 10–19. Extracapsular extension of a lymph node metastasis. The presence of extranodal or extracapsular spread of metastatic tumor had been claimed to be an ominous prognostic sign,[25] but it has not been confirmed by recent large studies to be an independent adverse factor in predicting survival[26] or recurrence.[27] This finding, nevertheless, should be included in the pathology report.

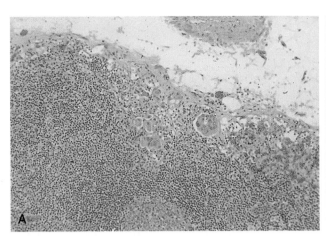

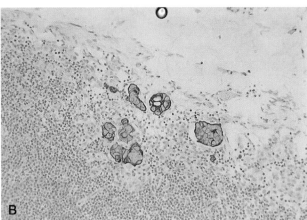

Figure 10–20. Micrometastases of mammary carcinoma. Several nests in the subcapsular location of this axillary lymph node *(A)* were confirmed by cytokeratin stain *(B)* to be a micrometastasis of mammary carcinoma. *Micrometastases,* or *occult metastases* (measuring ≤2 mm) can be detected by serial macroscopic slicing,[28] or by step-sectioning and immunohistochemistry using the cytokeratin cocktail.[29] By using additional techniques, occult lymph node metastases are found in 15%[30] to 25%[29] of apparently node-negative patients; this incidence goes up to 32% if intramammary lymphatic tumor emboli are included.[31] Interestingly, re-examination of the initial hematoxylin and eosin (H&E) sections led to finding of micrometastases in an additional 6% of cases, and when the remaining cases were subject to epithelial membrane antigen (EMA) immunostaining, micrometastases were identified in 7% more cases.[32] Using step-sectioning alone, additional micrometastases can be identified in up to 20% of patients.[33] There has been a claim that the tumor cells in subcapsular lymphatics or the subcapsular sinus have the same prognostic significance as overtly node-positive cases, whereas a micrometastasis growing within the lymphoid tissue does not have an adverse effect on prognosis.[30]

The prognostic significance of micrometastases is controversial; some authors claim that the survival of these patients does not differ from that of lymph node–negative patients.[31] In other studies micrometastases have been shown to indicate increased risk for local recurrence, but not to be a factor in overall survival.[28] Studies with longer follow-up show that there is a small but significant decrease in disease-free and overall survival.[34, 35] Micrometastases detected by immunohistochemistry alone do not constitute an adverse factor,[28, 36] and they are almost never found in >3 lymph nodes.[37] If micrometastasis is found, the pathology report should specify how this diagnosis was made (initial H&E, step-sections, or immunohistochemistry). Recently, the examination of *axillary sentinel node biopsy* specimens has become an important albeit so far unresolved issue. Most institutions use both step-sectioning and immunohistochemistry to evaluate these lymph nodes for micrometastases. If intraoperative consultation is requested on these specimens, it is preferable to perform only cytologic evaluation (scrape smear) in order to preserve the nodal tissue. It is important to note that only scrape intraoperative smears should be performed, and not touch imprints, as the latter technique is not optimal to evaluate for metastatic carcinoma and results in a significant number of false-negative diagnoses. When a frozen section is performed, ultrarapid immunohistochemistry for cytokeratin has been reported to be of value.[38] However, caution is warranted as to the reliability of intraoperative sentinel lymph node examination: in one recent study, it reliably identified macrometastases, but it had a significant false-negative rate of 25.8% for micrometastases.[39]

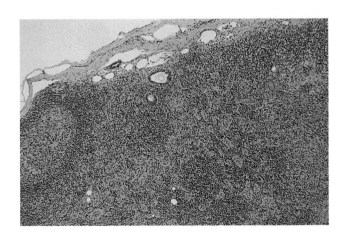

Figure 10–21. Benign epithelial inclusion in an axillary lymph node. The differential diagnosis of lymph node metastases includes rare benign epithelial inclusions that show cytologic and architectural features of benignity. Benign nevus cells in the lymph node capsule have also been reported; the incidence may be as high as 7.3% as detected by S-100 immunostain.[40]

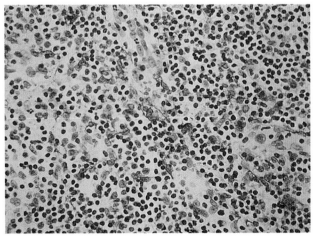

Figure 10–22. Cytokeratin-positive fibroblastic reticulum cells in an axillary lymph node. Another infrequent diagnostic pitfall (encountered when performing the cytokeratin stain on a lymph node) is the presence of so-called fibroblastic reticulum cells that stain positively for cytokeratin.[41] These cells should be readily recognizable due to their characteristic distribution in the lymph node.

VASCULAR AND PERINEURAL INVASION

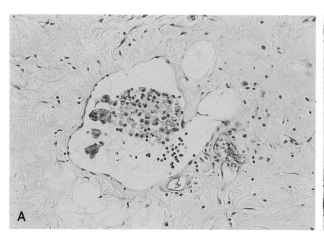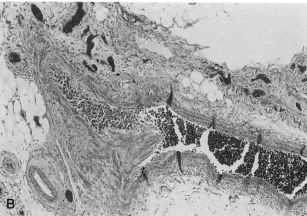

Figure 10–23. Vascular invasion. Lymphovascular space invasion is an unfavorable prognostic indicator. By convention, lymphatic or vascular tumor emboli are diagnosed only outside the invasive tumor mass, and tumor in spaces within the main mass is assumed to represent shrinkage artifact. The prognostic relevance of true intratumoral lymphatic or vascular tumor emboli has not been determined. Extratumoral lymphatic or vascular space invasion is seen in approximately 15% of infiltrating duct carcinomas. The majority of these patients also have lymph node metastases, but in node-negative patients the vascular space invasion worsens the prognosis[42, 43] and predisposes to local recurrence after breast conserving therapy.[44] Tumor emboli are most often found in thin-walled vessels (lymphatics, capillaries, or postcapillary venules) and, because the distinction between these vessels is impossible and not necessary, the general term of "vascular invasion" should be used. Strict diagnostic criteria need to be used to avoid overdiagnosis of vascular invasion. Tumor emboli must be seen within spaces with demonstrable endothelial lining *(A)*; in this case, there are lymphocytes in the lumen and adjacent small blood vessels, confirming the lymphatic nature of the vascular space involved. Rarely, a relatively large blood vessel is seen invaded by tumor *(B)*.

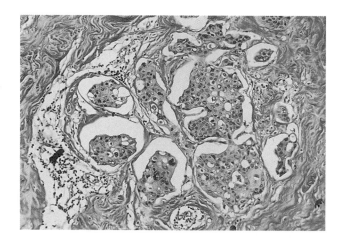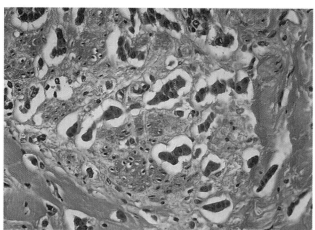

Figure 10–24. Retraction (shrinkage) artifact mimicking vascular invasion. Retraction artifact is the most common diagnostic pitfall in the diagnosis of vascular invasion. In addition to a lack of identifiable endothelial lining (sometimes problematic) or a characteristic topographic pattern of vessel involvement, there are other helpful features for confirming the presence of retraction artifact. In spaces created by retraction artifact, tumor nests are often attached to surrounding stroma, and these spaces most often are of the same shape as the tumor fragments seen within them. In contrast, true tumor emboli usually have a different configuration than the space within which they are seen.

In questionable cases, when all of the above criteria do not provide a satisfactory answer, one can resort to the use of immunohistochemical vascular markers (factor VIII related antigen, *Ulex europaeus,* CD31, and CD34).[43, 45] The caveat here is that the H&E impression is still the strongest evidence in favor of or against vascular space invasion because the immunostaining may fail to stain some vascular structures.

Figure 10–25. Perineural invasion. Perineural invasion is seen in up to 10% of invasive breast carcinomas and is seen more frequently in higher grade tumors.[1, p 287] It has not been shown to be an independent prognostic factor. This microphotograph shows predominantly intra-neural invasion.

EXTENSIVE INTRADUCTAL COMPONENT

Predominantly invasive

Predominantly DCIS with focal invasion

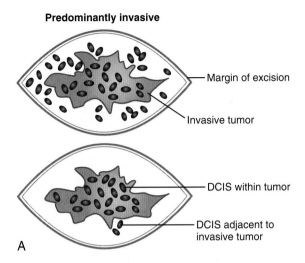

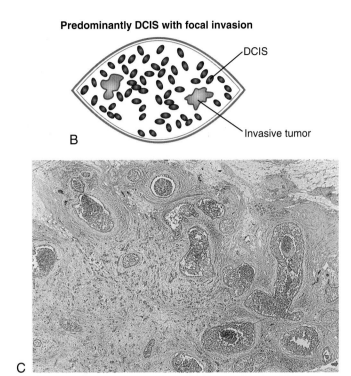

Figure 10–26. Extensive intraductal component. Extensive intraductal component (EIC) is defined as the amount of ductal carcinoma in situ (DCIS) within the invasive tumor that is ≥25% of the tumor mass and the presence of DCIS outside the main tumor mass[46] *(A)*. Tumors that consist predominantly of DCIS with one or more foci of microinvasion are also considered EIC positive *(B)*. EIC is seen in 10% of infiltrating duct carcinomas (IDC),[6] and is often associated with multiple foci of invasion. If the proportion of invasive component in the tumor mass is low, there seems to be an association with improved survival[47, 48]; however, if the invasive tumor grade is taken into account, this may not be true in all cases. An example of EIC is seen in *C*.

EIC predicts for the spread of the tumor in the breast[2] and is associated with positive surgical margins.[49] However, it is not an independent predictor of local recurrence or decreased survival in the presence of negative surgical margins,[49, 50] although a recent report showed an increased likelihood of local recurrence if the intraductal component of EIC is of high grade.[51] The presence or absence of EIC is used in making decisions about the extent of surgery.[52] (*A* and *B* from Connolly JL, Boyages J, Nixon AJ, et al: Predictors of breast recurrence after conservative surgery and radiation therapy for invasive breast cancer. Mod Pathol 11:134–139, 1998.)

MARGIN STATUS

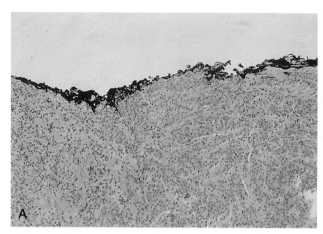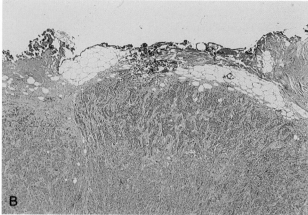

Figure 10–27. Infiltrating carcinoma and inked/cauterized margin. *A,* The tumor is transected in this section, directly abutting on the inked surgical margin (which also shows cautery artifact) and thus constituting a positive surgical margin. The microscopic margin status is among the most important pieces of information obtained from the pathologic examination of surgical breast specimens, although it is fraught with multiple technical and conceptual problems. Although the presence of tumor cells at the margin in a single low-power field is considered to constitute a positive margin, the definition of negative and close margins is far from being clear. Some pathologists define a negative margin as no tumor cells directly on the ink; others require a minimum 5-mm distance between tumor and inked margin. Other difficulties include fragmentation of the gross specimen, with leaking of the ink deeper into the breast tissue *(B)*, creating a falsely positive margin, and the notorious sampling problem—how much to sample and how to submit and examine the margins. A positive margin is associated with increased risk of local recurrence; this risk is further increased if the positive margin is associated with vascular space invasion.[51]

STROMAL HYALINIZATION

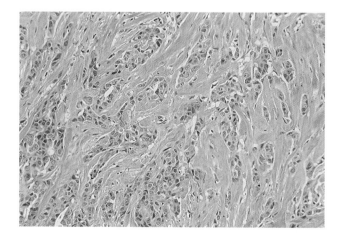

Figure 10–28. Hyalinized stroma in infiltrating duct carcinoma (IDC). Usually thought of as a feature that rules out invasion, stromal hyalinization can occasionally be seen in IDC. The prognostic significance of this feature is controversial, but it is associated with estrogen receptor expression and tumor response to hormonal therapy.[53, 54] This fact is most likely due to the association of stromal hyalinization with favorable tumor types (e.g., tubular, invasive cribriform carcinomas), which is not the case in this example.

TUMOR NECROSIS

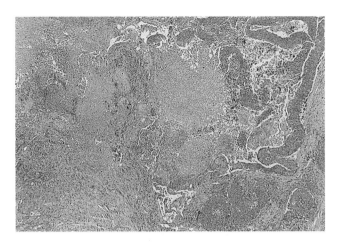

Figure 10–29. Extensive tumor necrosis in infiltrating duct carcinoma (IDC) of the breast. Confluent tumor necrosis has been shown to be a predictor of time to recurrence and a shortened survival. This effect, however, is only a factor during the first 2 years after the diagnosis and loses its significance with longer follow-up.[55]

ESTROGEN AND PROGESTERONE RECEPTORS

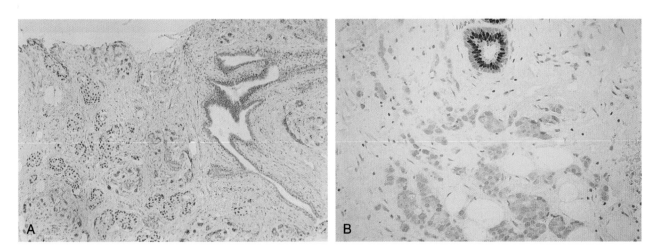

Figure 10–30. Estrogen receptor expression. Estrogen receptor (ER) expression, seen in 60% to 70% of breast carcinomas, is a weak favorable prognostic factor. It is used primarily to select patients for endocrine therapy, which confers a 20% to 30% survival and recurrence benefit in ER-positive patients. The traditional biochemical method of measuring ER expression has been replaced in most laboratories by immunohistochemical detection, which offers comparable and often more reliable results. There are several unresolved issues hindering complete clinical validation of the immunohistochemical method, such as a lack of consensus on the interpretation and reporting of results. There are several proposed methods that strive to make immunohistochemical detection more reproducible.[56] The figures show positive ER *(A)* and negative ER with positive internal control (benign duct) *(B)*. It is recommended that a percentage of immunoreactive cells be indicated in the report; the intensity score need not be included.[57]

Predictive Power of Combined ER and PR Phenotypes

Phenotype	Incidence (%)	Response Rate to Endocrine Therapy (%)
ER+/PR+	58	77
ER+/PR−	23	27
ER−/PR+	4	46
ER−/PR−	15	11

Figure 10–31. Predictive power of combined estrogen receptor (ER) and progesterone receptor (PR) phenotypes. Progesterone receptor expression is thought to be a test complementary to ER that increases the predictive power of ER. False-positive ER (ER-positive/PR-negative) results may indicate the existence of functionally inactive variants of ER. Conversely, ER-negative/PR-positive results may be false-negative, resulting from splice variants of ER that are not detected by the assays but are functional.[58] (From McGuire WL, Chamness GC, Fuqua SA: Estrogren receptor variants in clinical breast cancer. Mol Endocrinol 5: 1571–1577, 1991.)

OTHER COMMONLY USED PROGNOSTIC MARKERS

Proliferation Markers

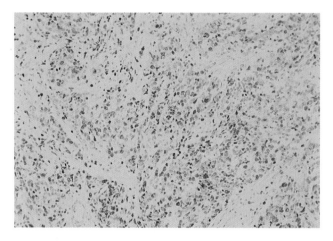

Figure 10–32. Ki-67 labeling of mammary carcinoma. Ki-67 antibody stains a high percentage of nuclei of this high-grade tumor. Many studies have demonstrated the prognostic importance of proliferation markers. These include mitotic index, S-phase fraction, thymidine labeling index, and Ki-67 (MIB1) index. Proliferation markers are also useful to predict response to chemotherapy.[59]

Although the mitotic index is a part of the histologic grading system, it has been shown to be an independent prognostic marker.[23, 60]

The Ki-67 (MIB1) labeling index is a statistically significant prognostic factor, but only in univariate analysis.[61]

S-phase fraction as assessed by flow cytometry has significance in multivariate analysis.[62] One of the shortcomings of this method, however, is that the suspension analyzed is not necessarily representative of the whole tumor and that adjacent benign tissue may be inadvertently analyzed.

Oncogenes and Tumor Suppressor Genes

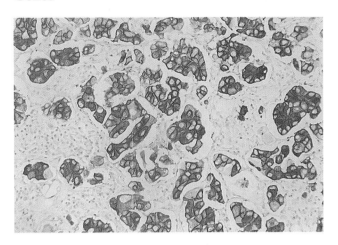

Figure 10–33. c-erbB-2 immunostaining of breast carcinoma. There is strong membranous staining of tumor cells, interpreted as "3+" expression. c-erbB2 (HER2/neu) is an oncogene that encodes for a growth factor receptor in the epidermal growth factor family. Its overexpression (seen in 20% to 30% of breast cancers) has been linked to poor outcome, especially in node-positive patients; its effect on prognosis in node-negative disease is controversial.[63, 64] More importantly, c-erbB-2 is a factor that can predict response to therapy; for example, new data are emerging that c-erbB-2 overexpression may correlate with enhanced response to anthracyclines, such as doxorubicin (Adriamycin).[65] While some reports indicate that c-erbB-2 overexpression confers resistance to adjuvant treatment with cyclophosphamide/methotrexate[66] and tamoxifen,[67] other studies have not confirmed these findings. In addition, a humanized monoclonal antibody directed against HER2/neu, Herceptin (trastuzumab) has been shown effective as a second-line treatment for patients with metastatic disease that failed first-line chemotherapy.[68]

The two most common assay methods used for detection of c-erbB-2 overexpression are immunohistochemistry (IHC) and fluorescent in situ hybridization (FISH).[57] While there are currently several FDA-approved IHC and FISH assays, a single test has not been proven to be the single best method to help determine eligibility for Herceptin or predict response to therapy and prognosis. It is not yet known whether FISH assays are superior to IHC, or whether FISH can be used as an adjunct to IHC as a corroborating test for borderline IHC results.

Because there is no single preferred method or reagent for c-erbB-2 testing, it is recommended that the method, primary reagent, and commercial supplier be reported with the assay result. Controls are to be used with each assay, with fixed embedded cell lines preferred. Only the invasive tumor should be scored (membranous staining only is recorded); the adjacent benign epithelium should not show strong membranous staining. The report should include an estimated percentage of staining cells and the scoring method used.

Other Prognostic Markers for Breast Cancer

Marker	Mechanism	Significance	References
p53	Tumor suppressor gene; involved in cell cycle arrest	Detects high-risk patients, especially if node-negative; mutations linked to poor prognosis, high grade and high proliferation rate, aneuploidy and steroid receptor negativity	56, 69, 70
Bcl-2	Oncogene; prevents apoptosis	Loss of expression associated with hormone receptor negativity, unfavorable morphology and poor prognosis	71
Angiogenesis markers	Prerequisite of tumor growth and metastasis	Associated with poor prognosis, but data are controversial	72–74
Cathepsins	Lysosomal enzymes involved in invasion and metastasis	Invasiveness markers; not an independent prognostic marker	75
Plasminogen activator (uPA)	Serine protease; determinant of tumor invasiveness	Claimed to be one of the strongest new prognostic factors significant in both uni- and multivariate analysis	61
Matrix metalloproteinases (interstitial collagenases, type IV collagenases, and stromelysins)	Invasiveness markers	Stromelysin-mRNA, detected by in situ hybridization, has been correlated with poor prognosis	76
c-erbB-3 and heregulin	c-erbB-3 gene encodes for transmembrane protein with homology to epidermal growth factor; heregulin is the growth factor ligand binding to c-erbB-3 receptor	Expressed in almost all breast cancers; prognostic significance is not clear	77
Breast cancer–associated genes	BRCA1 and BRCA2 genes implicated as predisposing to breast cancer	Morphology/prognosis	78, 79
DNA	Ploidy and S-phase measured by flow cytometry; DNA content measured by image cytometry		80

Figure 10–34. Other (nonconventional) prognostic markers. There are currently >100 putative markers that are being actively investigated for relevance in prognosis of breast cancer and treatment selection. This field is continuously in flux, as most proposed markers are sent into oblivion because they don't reach the statistically significant threshold; new markers constantly emerge and promise great breakthroughs in our understanding of breast cancer development and progression. Some of the most commonly cited putative indicators of breast cancer are listed in the figure.

Figure 10–35. Reporting guidelines (Association of Directors of Anatomic and Surgical Pathology [ADASP] recommendations). These guidelines are provided to help pathologists in communicating clinically useful and prognostically relevant information in the surgical pathology report. Use of these or any other guidelines is entirely optional and dependent on the individual pathologists and their institutional practices. (From Association of Directors of Anatomic and Surgical Pathology: Recommendations for the reporting of breast carcinoma. In Pathology Case Reviews, 3:241–247, 1998.)

Name: _____   SP _____

Breast	1) Left		2) Right	
Specimen	1) Excision (for palpable mass)		2) Mammographic localization	
	3) Incisional (includes core needle and FNA)			
	4) Re-excisional	5) Mastectomy	6) Chest wall	_____

Specimen size   _____

Tumor size(s)   _____

Tumor type	1) DCIS	5) Mixed NOS/ILC	9) Papillary
	2) LCIS	6) Tubular	10) Cribriform
	3) Infiltrating ductal (nos)	7) Mucinous	11) Other (specify)
	4) Infiltrating lobular	8) Medullary	_____

Grade of invasive carcinoma	1) I	2) II	3) III	_____
Gross margin	1) Free (specify distance)		2) Involved	_____
Margins invasive (specify type of margin evaluation)	1) Free (specify distance)	2) Focal	3) >Focal 4) Unevaluable	_____
Margins DCIS (specify type of margin evaluation)	1) Free (specify distance)	2) Focal	3) >Focal 4) Unevaluable	_____
DCIS nuclear morphology	1) High grade	2) Intermediate grade	3) Low grade	_____

DCIS patterns	1) Large areas of central necrosis (comedo)
	2) Small areas of central necrosis
	3) Cribiform 4) Solid 5) Micropapillary 6) Papillary
	(specify all that apply) _____

Calcification in situ	1) Absent	2) Prominent in DCIS	3) Focal in DCIS
	4) In LCIS	5) Prominent in benign breast tissue	
	6) Focal in benign breast tissue		

Peritumoral lymphatic invasion	1) Absent	2) Present	3) Dermal	_____
Peritumoral vascular invasion	1) Absent	2) Present		_____
Extent DCIS within invasive tumor	1) Absent	2) Slight	3) Moderate-marked	
	4) Tumor primarily DCIS with focal invasion			_____
Extent DCIS adjacent to invasive tumor	1) Absent	2) Slight	3) Moderate-marked	_____
EIC Status	1) EIC negative	2) EIC positive	3) EIC indeterminate	_____

NOTE: If a tumor is primarily DCIS with focal invasion or has a moderate or marked amount of DCIS within the infiltrating tumor and any in the adjacent tissue, it is EIC positive.

Skin	1) Not sampled	2) Free	3) Invasive	4) Dermal lymphatic _____
Nipple	1) Not sampled	2) Free	3) Invasive	4) Dermal lymphatic
	5) DCIS	6) Paget's		_____
Muscle	1) Not sampled	2) Free	3) Involved	

Mastectomy

Tumor location:	1) Central	2) UOQ	3) UIQ	4) LOQ	5) LIQ _____
Multiple areas involved	1) Central	2) UOQ	3) UIQ	4) LOQ	5) LIQ
	6) Only 1 area involved				_____

Lymph nodes (number of involved nodes in relation to total number examined)

Total	_____
Level I	_____
Level II	_____
Level III	_____
Other (specify)	_____

Extranodal extension	1) Absent	2) Present	_____

Metastatic cancer in other sites (specify)   _____

Nature of nontumorous breast tissue (describe):

Comments:

Ancillary studies (results and methodology used):

FNA, fine needle aspiration; DCIS, ductal carcinoma in situ; LCIS, lobular carcinoma in situ; NOS, not otherwise specified; ILC, infiltrating lobular carcinoma; EIC, extensive intraductal carcinoma; UOQ, upper outer quadrant; UIO, upper inner quadrant; LOQ, lower outer quadrant; LIQ, lower inner quadrant.

Figure 10–35. See legend on opposite page.

References

1. Rosen PP: Breast Pathology. Philadelphia, Lippincott-Raven. 1996.
2. Fisher ER, Gregorio RM, Fisher B, et al: The pathology of invasive breast cancer. A syllabus derived from findings of the National Surgical Adjuvant Breast Cancer Project (Protocol No. 4). Cancer 36:1–85, 1975.
3. Elston CW, Ellis IO (eds): The Breast. New York, Churchill Livingstone, 1998.
4. Pereira H, Pinder SE, Sibering DM, et al: Pathological prognostic factors in breast cancer. IV: Should you be a typer or a grader? A comparative study of two histological prognostic features in operable breast carcinoma. Histopathology 27:219–226, 1995.
5. Seidman JD, Schnapper LA, Aisner SC: Relationship of the size of the invasive component of the primary breast carcinoma to axillary lymph node metastasis. Cancer 75:65–71, 1995.
6. Fisher ER, Anderson S, Tan-Chiu, et al: Fifteen-year prognostic discriminants for invasive breast carcinoma. Cancer 91:1679–1687, 2001.
7. Gallager HS, Martin JE: An orientation to the concept of minimal carcinoma. Cancer 28:1505–1507, 1971.
8. Beahrs OH, Shapiro S, Smart C, et al: Summary report of the Working Group to Review the National Cancer Institute–American Cancer Society Breast Cancer Demonstration Projects. J Natl Cancer Inst 62:641–709, 1979.
9. Hartman WH: Minimal breast cancer: An update. Cancer 53:681–684, 1984.
10. Bedwani R, Vana J, Rosner D, et al: Management and survival of female patients with "minimal" breast cancer: As observed in the long-term and short-term surveys of the American College of Surgeons. Cancer 47:2769–2778, 1981.
11. Arnesson L-G, Hatschek T, Smeds S, Grontoft O: Histopathology grading in small breast cancer less than 10 mm: Results from an area with mammography screening. Breast Cancer Res Treat 44:39–46, 1997.
12. Lee AK, Loda M, Mackarem G, et al: Lymph node negative invasive breast carcinoma 1 cm or less in size (T1$_{A,B}$ N0 M0): Clinicopathologic features and outcome. Cancer 79:761–71, 1997.
13. Padmore RF, Fowble B, Hoffman J, et al: Microinvasive breast carcinoma: Clinicopathologic analysis of a single institution experience. Cancer 88:1403–1409, 2000.
14. Silver SA, Tavassoli FA: Mammary ductal carcinoma in situ with microinvasion. Cancer 82:2382–2390, 1998.
15. Elston CW, Ellis IO: Pathological prognostic factors in breast cancer. I: The value of histological grade in breast cancer: Experience from a large study with long-term follow-up. Histopathology 1991; 19:403–410, 1991.
16. Contesso G, Mouriesse H, Friedman S, et al: The importance of histologic grade in long-term prognosis of breast cancer. A study of 1,010 patients, uniformly treated at the Institut Gustave-Roussy. J Clin Oncol 5:1378–1386, 1987.
17. Parl FF, Dupont WD: A retrospective cohort study of histologic risk factors in breast cancer patients. Cancer 50:2410–2416, 1982.
18. Hopton DS, Thorogood J, Clayden AD, Mackinnon D: Histological grading of breast cancer: Significance of grade on recurrence and mortality. Eur J Surg Oncol 15:25–31, 1989.
19. Schumacher M, Schmoor C, Sauerbrei W: The prognostic effect of histological tumor grade in node-negative breast cancer patients. Breast Cancer Res Treat 25:235–245, 1993.
20. Henson DE, Ries L, Freedman LS, Carriaga M: Relationship among outcome, stage of disease, and histologic grade for 22,616 cases of breast cancer: The basis for a prognostic index. Cancer 68:2142–2149, 1991.
21. Kollias J, Elston CW, Ellis IO, et al: Early-onset breast cancer: Histopathological and prognostic considerations. Br J Cancer 75:1318–1323, 1997.
22. Bloom HJG, Richardson WW: Histological grading and prognosis in breast cancer. A study of 1409 cases of which 359 have been followed for 15 years. Br J Cancer 11:359–377, 1957.
23. Genestie C, Zafrani B, Asselain B, et al: Comparison of the prognostic value of Scarff-Bloom-Richardson and Nottingham histological grades in a series of 825 cases of breast cancer: Major importance of the mitotic count as a component of both grading systems. Anticancer Res 18:571–576, 1998.
24. Start RD, Flynn MS, Cross SS, et al: Is the grading of breast carcinomas affected by a delay in fixation? Virchows Arch A Pathol Anat Histopathol 419:475–477, 1991.
25. Clayton F, Hopkins CL: Pathologic correlates of prognosis in lymph node-positive breast carcinomas. Cancer 71:1780–1790, 1993.
26. Donegan WL, Stine SB, Samter TG: Implications of extracapsular nodal metastases for treatment and prognosis of breast cancer. Cancer 72:778–782, 1993.
27. Hetelekidis S, Shnitt SJ, Silver B, et al: The significance of extracapsular extension of axillary lymph node metastases in early-stage breast cancer. Int J Radiat Oncol Biol Phys 46:31–34, 2000.
28. de Mascarel I, Bonichon F, Coindre JM, Trojani M: Prognostic significance of breast cancer axillary lymph node micrometastases assessed by two special techniques: Reevaluation with longer follow-up. Br J Cancer 66:523–527, 1992.
29. McGuckin MA, Cummings MC, Walsh MD, et al: Occult axillary node metastases in breast cancer: Their detection and prognostic significance. Br J Cancer 73:88–95, 1996.
30. Hartveit F, Lilleng PK: Breast cancer: Two micrometastatic variants in the axilla that differ in prognosis. Histopathology 28:241–246, 1996.
31. Rosen PP, Saigo PE, Braun DW, et al: Occult axillary lymph node metastases from breast cancer with intramammary lymphatic tumor emboli. Am J Surg Pathol 6:639–641, 1982.
32. Lilleng PK, Hartveit F: "Missed" micrometastases—the extent of the problem. Acta Oncol 39:313–317, 2000.
33. Cohen LF, Breslin TM, Kuerer HM, et al: Identification and evaluation of axillary sentinel lymph nodes in patients with breast carcinoma treated with neoadjuvant chemotherapy. Am J Surg Pathol 24:1266–1272, 2000.
34. Rosen PP, Saigo PE, Braun DW, et al: Axillary micro- and macrometastases in breast cancer. Prognostic significance of tumor size. Ann Surg 194:585–591, 1981.
35. Yeatman TJ, Cox CE: The significance of breast cancer lymph node micrometastases. Surg Oncol Clin N Am 8:481–496, 1999.
36. Nasser IA, Lee AKC, Bosari S, et al: Occult axillary lymph node metastases in "node-negative" breast carcinoma. Hum Pathol 24:950–957, 1993.
37. Van Bogaert L-J: Immunohistochemical detection and significance of axillary lymph node micrometastases in breast carcinoma. Anal Quant Cytol Histol 17:75–76, 1995.
38. Nahrig J, Richter T, Kowolik J, et al: Comparison of different histopathological methods for the examination of sentinel lymph nodes in breast cancer. Anticancer Res 20:2209–2212, 2000.
39. Turner RR, Hansen NM, Stern SL, Giuliano AE: Intraoperative examination of the sentinel lymph node for breast carcinoma staging. Am J Clin Pathol 112:627–634, 1999.
40. Bautista NC, Cohen S, Anders KH: Benign melanocytic nevus cells in axillary lymph nodes. A prospective incidence and immunohistochemical study with literature review. Am J Clin Pathol 102:102–108, 1994.
41. Doglioni C, Dell'Orto P, Zanetti G, et al: Cytokeratin-immunoreactive cells of human lymph nodes and spleen in normal and pathological conditions. Virchows Archiv A Pathol Anat Histopathol 416:479–490, 1990.
42. Rosen PP: Tumor emboli in intramammary lymphatics in breast carcinoma: Pathologic criteria for diagnosis and clinical significance. Pathol Annu 18:215–232, 1983.
43. Pinder S, Ellis IO, O'Rourke S, et al: Pathological prognostic factors in breast cancer. III: Vascular invasion: Relationship with recurrence and survival in a large series with a long-term follow-up. Histopathology 24:41–47, 1994.
44. Clemente CG, Boracchi P, Andreola S, et al: Peritumoral lymphatic invasion in patients with node-negative mammary duct carcinoma. Cancer 69:1396–1403, 1992.
45. Saigo PE, Rosen PP: The application of immunohistochemical stains to identify endothelial-lined channels in mammary carcinoma. Cancer 59:51–54, 1987.
46. Schnitt SJ, Connolly JL, Harris JR, et al: Pathologic predictors of early local recurrence in stage I and stage II breast cancer treated by primary radiation therapy. Cancer 53:1049–1057, 1984.
47. Silverberg SG, Chitale AR: Assessment of the significance of the proportion of intraductal and infiltrating tumor growth in ductal carcinoma of the breast. Cancer 32:830–837, 1973.
48. Matsukuma A, Enjoji M, Toyoshima S: Ductal carcinoma of the

breast. An analysis of the proportion of intraductal and invasive components. Pathol Res Pract 187:62–67, 1991.

49. Gage I, Schnitt SJ, Nixon AJ, et al: Pathologic margin involvement and the risk of recurrence in patients treated with breast-conserving therapy. Cancer 78:1921–1928, 1996.

50. Hurd TC, Sneige N, Allen PK, et al: Impact of extensive intraductal component on recurrence and survival in patients with stage I or II breast cancer treated with breast conservation therapy. Ann Surg Oncol 4:119–124, 1997.

51. Voogd AC, Peterse JL, Crommelin MA, et al: Histological determinants for different types of local recurrence after breast-conserving therapy of invasive breast cancer. Dutch Study Group on local recurrence after breast conservation. Eur J Cancer 35:1828–1837, 1999.

52. Connolly JL, Boyages J, Nixon AJ, et al: Predictors of breast recurrence after conservative surgery and radiation therapy for invasive breast cancer. Mod Pathol 11:134–139, 1998.

53. Millis RR: Correlation of hormone receptors with pathological features in human breast cancer. Cancer 42:2869–2871, 1980.

54. Humeniuk V, Forrest APM, Hawkins RA, Prescott R: Elastosis and primary breast cancer. Cancer 52:1448–1452, 1983.

55. Gilchrist KW, Gray R, Fowble B, et al: Tumor necrosis is a prognostic predictor for early recurrence and death in lymph node-positive breast cancer: A 10-year follow-up study of 728 Eastern Cooperative Oncology Group patients. J Clin Oncol 11:1929–1935, 1993.

56. Allred DC, Harvey JM, Berardo M, Clark GM: Prognostic and predictive factors in breast cancer by immunohistochemical analysis. Mod Pathol 11:155–168, 1998.

57. Fitzgibbons PL, Page DL, Weaver D, et al: Prognostic factors in breast cancer. College of American Pathologists Consensus Statement 1999. Arch Pathol Lab Med 124:966–978, 2000.

58. Fuqua SA, Wolf DM: Molecular aspects of estrogen receptor variants in breast cancer. Breast Cancer Res Treat 35:233–241, 1995.

59. Stal O, Skoog L, Rutqvist LE, et al: S-phase fraction and survival benefit from adjuvant chemotherapy or radiotherapy of breast cancer. Br J Cancer 70:1258–1262, 1994.

60. Baak JPA, van Dop H, Kurver PHJ, Herman J: The value of morphometry to classic prognosticators in breast cancer. Cancer 56:372–382, 1985.

61. Harbeck N, Dettmar P, Thomssen C, et al: Prognostic impact of tumor biological factors on survival in node-negative breast cancer. Anticancer Res 18:2187–2198, 1998.

62. Hedley DW, Clark GM, Cornelisse CJ, et al: Consensus review of the clinical utility of DNA cytometry in carcinoma of the breast. Cytometry 14:482–485, 1993.

63. Tsuda HH: Prognostic and predictive value of c-erbB-2 (HER-2/neu) gene amplification in human breast cancer. Breast Cancer 8:38–44, 2001.

64. Ross JS, Fletcher JA: HER-2/neu (c-erbB-2) gene and protein in breast cancer. Am J Clin Pathol 112(Suppl 1):S53–S67, 1999.

65. Muss HB, Thor AD, Berry DA, et al: c-erbB-2 expression and response to adjuvant therapy in women with node-positive early breast cancer. N Engl J Med 330:1260–1266, 1994.

66. Stal O, Sullivan S, Wingren S, et al: c-erbB-2 expression and benefit from adjuvant chemotherapy and radiotherapy of breast cancer. Eur J Cancer 31A:2185–2190, 1995.

67. Carlomagno C, Perrone F, Gallo C, et al: c-erbB-2 overexpression decreases the benefit of adjuvant tamoxifen in early-stage breast cancer without axillary lymph node metastases. J Clin Oncol 14:2702–2708, 1996.

68. Cobleigh MA, Vogel CL, Tripathy D, et al: Efficacy and safety of Herceptin (humanized anti-HER2 antibody) as a single agent in 222 women with HER2 overexpression who relapsed following chemotherapy for metastatic breast cancer. Clin Oncol 17:2639–2648, 1999.

69. Thor AD, Moore DH, Edgerton SM, et al: Increased accumulation of the p53 suppressor gene product is an independent prognostic variable for breast cancer. J Natl Cancer Inst 84:845–855, 1992.

70. Molina R, Segui MA, Climent MA, et al: P53 oncoprotein as a prognostic indicator in patients with breast cancer. Anticancer Res 18:507–512, 1998.

71. Binder C, Marx D, Overhoff R, et al: Bcl-2 protein expression in breast cancer in relation to established prognostic factors and other clinicopathologic variables. Ann Oncol 6:1005–1010, 1995.

72. Folkman J: Angiogenesis and breast cancer [editorial]. J Clin Oncol 12:441–443, 1992.

73. Page DL, Jensen RA: Angiogenesis in human breast carcinoma: What is the question? Hum Pathol 26:1173–1174, 1995.

74. Weidner N: Tumoural vascularity as a prognostic factor in cancer patients: The evidence continues to grow. J Pathol 184(2):119–122, 1998.

75. Losch A, Tempfer C, Kohlberger P, et al: Prognostic value of cathepsin D expression and association with histomorphological subtypes in breast cancer. Br J Cancer 78:205–209, 1998.

76. Engel G, Heselmeyer K, Auer G, et al: Correlation between stromelysin-3 mRNA level and outcome in human breast cancer. Int J Cancer 58:830–835, 1994.

77. Travis A, Bell JA, Wencyk P, et al: C-erbB-3 in human breast carcinoma: Expression and relation to prognosis and established prognostic indicators. Br J Cancer 74:229–233, 1996.

78. Chappuis PO, Kapusta L, Begin LR, et al: Germline BRCA1/2 mutations and p27(Kip1) protein levels independently predict outcome after breast cancer. J Clin Oncol 18:4045–4052, 2000.

79. Silva JM, Gonzalez R, Provencio M, et al: Loss of heterozygosity in BRCA1 and BRCA2 markers and high-grade malignancy in breast cancer. Breast Cancer Res Treat 53:9–17, 1999.

80. Uyterlinde AM, Baak JP, Schipper NW, et al: Prognostic value of morphometry and DNA flow-cytometry features of invasive breast cancers detected by population screening: Comparison with control group of hospital patients. Int J Cancer 48:173–181, 1991.

CHAPTER 11

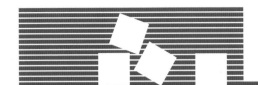

Infiltrating Carcinoma: Histologic Types Other Than Infiltrating Duct Carcinoma Not Otherwise Specified

Steven G. Silverberg
Olga B. Ioffe

INTRODUCTION

As discussed in the previous chapter, between 65% and 75% of invasive breast cancers in most published series are classified as infiltrating duct carcinoma not otherwise specified (IDC NOS). The remainder of the malignant tumors encountered are almost exclusively carcinomas, and they vary from histopathologic types that are relatively frequently encountered to others for which only a handful of case reports exist in the literature. Parenthetically, because the "NOS" in IDC NOS indicates that the diagnosis of this lesion is made by the lack of resemblance of a tumor to one of the less common specific types, this means that essentially two thirds of all breast carcinomas are diagnosed as IDC NOS by exclusion.

This rather strange circumstance has several important correlates. The first of these is that the criteria for the diagnosis of the various other histopathologic types should be very well defined, and should be rigorously adhered to in making the diagnosis of any one of these types. A malignant tumor that is not classifiable by these strict criteria as one of these types will then be diagnosed as IDC NOS. In fact, it is usually shown that, when a group of investigators performs a rigorous review of cases previously diagnosed as, for example, medullary carcinoma (but almost any other specific entity yields similar results), anywhere from 20% to 50% of the cases on file are reclassified as IDC NOS when strict criteria are applied.

The converse situation has not been studied as extensively. However, when Dr. Kazuei Hoshi and I (SGS) reviewed a series of 326 consecutive cases diagnosed as IDC NOS a few years ago, we confirmed the diagnosis in only 240 cases (74%). Tumors that were reclassified were most commonly lobular (38 cases) and cribriform (30 cases) carcinomas, but we also found 7 mucinous, 6 metaplastic, 2 tubular, and 1 papillary carcinoma that we believed had been inappropriately classified as IDC NOS.

Another implication of the fact that IDC NOS is diagnosed by exclusion is the assumption that in the future, as in the past, cases will continue to be carved out of this group and reclassified as new entities. Most of the tumors that are discussed in this chapter were once considered part of the IDC NOS group, and we have no doubt that new entities will continue to be identified in the future and be added to this list.

Clearly, the only reason for separating different types of invasive breast cancers is if there are important clinical differences—most importantly, those related to natural history and prognosis—between them and IDC NOS. It should be pointed out that Pereira and colleagues have made a rather convincing case that the variation observed clinically between different histopathologic variants of breast cancer is based more on grade than on type.[1] These authors recommend essentially that every invasive carcinoma of the breast be graded by the system originally applied to IDC NOS, and that accurate grading accounts for by far the greatest part of the prognostic differences reported between different histopathologic types.

Although there has been no comparably large and well executed study refuting these conclusions, there has not been another one confirming them, either. Even if we grant that the conclusion of Pereira and colleagues[1] may be generally correct, it seems to us that some elements of natural history specific to certain tumor types—for example, the fact that pure tubular carcinoma frequently metastasizes to axillary lymph nodes but almost never to distant viscera, the virtually invariable estrogen receptor negativity of adenoid cystic carcinoma, the relatively favorable prognosis of medullary carcinoma despite its definitional high tumor grade, as well as many others—suggest that accurate tumor typing will continue to be important, and that not all tumor types will necessarily need to be graded.

Major Types of Infiltrating Mammary Carcinoma
Grouped by Prognosis

Favorable	Intermediate	Unfavorable
Tubular	Infiltrating duct NOS	Inflammatory‡
Cribriform	Infiltrating lobular*	Carcinosarcoma
Mucinous (colloid)	Apocrine	Micropapillary
Medullary	Secretory (in adults)	Pleomorphic lobular
Adenoid cystic	Metaplastic†	Lipid-rich (?)
Secretory (in children)		Glycogen-rich (?)

Figure 11–1. In a summary of the material to follow, this table lists the more common types of invasive mammary carcinoma, and compares them prognostically with infiltrating duct carcinoma not otherwise specified (IDC NOS). Although different series have reported somewhat different results for some of these tumors, there is general consensus that infiltrating lobular carcinoma, which is the most common type after IDC NOS, has essentially the same survival rate, although other clinical features may be somewhat different, as will be discussed later in the chapter. Of the other relatively common histologic types, tubular, cribriform, mucinous (colloid), and medullary carcinoma are all considered to be prognostically favorable, as is the relatively rare adenoid cystic carcinoma. Histopathologic types established as prognostically unfavorable are less common, but they definitely include micropapillary carcinoma, pleomorphic lobular carcinoma, and carcinosarcoma (which is often classified as a variant of metaplastic carcinoma). Lipid-rich carcinoma and glycogen-rich clear cell carcinoma are probably also prognostically unfavorable, but very few cases of each of these entities have been described. Secretory carcinoma, which frequently occurs in children, seems to be favorable in this population but comparable in prognosis to IDC NOS in adults. Metaplastic carcinomas other than carcinosarcoma are also probably comparable to IDC NOS.

* Other than pleomorphic.   ‡ May be any histologic type.
† Other than carcinosarcoma.

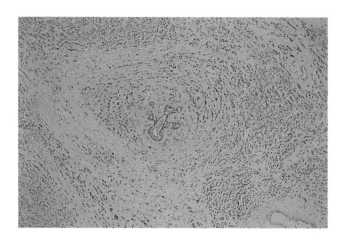

Figure 11–2. Infiltrating lobular carcinoma, classic pattern. Figures 11–2 and 11–3 illustrate the classic pattern of infiltrating lobular carcinoma, which for many years was the only pattern recognized. Figure 11–2 shows one low-power appearance of the classic pattern, in which tumor cells radiate in a "bull's eye" or "targetoid" pattern around residual benign ducts. Because this tumor is often paucicellular, particularly at its periphery, the boundaries of the tumor may be more difficult to establish radiographically and grossly than in cases of IDC NOS. The paucicellularity has often led to confusion with inflammatory lesions of the breast at low-power microscopic examination, particularly on frozen sections. See also Chapter 9 for additional discussion of infiltrating lobular carcinoma.

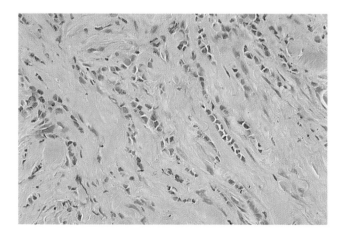

Figure 11–3. Infiltrating lobular carcinoma (ILC), classic type. At higher magnification than in Figure 11–2, we see one of the other typical manifestations of this tumor type, with tumor cells growing in a single-file pattern, separated by a fibrotic stroma. The individual tumor cells are small and uniform, and mitotic figures are rare. About 50% of cases of ILC are accompanied by lobular carcinoma in situ. The tumor is frequently multifocal and bilateral. Although the overall prognosis is similar to that of IDC NOS, ILC differs by having a higher proportion of estrogen receptor–rich tumors, by showing a sinus catarrh pattern of lymph node metastases, and by metastasizing with some predilection to the ovaries, uterus, gastrointestinal tract, and peritoneal surfaces.[2, 3]

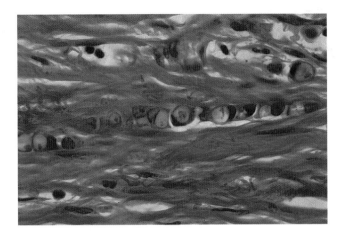

Figure 11–4. Infiltrating lobular carcinoma (ILC), classic type. In this high-power photomicrograph, we see another typical feature of infiltrating lobular carcinoma—the presence of numerous intracellular lumens giving the appearance of signet ring cells. Although these cells may also be seen in ductal carcinomas, they are far more frequent in the lobular types, and appear to be prognostically significant, in that tumors with more than 10% signet ring cells have a less favorable prognosis.[4] The "targetoid" appearance of the intracellular lumens, with an eosinophilic dot within a clear space, is quite different from the large globules forming the signet ring cells of a gastric or other extramammary signet ring cell carcinoma.

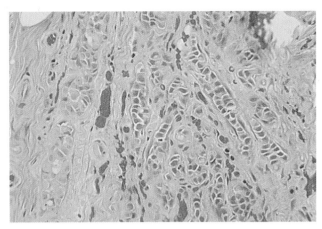

Figure 11–6. Infiltrating lobular carcinoma (ILC), solid type. The solid pattern of ILC is characterized by either a sheetlike pattern or irregularly shaped nests of lobular carcinoma–type cells. In this figure, the irregular nesting pattern is seen.

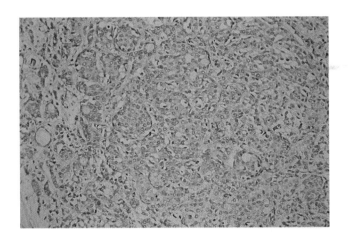

Figure 11–5. Infiltrating lobular carcinoma (ILC), alveolar type. The nonclassic architectural patterns of ILC were recognized only about 2 decades ago,[5] and the pleomorphic pattern was recognized only within the past decade.[6, 7] Prior to this recognition, these tumors were all classified as infiltrating duct carcinoma not otherwise specified (IDC NOS). The lobular nature of these variants can be confirmed by the fact that they frequently occur in combination with the classic pattern (so-called mixed pattern of ILC), they tend to be associated with lobular carcinoma in situ (LCIS) more than with ductal carcinoma in situ (DCIS), and they are immunohistochemically nonreactive for E-cadherin, while tumors showing ductal differentiation are strongly reactive.[8] Alveolar ILC is defined as a tumor characterized by globular arrangements of ≥20 cells with the same cytologic features as those seen in the classic pattern of ILC. Each globular aggregate may resemble LCIS, but the number of aggregates crowded into one field and the lack of a lobular architecture clearly indicate that this is an infiltrating tumor.

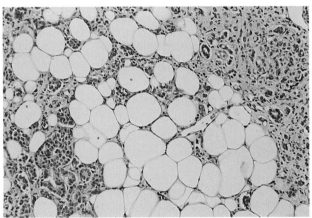

Figure 11–7. Infiltrating tubulolobular carcinoma. In the tubulolobular variant of infiltrating lobular carcinoma (ILC), some of the small uniform tumor cells aggregate to form small tubules, as well as the other classic lobular structures described and illustrated previously. It should be noted that this is not a "collision tumor" composed of separate lobular and tubular elements, but rather an intimate admixture within one tumor, as shown in the figure. The cytologic appearance of the cells forming the tubules should be identical to that of the cells forming other structures. This pattern is distinctly uncommon, but there is some evidence that it may have the most favorable prognosis among the subtypes of ILC. On the other hand, the prognostic significance of the other subtypes is argued in the literature, with some authors suggesting a less favorable prognosis for the nonclassic patterns,[9] a finding not confirmed by others.[10] In our own studies, the only statistically significant prognostic markers among the subtypes of ILC discussed thus far are a high proportion (>10%) of signet ring cells and a high S-phase fraction, both of which are prognostically unfavorable.[4, 11]

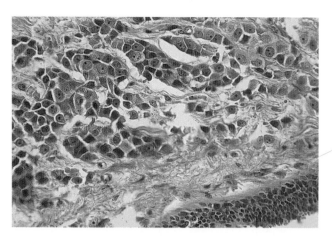

Figure 11-8. Infiltrating pleomorphic lobular carcinoma. This variant of infiltrating lobular carcinoma (ILC) was described in 1992, and is characterized by typical lobular carcinoma architecture (any one or more of the forms described previously) combined with a high nuclear grade and brightly eosinophilic cytoplasm that can be demonstrated to be of apocrine type by gross cystic disease fluid protein-15 (GCDFP-15) immunoreactivity[6, 12]; of note, most classic lobular carcinomas are GCDFP-15 negative. In the case illustrated here, the large size of the tumor cells can be compared with the benign ductal cells at the lower right. These cells are much larger than typical ILC cells and their nuclei are more bizarre, but the solid growth pattern and the lack of cohesiveness between the cells are typical of ILC. The lobular nature of this tumor can be confirmed by negative E-cadherin immunostaining. If not correctly diagnosed as pleomorphic lobular carcinoma, cases of this sort would probably be categorized as grade 3 infiltrating duct carcinoma not otherwise specified (IDC NOS); however, the prognosis of pleomorphic lobular carcinoma is even worse, with an average 5-year survival of around 20% in reported series.[6, 13]

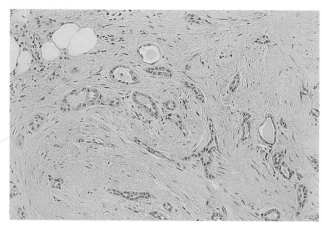

Figure 11-10. Tubular carcinoma. This figure represents the sclerosing pattern of tubular carcinoma, in which dense stroma surrounds the haphazardly arranged tubules. Note that the tubules are often teardrop-shaped rather than uniformly round. At this magnification, we begin to see that the tubules are lined by a single layer of rather uniform small tumor cells.

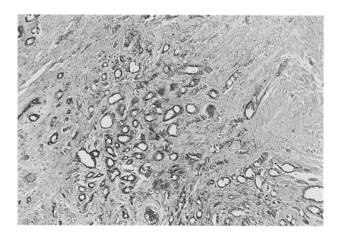

Figure 11-9. Tubular carcinoma. Tubular carcinoma is essentially a very well differentiated infiltrating duct carcinoma of the breast, but with specific features that define its natural history.[14] Grossly, it resembles typical infiltrating duct carcinoma not otherwise specified (IDC NOS), presenting as a hard lesion with stellate margins, but it is usually quite small. It comprises from 1% to 10% of all breast carcinomas in different series, and is characterized by the presence of well formed regular tubules lined by a single layer of cuboidal cells and separated by a desmoplastic or hyalinized stroma. The tubules appear to be distributed at random rather than arranged in any particular pattern, and they may be seen infiltrating into fat without any surrounding reactive stroma. More than 50% of cases are associated with ductal carcinoma in situ (DCIS), and many contain microcalcifications, often within the foci of DCIS.

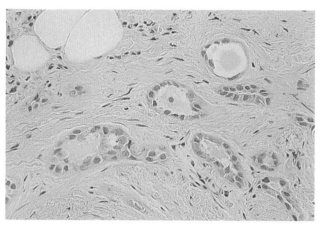

Figure 11-11. Tubular carcinoma. At somewhat higher magnification than in Figure 11-10, the low cytologic grade of the tumor cells and the absence of a surrounding myoepithelial layer are seen more clearly. The diagnosis of tubular carcinoma should be made only when the classic histopathologic features described and illustrated in Figures 11-9 to 11-11 are present. Stratification of the cells within the tubules to more than a single layer and solid nests of tumor cells should suggest the diagnosis of a low-grade infiltrating duct carcinoma not otherwise specified (IDC NOS). This distinction is important because of the extremely favorable prognosis of this tumor when classic tubular elements comprise ≥75% of the tumor.[15, 16] In this situation, although axillary lymph node metastases occur in up to 30% of cases, distant metastases and tumor-related death are extremely rare. It is not clear whether this extremely favorable prognosis is correlated with the tubular morphology or with the usual small size of these tumors. Careful perusal of published studies fails to reveal whether the larger (>2 cm) tubular carcinomas are those that are associated with the rare distant metastases, and also does not permit correlation of the status of the axilla with subsequent behavior.

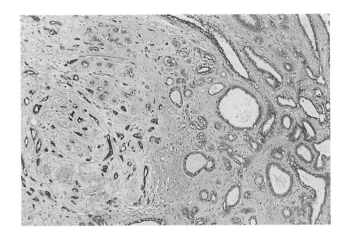

Figure 11–12. Tubular carcinoma and adjacent sclerosing adenosis. In addition to infiltrating duct carcinoma not otherwise specified (IDC NOS), the main differential diagnoses of tubular carcinoma are benign lesions such as sclerosing and microglandular adenosis and radial scar. In this figure, a tubular carcinoma is seen on the left and sclerosing adenosis on the right. Note the uniform size and haphazard distribution of the tubular carcinoma, which at higher magnification could be seen to be composed of tubules lined by a single cell layer. In sclerosing adenosis, on the other hand, the size and shape of the tubular structures are quite variable, usually being most sclerosed in the center of the lesion and more dilated around the periphery. The entire lesion maintains a lobular configuration with a well defined periphery, unlike the infiltrative margins of tubular carcinoma. In addition, even at this magnification, the double cell lining (epithelial cells surrounded by myoepithelial cells) can be appreciated within the sclerosing adenosis, and if necessary, the presence of myoepithelial cells can be confirmed by an actin immunostain.

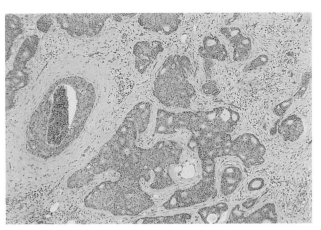

Figure 11–14. Infiltrating cribriform carcinoma. Infiltrating cribriform carcinoma is another type of mammary cancer separated from infiltrating duct carcinoma not otherwise specified (IDC NOS) only within the past 2 decades.[18, 19] It is thought to comprise 3% to 5% of all invasive breast cancers, and tends to be intermediate in size between the smaller tubular carcinoma and the larger IDC NOS. Because it often coexists with one or both of these other patterns, it may represent a transition stage between the two. As seen in the figure, this tumor displays islands of cells with uniform punched-out spaces, identical to the picture of the cribriform pattern of ductal carcinoma in situ (DCIS). However, the irregular shapes and sizes of the islands, as well as reactive stroma, indicate that this is an invasive tumor. In this figure, the more rounded nest of cells with central necrosis at the 9 o'clock position probably represents DCIS, while the remainder of the tumor in this field is infiltrating cribriform carcinoma. The presence of DCIS, often but not necessarily or exclusively of cribriform type, is quite characteristic.

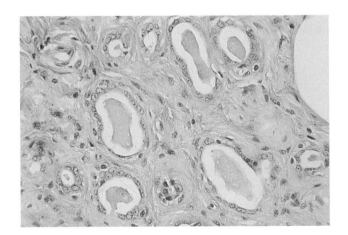

Figure 11–13. Microglandular adenosis. A more difficult—but fortunately rarer—mimic of tubular carcinoma is the entity known as microglandular adenosis.[17] The average pathologist is likely to see 100 cases of sclerosing adenosis for each case of tubular carcinoma and 100 cases of tubular carcinoma for each case of microglandular adenosis, pointing out the extreme rarity of the last-mentioned lesion. The differential diagnostic problem arises, however, because microglandular adenosis is also composed of tubules that lack a myoepithelial cell layer. Fortunately for the pathologist facing this differential diagnostic problem, microglandular adenosis also lacks the reactive stroma of tubular carcinoma, usually contains tubules that are less teardrop-shaped than those of tubular carcinoma, and features tubules lined by even less atypical cells and containing prominent intraluminal colloid-like secretory material.

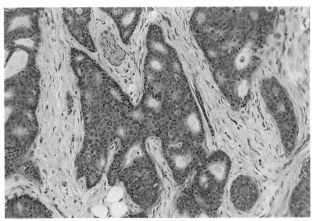

Figure 11–15. Infiltrating cribriform carcinoma. At higher magnification, the features seen in Figure 11–14 are again noted, and the uniformity and small size of the nuclei—which are virtually always of nuclear grade 1 or 2—are more apparent. Focally in these tumors, the cribriform spaces may be replaced by solid nests of tumor cells, but the well differentiated appearance of the nuclei is constant. The tumor is almost always diploid and rich in estrogen receptor. The prognosis is excellent as long as the infiltrating cribriform pattern comprises >50% of the invasive component of a breast cancer. As with tubular carcinoma, axillary lymph node metastases may be present, but distant metastases and death are extremely rare. The differential diagnosis includes tubular carcinoma, low-grade infiltrating duct carcinoma not otherwise specified (IDC NOS), and cribriform ductal carcinoma in situ (DCIS) all of which have been discussed previously. Another major differential diagnostic possibility is adenoid cystic carcinoma, which is discussed later (see Fig. 11–32).

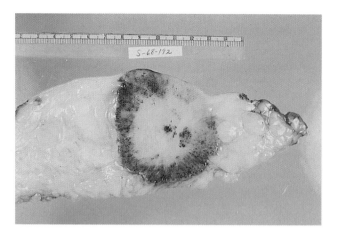

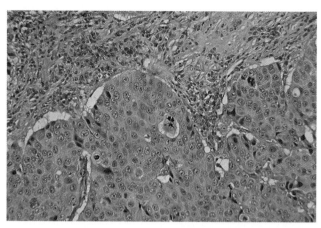

Figure 11–16. Medullary carcinoma. Medullary carcinoma of the breast represents a conundrum that has been known for many years—an extremely poorly differentiated breast carcinoma with (in the great majority of, but not all, published series) a relatively favorable prognosis.[20-22] The diagnosis of medullary carcinoma can be suspected at the gross level by the observation of a very well demarcated, generally soft rather than firm or hard, usually white rather than yellow tumor, as shown in this figure. As in this case, in the past these tumors often grew to a large size before being detected clinically, although—like other breast cancers—they are now being seen earlier in their natural history.

Figure 11–18. Medullary carcinoma. At higher magnification than in Figure 11–17, the additional diagnostic features of medullary carcinoma are revealed. This section, taken from the center of the tumor, shows both the prominent lymphoplasmacytic infiltrate as well as the sheetlike growth of large, pleomorphic, poorly differentiated cells with vesicular nuclei and prominent nucleoli. Numerous apoptoses and mitoses are easily seen. Not seen in Figures 11–16 to 11–18 but relatively common in medullary carcinomas are multinucleate giant cells and foci of squamous metaplasia. In the typical case, no intraductal component is present. It is apparent from the description of the typical histopathologic features of these tumors that they are invariably assigned a grade of 3 by the Nottingham system; they are also almost always aneuploid and both estrogen receptor and progesterone receptor negative. However, despite these factors which would predict an unfavorable prognosis, in most series the survival rate has been better than that for infiltrating duct carcinoma not otherwise specified (IDC NOS), and certainly much better than that for grade 3 IDC NOS. The reason for this has been somewhat obscure, but it may be related to host immune response manifested histologically by the prominent inflammatory cell infiltrate.

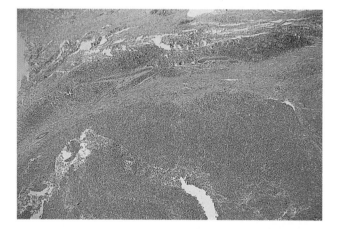

Figure 11–17. Medullary carcinoma. Although the diagnostic criteria for medullary carcinoma have varied somewhat in different series over the years, there is general agreement that the tumor should be well circumscribed, as seen in this low-power photomicrograph. The tumor must also maintain the so-called syncytial growth pattern, that is, solid sheets and nests with no tubular or papillary growth. In this figure, a lymphoplasmacytic infiltrate is seen around the periphery of the tumor, but more important is a moderate to marked infiltrate within the tumor stroma itself.

PROPOSED HISTOLOGIC CRITERIA FOR THE DIAGNOSIS OF MEDULLARY CARCINOMA

PRIMARY*

    1. Predominantly circumscribed border

    2. Syncytial growth ≥75%

    3. Presence of admixed stromal mononuclear infiltrate

    4. Grade 2 or 3 nuclei

    5. Absence of glandular features

SECONDARY†

    1. Microscopically completely circumscribed

    2. 2+ to 3+ mononuclear infiltrate

    3. Absence of in situ carcinoma

*Diagnosis of IDC is mandatory if any one of these criteria is not met.

†Diagnosis of IDC is mandatory if two or more of these criteria are not met.

Figure 11–19. Criteria for diagnosis of medullary carcinoma. The criteria for the histopathologic diagnosis of medullary carcinoma have varied in different series published over a period of many years. Several of these have included both "typical medullary" and "atypical medullary" categories, with the latter having a somewhat poorer prognosis than the former, but still better than that of a controlled series of infiltrating duct carcinoma not otherwise specified (IDC NOS). In the report of Wargotz and Silverberg, which we quote here, the category of atypical medullary carcinoma was eliminated, and the criteria for the diagnosis of medullary carcinoma were made more specific, so that any tumor that does not satisfy these criteria is diagnosed as IDC NOS (perhaps with the designation "medullary-like").[21] Note that the diagnostic criteria are divided into those of primary and secondary importance, with less strict reliance on the presence of all of the latter than the former. In our experience, if this diagnostic schema is followed strictly, many cases previously classified as medullary carcinoma will be reassigned to the category of medullary-like IDC NOS. The cases retained as medullary carcinoma will continue to display the paradoxically favorable survival.

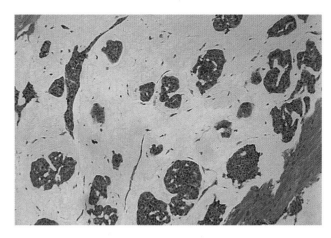

Figure 11–21. Mucinous carcinoma. Microscopically, pure mucinous carcinoma is characterized by nests and single cells of generally well differentiated carcinoma, floating in large pools of extracellular mucin. The mucin should comprise at least 50% of the entire tumor volume, and often comprises considerably more.

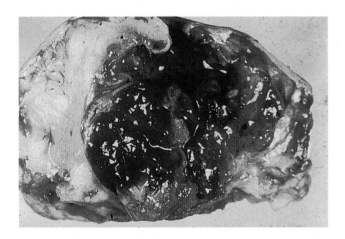

Figure 11–20. Mucinous (colloid, gelatinous) carcinoma. Although variable degrees of mucin may be produced by many mammary carcinomas, massive deposition of extracellular mucin is an unusual phenomenon that characterizes the subtype of breast cancer known as mucinous carcinoma.[14, 23] This type, which is frequently admixed with infiltrating duct carcinoma not otherwise specified (IDC NOS), comprises about 2% to 3% of all breast carcinomas. The gross appearance, as seen in this photograph, is represented by a usually well circumscribed and often large, gelatinous mass. The main differential diagnosis at the macroscopic level is with a myxoid fibroadenoma.

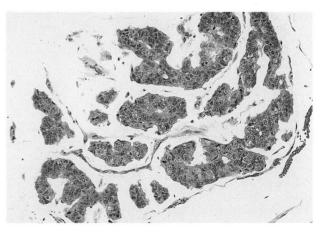

Figure 11–22. Mucinous carcinoma. At higher magnification, the relative uniformity of the tumor cells and the low nuclear grade are characteristic. The tumor cells are frequently arranged as small glands with central lumens, which may contain mucin. Mucin may also be encountered as globules within the cytoplasm. Mitotic figures are encountered, but usually they are not numerous. A common finding is the presence of argyrophilic granules that stain immunohistochemically for neuroendocrine markers in few or many of the tumor cells. The prognosis is generally favorable for this tumor, although distant metastases certainly do occur. When the tumor is mixed with infiltrating duct carcinoma not otherwise specified (IDC NOS), the survival rate is lower, and metastatic disease usually consists of the IDC NOS component.

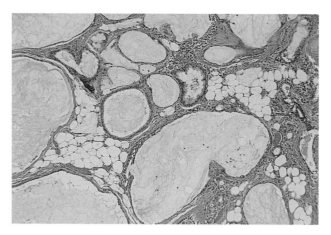

Figure 11–23. Mucocele-like lesion (differential diagnosis of mucinous carcinoma). Although other primary carcinomas of the breast can secrete mucin, they are unlikely to be confused with a typical mucinous carcinoma. The most problematic differential diagnosis is with the so-called mucocele-like lesion (pictured here), which is a mass composed of multiple cysts containing mucin, with rupture and discharge of generally acellular mucin into surrounding parenchyma. If the mucin is entirely acellular, confusion with mucinous carcinoma is unlikely, but not infrequently the cysts filled with mucin may be lined by a thin epithelial layer or even by proliferated and atypical cells, reflecting the recent observation that about half of mucocele-like lesions actually represent in situ or even invasive mucinous carcinoma.[24, 25] Thus, careful search should be made within these lesions for foci diagnosable as carcinoma. When the diagnosis of carcinoma is made in a mucocele-like lesion, the prognosis is at least as favorable as, and probably more so than, the usual mucinous carcinoma.

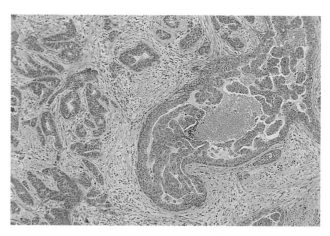

Figure 11–25. Micropapillary ductal carcinoma in situ with infiltrating duct carcinoma not otherwise specified (IDC NOS). Lesions of this sort are also likely to be reported as infiltrating papillary carcinoma, even though the infiltrating component is not particularly papillary. We believe that true infiltrating papillary carcinoma of the breast is an extremely rare lesion, and we are sure of neither its natural history nor its prognosis, since the majority of cases reported under this title are—as illustrated in Figures 11–24 and 11–25—either noninfiltrating or nonpapillary (if not both).

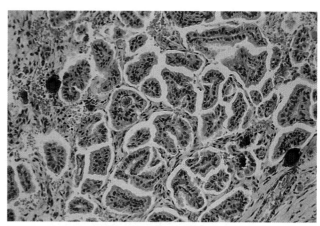

Figure 11–26. Infiltrating micropapillary carcinoma. The one type of mammary carcinoma that is both infiltrating and papillary is the recently described micropapillary carcinoma, which is shown here and in Figure 11–27. In contradistinction to the confused literature on "papillary carcinoma of the breast," which implies a favorable prognosis, invasive micropapillary carcinoma is one of the most aggressive types of mammary carcinoma.[27] Too few cases have been reported to establish a classic clinical profile or gross appearance, and the micropapillary pattern is not infrequently admixed with other histopathologic tumor types. From the few reports published to date, micropapillary carcinoma appears to be associated with an increased incidence of lymph node metastases, high tumor grade, aneuploidy, and larger tumor size[27, 28]; however, the adverse effect on survival may not be significant on multivariate analysis.[28] The characteristic microscopic appearance is one of small glandular and papillary spaces, often with microcalcifications in the form of psammoma bodies, characteristically surrounded by cleftlike spaces. A serrated peripheral border of the cell clusters is a common but not invariable finding. An accompanying ductal carcinoma in situ, often of micropapillary type, is frequently present, and helps to distinguish this tumor from a metastatic serous carcinoma derived from the ovary or elsewhere in the female genital system, the microscopic appearance of which is quite similar. Metastatic serous carcinomas also tend to be multifocal, and to demonstrate lymphatic or vascular space invasion.

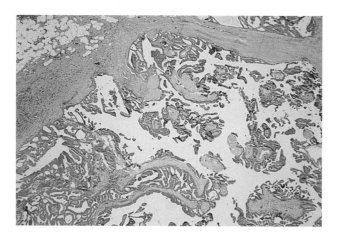

Figure 11–24. Intracystic papillary carcinoma. The subject of papillary carcinoma of the breast is an extremely difficult one to approach from the point of view of a literature review. There is no doubt in our minds that the vast majority of cases reported as "papillary carcinoma" are noninvasive lesions, composed of either the micropapillary or stratified spindle cell papillary ductal carcinoma in situ or intracystic papillary carcinoma, as in this figure.[26] Areas of pericystic sclerosis with pseudoinvasion of the papilloglandular component (as seen at the 12 o'clock position in the figure) can often lead to a mistaken diagnosis of infiltrating carcinoma. On the other hand, true foci of invasion are occasionally seen in this lesion and signify the ability to metastasize, although the prognosis is generally still good.

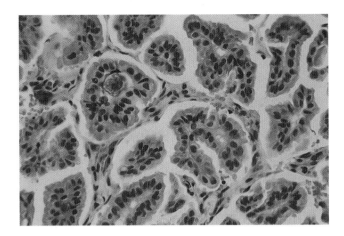

Figure 11–27. Infiltrating micropapillary carcinoma. At higher magnification, the tumor cells are small and well differentiated. Mitotic figures are not numerous, and this tumor will be graded as well differentiated (Nottingham grade 1), belying its highly aggressive nature. However, some series report the majority of these tumors to be of high nuclear grade.[27, 29]

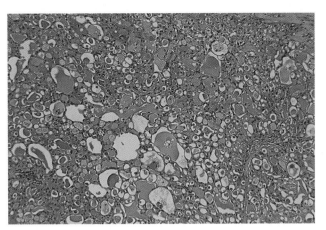

Figure 11–29. Secretory carcinoma. This rare tumor is also known as juvenile carcinoma, because of its original description in young girls and adolescents, but most of the cases we have seen (including the one illustrated here) have occurred in adults.[33, 34] The tumor is frequently grossly circumscribed and has a gray or yellow, relatively soft cut surface. The tumor cells grow in large nests, in which even at low magnification the voluminous intracellular and extracellular secretory material (predominantly sulfated acid mucopolysaccharide) is evident.

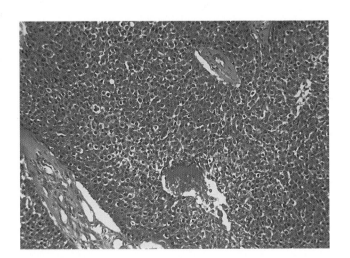

Figure 11–28. Solid papillary carcinoma with neuroendocrine features. These tumors consist of a solid proliferation of relatively uniform cells with fibrovascular cores that have an expansile and focally invasive outline at low-power examination.[30] A proportion of solid papillary carcinomas exhibit neuroendocrine differentiation evidenced by electron microscopy and positive immunostains for various neuroendocrine markers.[31] These tumors appear to behave as low-grade carcinomas although distant metastases have been reported.[32]

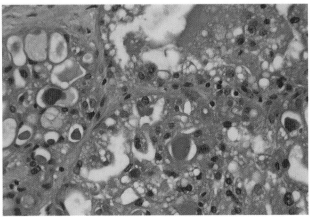

Figure 11–30. Secretory carcinoma. At higher magnification, the cells may form tubular, papillary, or solid structures architecturally, and the individual cells exhibit abundant clear or amphophilic cytoplasm. In addition to the large eosinophilic globules, intracellular microvesicles are present. Tumor cell nuclei tend to be small and uniform. The prognosis of this tumor is excellent in children, but less favorable in adults, and probably not markedly different from that of other infiltrating carcinomas. The main differential diagnosis is with lipid-rich and glycogen-rich carcinomas.

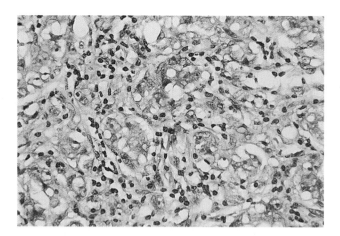

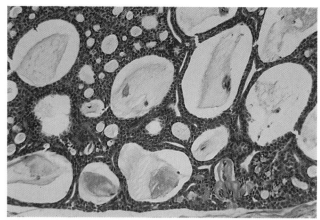

Figure 11–31. Lipid-rich and glycogen-rich carcinoma. Lipid-rich carcinoma, illustrated in this figure, is an extremely rare variant of infiltrating mammary carcinoma, composed of cells containing abundant lipid.[35] With the usual processing techniques, lipid is manifested in hematoxylin and eosin–stained sections by vacuolated cytoplasm. The presence of lipid can be demonstrated in frozen sections or imprints of fresh tissue, by electron microscopy, or by other techniques that preserve lipid material. The similarity to secretory carcinoma (see Figs. 11–29 and 11–30) is apparent, and in some cases which have been fixed entirely in formalin, negative periodic acid–Schiff (PAS) and mucin stains are necessary to rule out that diagnosis. The largest series of lipid-rich carcinomas reported comprised only 13 examples, 11 of which had axillary lymph node metastases, and 8 of which had either killed their hosts or recurred.[36] Thus, on the basis of this somewhat limited evidence, lipid-rich carcinoma is thought to be a prognostically unfavorable tumor type.

Glycogen-rich clear cell carcinoma. Although various investigators have reported that between 1% and 3% of mammary carcinomas are of this type, it has been extremely rare in our own experience, and fewer than 50 examples have been reported in the literature.[37] The tumor has the architectural features of intraductal and/or infiltrating duct carcinoma, but is characterized cytologically by voluminous clear (occasionally foamy or finely granular) cytoplasm. Apocrine features are sometimes also present, and it has been suggested that glycogen-rich carcinoma may be a variant of apocrine carcinoma (which itself is a variant of infiltrating duct carcinoma not otherwise specified [IDC NOS] with no particular prognostic significance). As expected, at both the histochemical and electron microscopic levels, the cytoplasmic contents can be demonstrated to be predominantly glycogen. The prognosis among cases reported in the literature has been slightly (but perhaps not significantly) worse than that of IDC NOS. The differential diagnosis, as mentioned previously, includes both secretory and lipid-rich carcinomas, and also must include the rare possibility of an extramammary clear cell adenocarcinoma metastatic to the breast.

Figure 11–32. Adenoid cystic carcinoma. Adenoid cystic carcinoma belongs to a group of tumors that are considered salivary or sweat gland–like neoplasms. These also include subareolar papillomatosis/nipple adenoma, syringomatous adenoma of the nipple, benign mixed tumor (pleomorphic adenoma), adenomyoepithelioma, and myoepithelial carcinoma, as well as even rarer lesions such as acinic cell carcinoma. Adenoid cystic carcinoma is probably the most common of the malignant variants, but it is still a rare tumor, comprising <0.1% of mammary carcinomas.[38] Adenoid cystic carcinomas have no particular distinguishing clinical or gross features, although they tend to be well circumscribed. Histologically, they are identical to their far more common salivary gland counterparts, and are characterized by a cylindromatous pattern which may resemble that of infiltrating cribriform carcinoma (see Figs. 11–14 and 11–15). Unlike cribriform carcinoma, however, the material within the cystic spaces consists of stromal and basement membrane elements rather than secretions. A similar pattern is encountered in collagenous spherulosis, a benign lesion that also enters the differential diagnosis.[39] Adenoid cystic carcinoma is usually composed of low-grade cells, but despite this, it is almost invariably both estrogen receptor and progesterone receptor negative.[40] This is another differentiating feature from infiltrating cribriform carcinoma. Additionally, infiltrating cribriform carcinoma usually contains an intraductal component, whereas adenoid cystic carcinoma virtually never does. An additional diagnostic problem in adenoid cystic carcinoma is the occasional presence of a more poorly differentiated component composed of solid elements, sometimes consisting of basaloid cells. For a definitive diagnosis of adenoid cystic carcinoma, a classic cylindromatous component should be found at least somewhere in the tumor. The prognosis of adenoid cystic carcinoma is excellent, and it virtually never metastasizes to axillary lymph nodes,[41] although rare cases with distant metastases—often after many years—have been reported.

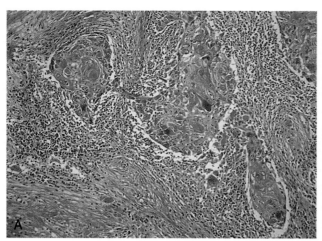
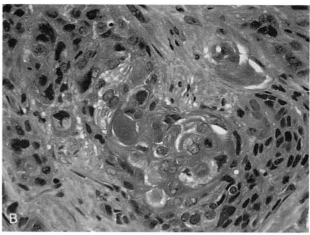

Figure 11–33. *A, B,* Squamous carcinoma. Although the prototype of mammary carcinoma is adenocarcinoma, rare tumors show metaplasia of various types. These have been classified differently by different authors. For example, Wargotz and Norris, reporting the material of the Armed Forces Institute of Pathology, divided metaplastic carcinomas into spindle cell carcinoma, carcinosarcoma, matrix-producing carcinoma, pure squamous cell carcinoma, and metaplastic carcinoma with osteoclast-like giant cells.[42] Rosen, on the other hand, includes a squamous type of metaplastic carcinoma, but also has a separate category of pure squamous carcinoma.[43] Rosen also does not include carcinosarcoma (the most aggressive variant in the Wargotz series) among his carcinomas with metaplasia, but he does include two variants not mentioned by Wargotz—a choriocarcinoma type, in which syncytiotrophoblastic giant cells are present, and a low-grade adenosquamous carcinoma, a rare tumor in the breast resembling a syringomatous squamous tumor of the skin, and therefore classified by us among the salivary and sweat gland–like tumors of the breast. In any event, squamous differentiation, as illustrated here, is relatively easy to recognize, but it must be distinguished from squamous carcinoma arising in the skin of the breast rather than in mammary parenchyma per se, from foci of squamous differentiation which are fairly common within medullary carcinomas, and from benign squamous metaplasia which often occurs at the periphery of a mammary infarct. Metastatic squamous cell carcinomas to the breast also occur, and the presence of an intraductal component (squamous or otherwise) will help to rule out that possibility.

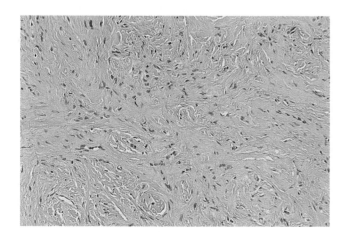
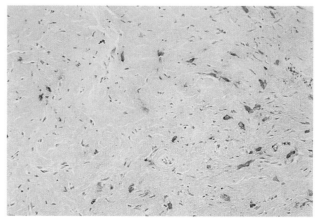

Figure 11–34. Metaplastic carcinoma, spindle cell type. This is the most common type of metaplastic carcinoma of the breast, and it is often the most difficult to recognize. As in the case illustrated here, the spindle cells may be deceptively lacking in atypia, leading to confusion with benign lesions such as fibromatosis and even nonspecific scars. It is important in such cases to perform immunostains for cytokeratins or epithelial membrane antigen, or to use electron microscopy to demonstrate the epithelial nature of the tumor cells.

Figure 11–35. Metaplastic carcinoma, spindle cell type, cytokeratin immunostain. In this immunostain for AE1/AE3, performed on the tumor shown in Figure 11–34, strong staining of many of the bland-appearing tumor cells is seen. We make it a rule to investigate any mammary mass composed of bland spindle cells without any other explanation, such as scarring after a previous needle or excisional biopsy. In one series, tumors with fibromatosis-like phenotype had a high risk of local recurrence, but were not demonstrated to metastasize,[44] much like fibromatosis. However, in other reports, they behave like carcinomas, metastasizing to axillary lymph nodes or beyond in anywhere from 6% to 54% of reported cases.[45,59]

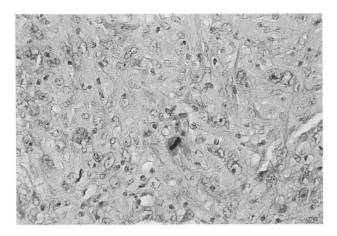

Figure 11–36. Metaplastic carcinoma, spindle cell type. This spindle cell carcinoma is considerably easier to diagnose as a malignant tumor, because it is composed of highly atypical cells with numerous mitotic figures. The main diagnostic problem here would be to make the distinction from a mammary sarcoma, and again immunohistochemistry and electron microscopy can be helpful to demonstrate the epithelial nature of the tumor cells. The malignant phenotype of the spindle cells present in this case is similar to that seen in the carcinosarcomas reported by Wargotz and Norris,[47] and suggests that a careful search for a malignant glandular or squamous component should be undertaken.

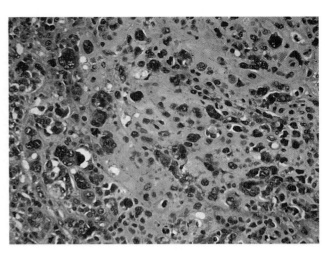

Figure 11–38. Metaplastic matrix-producing carcinoma. At higher power, the malignant cytologic features of metaplastic chondroid cells can be appreciated. These cells can demonstrate loss of epithelial markers by immunohistochemistry, a phenomenon that should be considered when evaluating sentinel lymph nodes for micrometastases using cytokeratin stains.

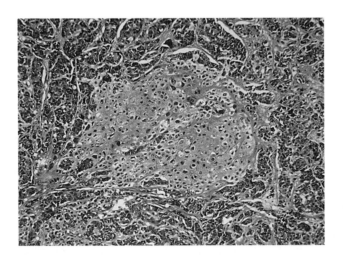

Figure 11–37. Metaplastic matrix-producing carcinoma. Islands of malignant cartilaginous tissue are seen within this high-grade infiltrating duct carcinoma. Note absence of a transition zone between malignant epithelium and chondroid matrix (Figs. 11–37 and 11–38). Matrix-producing carcinoma is a variant of metaplastic carcinoma that shows a direct transition between malignant epithelial cells and a cartilaginous or osseous stromal matrix without an intervening spindle cell zone[46]; tumors that show a transitional spindle cell sarcoma zone between malignant epithelium and matrix are termed carcinosarcomas.[47]

If all metaplastic carcinomas are grouped together, the reported disease-free and overall survival are decreased compared with typical mammary carcinoma, despite the fact that they metastasize to axillary lymph nodes less frequently.[48] If these tumors are separated by type of metaplasia, carcinosarcoma appears to be the only unfavorable prognostic type compared with infiltrating duct carcinoma (IDC NOS) or all other types of metaplastic carcinoma, including matrix-producing tumors.[47] A recent series of 32 matrix-producing carcinomas showed a better survival than IDC NOS when adjusted for stage.[49]

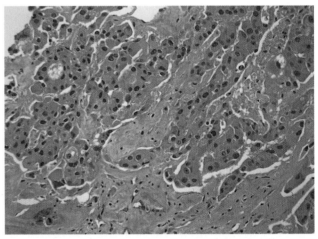

Figure 11–39. Infiltrating apocrine carcinoma. This tumor is composed of cords and nests of cells with abundant eosinophilic granular cytoplasm, reminiscent of apocrine metaplasia.[14] The apocrine variant of breast carcinoma constitutes up to 4% of all breast carcinomas in some series[50]; it is very similar in its manifestations and prognostic profile to infiltrating duct carcinoma not otherwise specified (IDC NOS),[51] and is not considered by many to be a special type of breast cancer. Apocrine carcinomas (as all other apocrine breast lesions) express androgen receptor and are negative for estrogen and progesterone receptors.[52] In addition, most apocrine lesions express gross cystic disease fluid protein-15.[53]

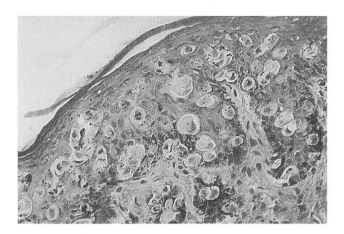

Figure 11–40. Paget's disease of the nipple. Although not a specific type of mammary carcinoma, Paget's disease of the nipple is important to recognize because it occasionally represents the first pathologic manifestation of an underlying intraductal or infiltrating duct carcinoma[54]; invasive cancer is found in over half of patients.[55] The underlying ductal carcinoma in situ is always of high grade.[56] The clinical manifestations include crusting and erosion of the nipple, pruritus, and bloody discharge. The lesion generally first presents to the pathologist as a skin biopsy of the involved nipple. The nipple epidermis is infiltrated by large, round to ovoid cells with a round malignant-appearing nucleus and voluminous clear cytoplasm. Mitotic figures may be seen in these cells. These large cells are generally separated by residual normal squamous cells of the epidermis, but they may focally or completely replace normal squamous cells and form large masses of malignant cells. The tumor cells are immunoreactive for cytokeratins and usually for carcinoembryonic antigen, and also are periodic acid–Schiff (PAS) positive before and after diastase digestion. The differential diagnosis is with in situ squamous carcinoma and melanoma. The finding of very high incidence (>90% of cases) of c-erbB-2 positivity in mammary Paget's disease could also be of potential help in the diagnosis.[57]

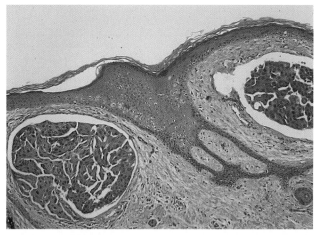

Figure 11–41. Inflammatory carcinoma. This tumor is not a special subtype of mammary carcinoma but rather a clinical presentation, characterized by erythema of the skin overlying the breast and *peau d'orange* changes; skin biopsy reveals tumor emboli in dermal lymphatics, and dilated lymphatic vessels. Women with this complication tend to be younger, and the tumor in these cases tends to be steroid receptor negative and c-erbB-2 positive.[58] Inflammatory carcinoma used to be almost uniformly lethal, but with the advent of neoadjuvant therapy 5-year survival ranges from 25% to 48%, still significantly worse than with noninflammatory carcinoma.

References

1. Pereira H, Pinder SE, Sibering DM, et al: Pathological prognostic factors in breast cancer. IV: Should you be a typer or a grader? A comparative study of two histological prognostic features in operable breast carcinoma. Histopathology 27:219–226, 1995.
2. Borst MJ, Ingold JA: Metastatic patterns of invasive lobular versus invasive ductal carcinoma of the breast. Surgery 114:637–642, 1993.
3. Winston CB, Hadar O, Teitcher JB, et al: Metastatic lobular carcinoma of the breast: Patterns of spread in the chest, abdomen, and pelvis on CT. AJR Am J Roentgenol 175:795–800, 2000.
4. Frost AR, Terahata S, Yeh IT, et al: The significance of signet ring cells in infiltrating lobular carcinoma of the breast. Arch Pathol Lab Med 119:64–68, 1995.
5. Martinez V, Azzopardi JG: Invasive lobular carcinoma of the breast: Incidence and variants. Histopathology 3:467–488, 1979.
6. Eusebi V, Magalhaes F, Azzopardi JG: Pleomorphic lobular carcinoma of the breast: An aggressive tumor showing apocrine differentiation. Hum Pathol 23:655–662, 1992.
7. Weidner N, Semple JP: Pleomorphic variant of the invasive lobular carcinoma of the breast. Hum Pathol 23:1167–1171, 1992.
8. Acs G, Lawton TJ, Rebbeck TR, et al: Differential expression of E-cadherin in lobular and ductal neoplasms of the breast and its biologic and diagnostic implications. Am J Clin Pathol 2001;115:85–98, 2001.
9. DiCostanzo D, Rosen PP, Gareen I, et al: Prognosis in infiltrating lobular carcinoma: An analysis of "classical" and variant tumors. Am J Surg Pathol 14:12–23, 1990.
10. Frost AR, Terahata S, Yeh IT, et al: An analysis of prognostic features in infiltrating lobular carcinoma of the breast. Mod Pathol 8:830–836, 1995.
11. Frost AR, Karcher DS, Terahata S, et al: DNA analysis and S-phase fraction determination by flow cytometric analysis of infiltrating lobular carcinoma of the breast. Mod Pathol 9:930–937, 1996.
12. Radhi JM: Immunohistochemical analysis of pleomorphic lobular carcinoma: Higher expression of p53 and chromogranin and lower expression of ER and PgR. Histopathology 36:156–160, 2000.
13. Bentz JS, Yassa N, Clayton F: Pleomorphic lobular carcinoma of the breast: Clinicopathologic features of 12 cases. Mod Pathol 11:814–822, 1998.
14. World Health Organization: Histological Typing of Breast Tumours, 2nd ed. (International Histological Classification of Tumours No. 2). Geneva, World Health Organization, 1981, p 19.
15. Rosen PP, Groshen S, Saigo PE, et al: A long-term follow-up study of survival in Stage I (T1N0M0) and Stage II (T1N1M0) breast carcinoma. J Clin Oncol 7:355–366, 1989.
16. Stalsberg H, Hartmann WH: The delimitation of tubular carcinoma of the breast. Hum Pathol 31:601–607, 2000.
17. Rosen PP: Microglandular adenosis. A benign lesion simulating invasive mammary carcinoma. Am J Surg Pathol 7:137–144, 1983.
18. Page DL, Dixon JM, Anderson TJ, et al: Invasive cribriform carcinoma of the breast. Histopathology 7:525–536, 1983.
19. Venable JG, Schwartz AM, Silverberg SG: Infiltrating cribriform carcinoma of the breast: A distinctive clinicopathologic entity. Hum Pathol 21:333–338, 1990.
20. Ridolfi RL, Rosen PP, Port A, et al: Medullary carcinoma of the

breast: A clinicopathologic study with 10 year follow-up. Cancer 40:1365–1385, 1977.

21. Wargotz ES, Silverberg SG: Medullary carcinoma of the breast. A clinicopathologic study with appraisal of current diagnostic criteria. Hum Pathol 19:1340–1346, 1988.

22. Pedersen L, Zedeler K, Holck S, et al: Medullary carcinoma of the breast. Prevalence and prognostic importance of classical risk factors in breast cancer. Eur J Cancer 31A:2289–2295, 1995.

23. Clayton F: Pure mucinous carcinomas of the breast: Morphologic features and prognostic correlates. Hum Pathol 17:34–38, 1986.

24. Hamele-Bena D, Cranor ML, Rosen PP: Mammary mucocele-like lesions. Benign and malignant. Am J Surg Pathol 20:1081–1085, 1996.

25. Weaver MG, Abdul-Karim FW, al-Kaisi N: Mucinous lesions of the breast. A pathological continuum. Pathol Res Pract 189:873–876, 1993.

26. Lefkowitz M, Lefkowitz W, Wargotz ES: Intraductal (intracystic) papillary carcinoma of the breast and its variants: A clinicopathological study of 77 cases. Hum Pathol 25:802–809, 1994.

27. Tresserra F, Grases PJ, Fabregas R, et al: Invasive micropapillary carcinoma. Distinct features of a poorly recognized variant of breast carcinoma. Eur J Gynaecol Oncol 20:205–208, 1990.

28. Paterakos M, Watkin WG, Edgerton SM, et al: Invasive micropapillary carcinoma of the breast: A prognostic study. Hum Pathol 30:1459–1463, 1999.

29. Middleton LP, Tresserra F, Sobel ME, et al: Infiltrating micropapillary carcinoma of the breast. Mod Pathol 12:499–504, 1999.

30. Rosen PP. Breast Pathology. Philadelphia, Lippincott-Raven, 1996, p 345.

31. Dickersin GR, Maluf HM, Koerner FC: Solid papillary carcinoma of breast: An ultrastructural study. Ultrastruct Pathol 21:153–161, 1997.

32. Maluf HM, Koerner FC: Solid papillary carcinoma of the breast. A form of intraductal carcinoma with endocrine differentiation frequently associated with mucinous carcinoma. Am J Surg Pathol 19:1237–1244, 1995.

33. Tavassoli FA, Norris HJ: Secretory carcinoma of the breast. Cancer 45:2404–2413, 1980.

34. Oberman HA: Secretory carcinoma of the breast in adults. Am J Surg Pathol 4:465–470, 1980.

35. Wrba F, Ellinger A, Reiner G, et al: Ultrastructural and immunohistochemical characteristics of lipid-rich carcinoma of the breast. Virchows Arch A Pathol Anat Histopathol 413:381–385, 1988.

36. Ramos CV, Taylor HB: Lipid-rich carcinoma of the breast. A clinicopathologic analysis of 13 examples. Cancer 33:812–819, 1974.

37. Hayes MM, Seidman JD, Ashton MA: Glycogen-rich clear cell carcinoma of the breast. A clinicopathologic study of 21 cases. Am J Surg Pathol 19:904–911, 1995.

38. Lamovec J, Us-Krasovec M, Zidar A, Kljun A: Adenoid cystic carcinoma of the breast: A histologic, cytologic, and immunohistochemical study. Semin Diagn Pathol 6:153–164, 1989.

39. Clement PB, Young RH, Azzopardi JG: Collagenous spherulosis of the breast. Am J Surg Pathol 11:411–417, 1987.

40. Trendell-Smith NJ, Peston D, Shousha S: Adenoid cystic carcinoma of the breast: A tumour commonly devoid of oestrogen receptors and related proteins. Histopathology 35:241–248, 1999.

41. Kleer CG, Oberman HA: Adenoid cystic carcinoma of the breast: Value of histologic grading and proliferative activity. Am J Surg Pathol 22:569–575, 1998.

42. Wargotz ES, Norris HJ: Metaplastic carcinoma of the breast. IV: Squamous carcinoma of ductal origin. Cancer 65:272–276, 1990.

43. Rosen PP: Breast Pathology. Philadelphia, Lippincott-Raven, 1996, p 397.

44. Gobbi H, Simpson JF, Borowsky A, et al: Metaplastic breast tumors with a dominant fibromatosis-like phenotype have a high risk of local recurrence. Cancer 85:2170–2182, 1999.

45. Wargotz ES, Deos PH, Norris HJ: Metaplastic carcinomas of the breast. II: Spindle cell carcinoma. Hum Pathol 20:732–740, 1989.

46. Wargotz ES, Norris HJ: Metaplastic carcinomas of the breast. I: Matrix-producing carcinoma. Hum Pathol 20:628–636, 1989.

47. Wargotz ES, Norris HJ: Metaplastic carcinomas of the breast. III: Carcinosarcoma. Cancer 64:1490–1499, 1989.

48. Rayson D, Adjei AA, Suman VJ, et al: Metaplastic breast cancer: Prognosis and response to systemic therapy. Ann Oncol 10:413–419, 1999.

49. Chhieng C, Cranor M, Lesser ME, Rosen PP: Metaplastic carcinoma of the breast with osteocartilaginous heterologous elements. Am J Surg Pathol 22:188–194, 1998.

50. Eusebi V, Millis RR, Cattani MG, et al: Apocrine carcinoma of the breast. A morphologic and immunocytochemical study. Am J Pathol 123(3):532–541, 1986.

51. Abati AD, Kimmel M, Rosen PP: Apocrine mammary carcinoma. A clinicopathologic study of 72 cases. Am J Clin Pathol 94:371–377, 1990.

52. Gatalica Z: Immunohistochemical analysis of apocrine breast lesions. Consistent over-expression of androgen receptor accompanied by the loss of estrogen and progesterone receptors in apocrine metaplasia and apocrine carcinoma in situ. Pathol Res Pract 193:753–758, 1997.

53. Pagani A, Sapino A, Eusebi V, et al: PIP/GCDFP-15 gene expression and apocrine differentiation in carcinomas of the breast. Virchows Arch 425:459–465, 1994.

54. Chaudary MA, Millis RR, Lane EB, Miller NA: Paget's disease of the nipple: A ten year review including clinical, pathological, and immunohistochemical findings. Breast Cancer Res Treat 8:139–146, 1986.

55. Kollmorgen DR, Varanasi JS, Edge SB, et al: Paget's disease of the breast: A 33-year experience. J Am Coll Surg 187:171–177, 1998.

56. Bobrow LG, Happerfield LC, Gregory WM, et al: The classification of ductal carcinoma in situ and its association with biological markers. Semin Diagn Pathol 11:199–207, 1994.

57. Hitchcock A, Topham S, Bell J, et al: Routine diagnosis of mammary Paget's disease. A modern approach. Am J Surg Pathol 16:58–61, 1992.

58. Charpin C, Bounier P, Khouzami A, et al: Inflammatory breast carcinoma: An immunohistochemical study using monoclonal anti-pHER-2/neu, pS2, cathepsin, ER and PR. Anticancer Res 12:591–598, 1992.

59. Kurian KM, Al-Nafussi A: Sarcomatoid/metaplastic carcinoma of the breast: a clinicopathological study of 12 cases. Histopathology 40:58–64, 2002.

CHAPTER 12

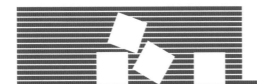

Stromal and Vascular Tumors

Syed A. Hoda

INTRODUCTION

The stroma of the breast comprises blood vessels, fibroblasts, myofibroblasts, smooth muscle, peripheral nerves and, last but certainly not the least, adipose tissue. As can be expected from such a heterogeneous group, the spectrum of non-neoplastic and neoplastic lesions arising from these tissues is remarkably varied. However, in terms of incidence, malignances of epithelial origin vastly outnumber those of stromal origin, the latter comprising <1% of all breast cancers.[1]

Most stromal and vascular tumors, regardless of intra- or extramammary origin, are strikingly similar with respect to clinical and pathologic features, for example, an intramammary lipoma requires the same diagnostic criteria as an extramammary lipoma, that is, a capsule and a monotonous population of mature adipocytes. There are, of course, several noteworthy pathologic differences in stromal and vascular tumors arising in the breast, for example, pseudoangiomatous stromal hyperplasia is an entity virtually unique to the breast[2] and hemangiopericytoma of the breast generally behaves in a less malignant fashion in the breast than elsewhere.[3]

A complete list of all possible stromal and vascular tumors of the breast would be virtually endless: alveolar soft part sarcoma, amyloidoma, epithelioid leiomyoma, malignant fibrous histiocytoma, mesenchymoma (including malignant variants), mucinosis, myxomatosis, osteosarcoma, pleomorphic adenoma, etc. Many of the aforementioned lesions are exceptionally unusual in the breast. Several reports of these rarer forms of sarcoma predate immunohistochemistry and do not describe electron microscopic findings. It is also likely that reports of at least some rarer forms of mammary sarcoma, including liposarcoma, chondrosarcoma, and rhabdomyosarcoma, may represent relative overgrowth of a particular component in a malignant cystosarcoma phyllodes.

Some uncommon stromal tumors, including carcinosarcoma and stromal sarcoma, have generated controversy (quite out of proportion to their incidence). Most, but not all, authorities would concede that carcinosarcoma en-compasses two tumor categories: carcinomas arising in cystosarcoma phyllodes, and biphasic malignant tumors that do not originate in cystosarcoma phyllodes. Stromal sarcoma is a loose diagnostic term that has been used to include (1) all sarcomas that do not qualify as cystosarcoma or angiosarcoma[4] and (2) sarcomas arising from hormonally responsive periductal and perilobular specialized stroma.[5]

An excisional biopsy usually suffices for most benign stromal and vascular tumors of the breast. Mastectomy is the usual treatment for most forms of mammary sarcomas. Routine axillary dissection is not indicated because nodal metastases are uncommon. Breast conservation may be appropriate for low-grade sarcomas or for smaller sarcomas. The role of radiation therapy and chemotherapy in the management of mammary sarcoma remains largely controversial.[6] As an early event, recurrences are primarily local, and metastases to the lung are a later event in the course of most breast sarcomas.[1] The role of the pathologist in assessing the prognosis of mammary mesenchymal tumors is paramount, and it is important that pathologists interact with clinicians in the appropriate planning of the management of these mammary tumors.

In this chapter, the essential pathologic characteristics of 12 of the most common stromal and vascular neoplasms (including 2 non-neoplastic "tumoral" lesions) are illustrated. In addition, two types of tumors, metaplastic and metastatic, are discussed, both of which are in the differential diagnosis of spindle cell lesions of the breast. Neither myoepithelial neoplasms (which are not truly stromal in origin) nor Stewart-Treves syndrome (which is not truly a mammary neoplasm, but one of the ipsilateral lymphedematous upper limb arising postmastectomy) are discussed here. Fibroepithelial neoplasms (including cystosarcoma phyllodes) are discussed elsewhere. Readers wishing to delve into the clinical, pathologic, nosologic (and other controversial) intricacies of rarer forms of stromal and vascular tumors may wish to peruse some of the excellent reviews of the topic.[7, 8]

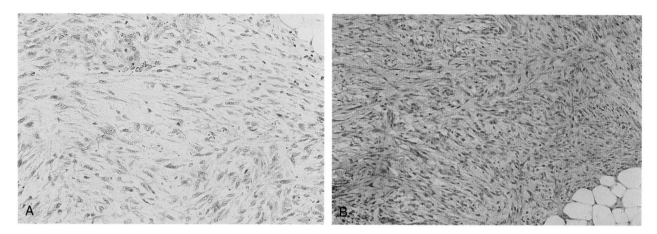

Figure 12–1. Nodular fasciitis. This form of "pseudosarcomatous" fasciitis is a rapidly developing myofibroblastomatous lesion of soft tissue that is often mistaken for a spindle cell sarcoma. Nodular fasciitis may occur in the superficial or the deep soft tissues of the breast. The histologic features of mammary nodular fasciitis include spindle cell myofibroblastic proliferation and abundant mitotic activity *(A)*, which are similar to those observed in extramammary nodular fasciitis. The lesion may be associated with trauma and consequent fat necrosis. Smooth muscle actin *(B)*, but not cytokeratin, is expressed by the proliferating myofibroblasts.

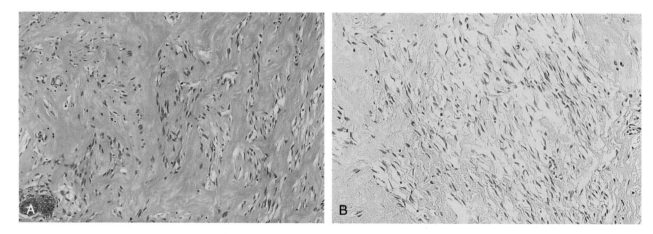

Figure 12–2. Pseudoangiomatous stromal hyperplasia (PASH). This is a "tumoral" lesion formed by myofibroblasts with variable expression of myoid and fibroblastic features.[2] PASH is characterized by anastomosing slitlike spaces, lined by myofibroblasts, in dense collagenous stroma *(A)*. Unlike angiosarcoma, PASH displays neither cytologic atypia nor mitotic activity. The pseudoangiomatous appearance may be absent in the relatively more cellular areas of the lesion *(B)*. Although PASH is usually an incidental focal finding associated with either a benign or malignant breast biopsy, it may rarely present as a well demarcated, firm lesion with a smooth contour. Immunohistochemically, the myofibroblasts are reactive with CD34, but nonreactive with CD31, factor VIII, and *Ulex.* It may be appropriate to think of myofibroblastoma and PASH as related myofibroblastic lesions—the more cellular of the two being designated as myofibroblastoma. The predilection of PASH for premenopausal women, massive increase of PASH lesions during pregnancy, positivity for progesterone receptors, and negativity for estrogen receptors are all indicative of a hormonal relationship.

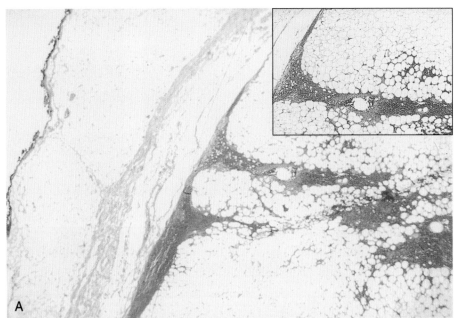

Figure 12–3. Lipoma and angiolipoma. Lipoma is a ubiquitous benign neoplasm of mature adipose tissue and is uncommonly recognized in the breast—often blending imperceptibly with mammary stromal adipose tissue, on gross as well as microscopic examination. When recognized, the tumor is well demarcated, soft, and mobile. Cut section shows a lobulated, tan mass. Breast glandular elements are not present within the lesion. The presence of a soft tissue density on mammography may prompt a biopsy following a needle localization procedure (with accompanying hemorrhage along the needle tract, seen in *A* [and *inset*]).

More commonly identified than a lipoma is angiolipoma, characterized by the presence of branching capillary channels that are particularly prominent in the periphery of the lesion. Minute intraluminal fibrin thrombi are present within these capillary channels *(B)*. Mammary angiolipomas may not be painful in contradistinction to angiolipomas occurring at other sites, and may occasionally be "cellular."[9]

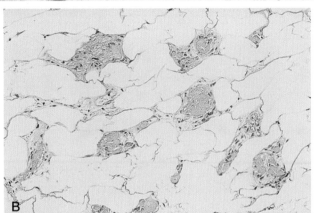

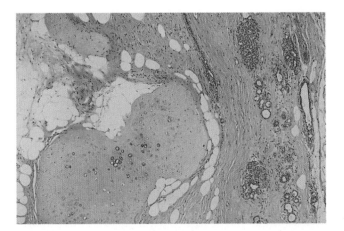

Figure 12–4. Chondrolipoma. Chondrolipoma presents as a palpable, discrete mass composed of mature adipocytes with admixed islands of mature hyaline cartilage.[10] Benign cartilaginous elements may be observed in a variety of other stromal lesions of the breast, including pleomorphic adenoma. It ought to be remembered that cartilaginous elements, even those that appear histologically benign, are also a common metaplastic element in mammary carcinoma.

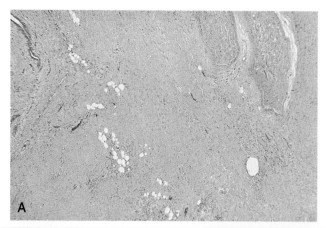

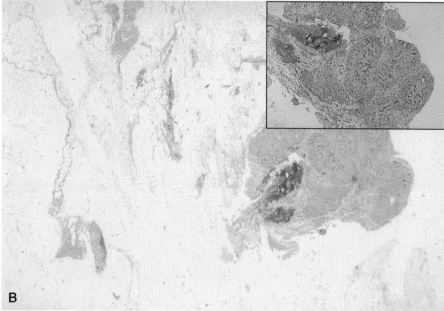

Figure 12–5. Neurofibroma and schwannoma. Neurofibroma *(A)* and schwannoma *(B,* detail in inset) are rare in the breast, and malignant peripheral nerve sheath tumors are even rarer. These lesions are grossly and microscopically similar to those occurring elsewhere in the body.[11] Von Recklinghausen's disease is associated with approximately one third of peripheral nerve sheath tumors in the breast, wherein multiple neurofibromas are evident not only in the mammary skin but also in the breast parenchyma.

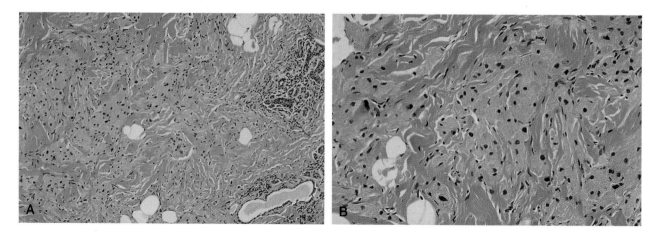

Figure 12–6. Granular cell tumor. Granular cell tumor (the erstwhile myoblastoma) may be seen in a wide variety of sites, but the female breast is one of its more common locations. Intramammary granular cell tumor may be mistaken clinically, radiographically, and even on gross appearance for an invasive carcinoma. The tumor is firm and has a deceptively infiltrating gross appearance. Microscopically, uniform polygonal cells bearing coarse granules and centrally placed innocuous nuclei are seen *(A, B).* Immunoreactivity with S-100 protein is confirmatory. The rare metastatic granular cell tumor may not be histologically exceptional.[12]

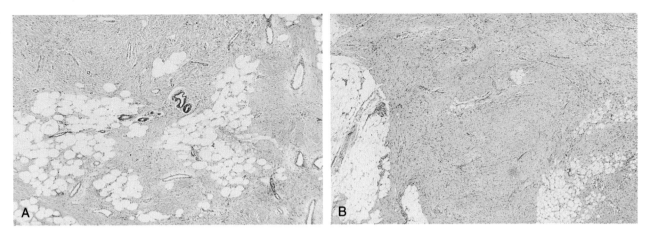

Figure 12–7. Fibromatosis. Fibromatosis (desmoid tumor) is an uncommon locally aggressive lesion of the mammary stroma.[13] Unlike abdominal fibromatosis, mammary fibromatosis is not associated with pregnancy. Mammary fibromatosis generally arises de novo, but it may follow augmentation procedures.[14] The tumor presents as a palpable, firm, ill defined mass with infiltrative edges on cut section. The overlying skin or the nipple may be retracted. Microscopically, the lesion is composed of spindle cells and collagen. The spindle cells are rather uniformly slender with bland cytologic features, and they are arranged in fascicles that circumvent the native glandular elements of the breast *(A)*. Cellularity is generally uniform within a particular lesion *(B)*, but it may be variable. Mitoses are present but scanty (<3 per 10 high-power fields). Wide local excision, with negative margins, is usually curative, but mastectomy may be indicated for larger or recurrent lesions.[15] Fibrosarcoma is relatively more cellular, more mitotically active, and composed of pleomorphic cells that typically form a "herringbone" pattern.

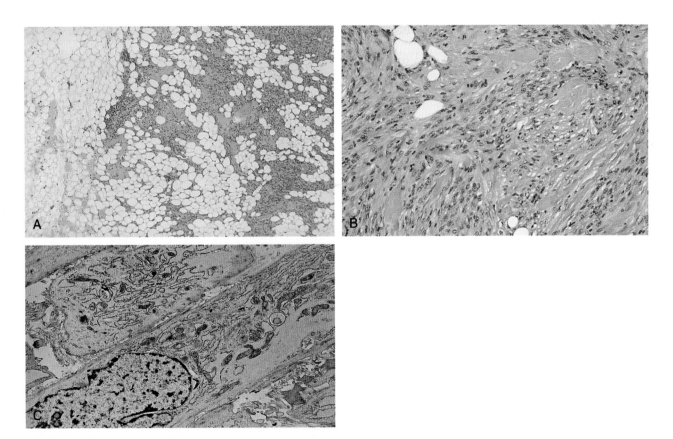

Figure 12–8. Myofibroblastoma. Myofibroblasts are ubiquitous stromal cells that defy precise characterization because of their uncertain position in the morphologic and functional spectrum between fibroblasts and smooth muscle cells.[16] Morphologically, myofibroblasts are characterized by spindle-shaped cells with ill defined cytoplasm and nuclei that are tapered at both poles and possess minute nucleoli. Immunohistochemically, myofibroblasts are generally positive for vimentin, smooth muscle actin, and CD 34 and they are negative for desmin, laminin, and collagen type IV.

Myofibroblastoma is usually a benign entity that is seen commonly, but by no means exclusively, in the male breast. The lesion is rare and presents as a discrete, firm, mobile mass. The tumor is composed of spindle cells and may, or may not *(A)*, have a circumscribed edge. The spindle cells are arranged in fascicles within relatively broad bands of dense collagenized stroma *(B)*. These spindle cells have ovoid nuclei and relatively pale cytoplasm. Ultrastructurally *(C)*, the lesional cells show prominent branching rough endoplasmic reticulum (seen best in the right half of *C*) and subplasmalemmal arrays of actin microfilaments with interspersed fusiform densities (seen best in the center of *C*), all characteristic of myofibroblastic differentiation. A few cases of the malignant counterpart of myofibroblastic tumor have been reported.[16]

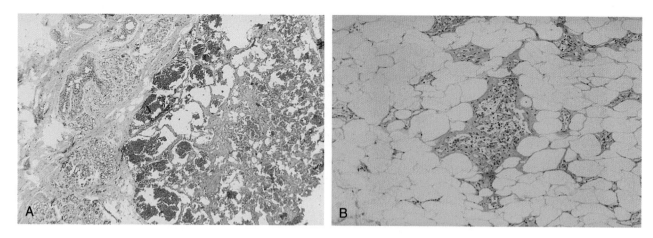

Figure 12–9. Hemangioma and its variants. A wide variety of hemangiomatous lesions occur within the mammary stroma.[17] An aggregate of histologically unremarkable capillaries in the periductal or perilobular region, evident only on microscopy, is generally referred to as a hemangioma but is of no clinical importance. Palpable hemangiomas are stromal lesions that are generally located around, but not necessarily within, breast glandular parenchyma. These are generally of the cavernous type and are well circumscribed. The vascular channels are lined by bland endothelial cells that completely lack cytologic atypia, pleomorphism, and mitotic activity (A; Table 12–1). "Atypical" hemangiomas encompass a group of extremely uncommon benign vascular lesions that are <2 cm in greatest dimension and are characterized by relative circumscription, anastomosing channels, and endothelial proliferation (B). In the only series of such cases reported to date,[18] more than half of these lesions were detected mammographically.

Table 12–1

HEMANGIOMA VS. LOW-GRADE ANGIOSARCOMA

Pathologic Feature	Hemangioma	Low-Grade Angiosarcoma
*"Critical diagnosis requires experience transcending tabular guidelines."**		
Size	Usually <2 cm	Usually >2 cm
Margins	Circumscribed	Ill-defined
Architecture	Lobulated	Lacks lobulation
Vascular channels	Generally unconnected	Interanastomosing†

*From McDivitt RW, Stewart FW, Berg JW: Tumors of the breast. In Atlas of Tumor Pathology, 2nd series. Washington, DC, Armed Forces Institute of Pathology, 1967, p 28.

† Rule 1: Freely anastomosing vascular channels are the histologic hallmark of angiosarcoma, and are apparent in even better differentiated areas. Rule 2: There are exceptions to every rule!

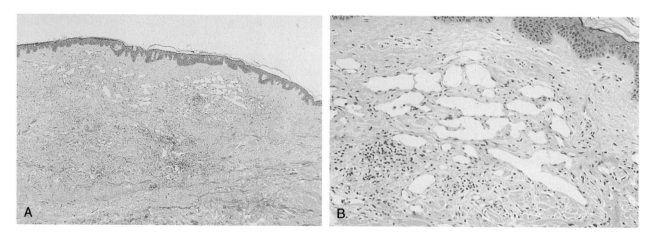

Figure 12–10. Postradiation "atypical" vascular lesions. A variety of sarcomas following radiation therapy to the breast have been reported.[19, 20] However, the category of atypical vascular lesions (AVL) that occur after radiation therapy has been described only recently.[21] Most AVLs measure about 5 mm and are located in the dermis. Histologic examination shows enlarged vascular channels that are lined by cytologically atypical (but not frankly malignant) endothelial cells (Table 12–2). There is usually no accompanying hemorrhage. A few lymphocytes may be present in the stroma in the immediate vicinity of the lesion. Based on currently available data, AVL does not seem to progress to angiosarcoma.

Table 12–2

POSTRADIATION ATYPICAL VASCULAR LESION (AVL)
VS. LOW-GRADE ANGIOSARCOMA (LGA)

Pathologic Feature	AVL	LGA
Subcutaneous involvement	−	+
Papillary endothelial hyperplasia	−	+
Prominent nucleoli	−	+
Mitoses	−	+
Cytologic atypia	−	+
"Blood lakes" (Fig. 12–11*D*)	−	+
Circumscription	+	−
Stromal projection into lumen	+	−
Dissection of dermal collagen	+	+
Endothelial hyperchromasia	+	+
Lymphocytic infiltrate	+	+

Modified from Fineberg S, Rosen PP: Cutaneous angiosarcoma and atypical vascular lesions of the skin and breast after radiation therapy for breast carcinoma. Am J Clin Pathol 102:757–763, 1994.

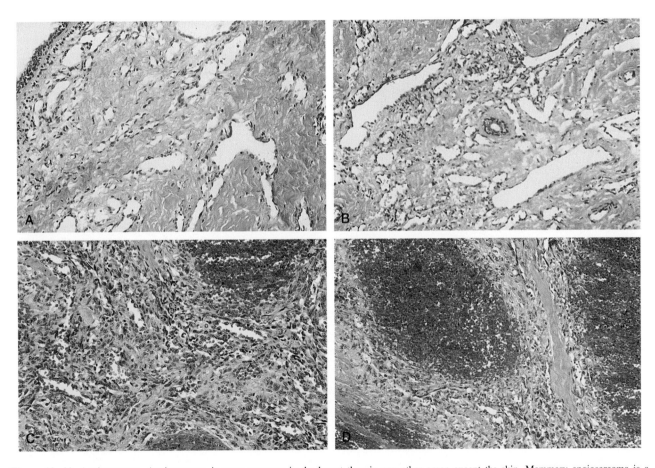

Figure 12–11. Angiosarcoma. Angiosarcoma is more common in the breast than in any other organ except the skin. Mammary angiosarcoma is a heterogeneous group of lesions in which prognosis is dictated by pathologic grading.[22] Angiosarcomas may be associated with prior radiation therapy, arise in the lymphedematous arm following ipsilateral mastectomy, or arise de novo. The latter group of tumors are variable in size, grossly heterogeneous, and have friable, spongy, or frankly hemorrhagic areas. For the diagnosis of mammary angiosarcoma to be clinically meaningful, the lesion is best classified into histologic grades (Table 12–3). It is imperative that the entire lesion be sampled thoroughly before the lesion is graded, as there may be wide histologic variations of pattern. Low-grade angiosarcoma *(A, B)* is by no means a negligible tumor, notwithstanding its subtle histologic features,[23] and these tumors may develop local and systemic recurrences. Angiosarcoma may arise at any age; however, higher grade tumors *(C, D)* generally occur in the fourth decade of life. Recurrent angiosarcomas may be of a higher grade than the original tumor.

Table 12–3

GRADING OF MAMMARY ANGIOSARCOMA

Type	Differentiation	Pathologic Features
Type I	Well (Fig. 12–11A, B)	Interanastomosing vascular channels Endothelial cells inconspicuous Occasional endothelial "tufting"

Type II	Moderate	Lesion composed of type I angiosarcoma with
		  scattered capillary endothelial proliferation
		  scattered solid areas, occasional mitoses

Type III	Poor (Fig. 12–11C, D)	Lesion with or without features of Type I/II angiosarcoma with sarcomatous areas and necrosis

Modified from Donnell RM, Rosen PP, Lieberman PH, et al: Angiosarcoma and other vascular tumors of the breast. Pathologic analysis as a guide to prognosis. Am J Surg Pathol 5:629–642, 1981.

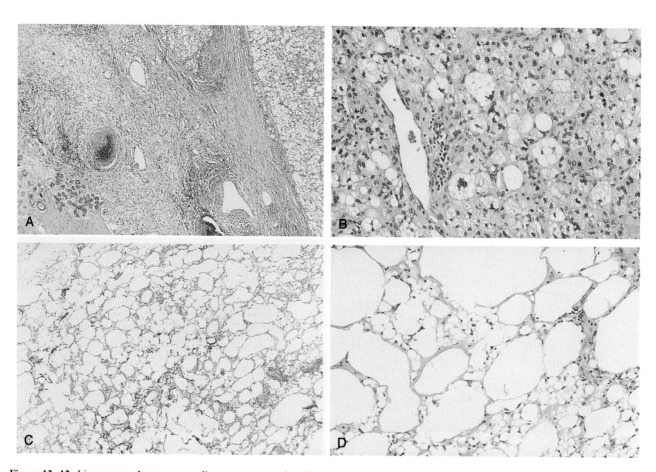

Figure 12–12. Liposarcoma. Intramammary liposarcoma may arise either de novo or from a cystosarcoma phyllodes. The gross features are variable (circumscribed or infiltrative), and the histologic features are similar to the types arising elsewhere in the body (myxoid, well differentiated, pleomorphic, etc). The finding of characteristic lipoblasts is essential for the diagnosis (A, B). So-called silicone mastitis may superficially resemble liposarcoma. The latter is caused by either liquid silicone or leakage from prosthetic devices (see Chapter 13). A diffuse granulomatous reaction to silicone is present, admixed with fat necrosis and clear vacuolated spaces of varying sizes (C, D). The clear spaces represent dissolution of foreign material in tissue processing.

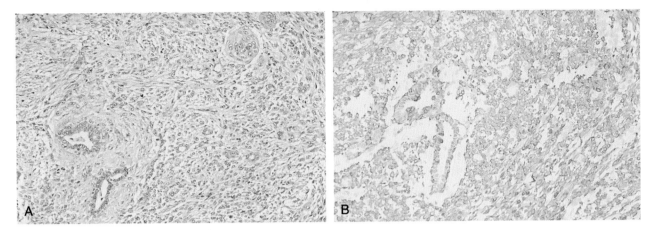

Figure 12–13. Metaplastic carcinoma. Metaplastic tumors ought to be considered in the differential diagnosis of mesenchymal neoplasms of the breast. In general, there are basically two types of metaplastic tumors: (1) infiltrating duct carcinoma that develops areas of spindle cell (squamoid) differentiation and (2) matrix-producing carcinoma in which there is a direct transition from gland-forming carcinoma to a matrix of either cartilaginous or osseous stroma. Some metaplastic carcinomas are exceedingly spindly (A), and they may be immunoreactive with only high-molecular-weight cytokeratin 903 (B).

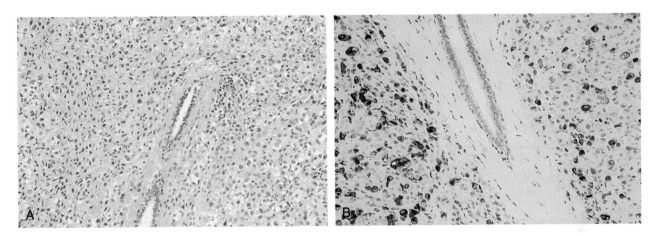

Figure 12–14. Metastatic tumors. Before the diagnosis of primary mammary sarcoma is rendered, metastatic sarcoma should be excluded. It is important to remember that immunohistochemical reactivity may be misleading as some sarcomas may exhibit cytokeratin positivity, and clinical correlation is always necessary. Metastatic melanoma is the great masquerader in breast pathology, and it may be confused with primary or metastatic sarcoma (A). It is notable that some breast carcinomas are S-100 protein positive, and hence an HMB-45 stain is of added value in melanoma (B). Even positivity with the latter may still not be diagnostic of melanoma.[24] Clinical and histologic correlation is always prudent.

References

1. Moore MP, Kinne DW: Breast sarcoma. Surg Clin North Am 76: 383–392, 1996.
2. Powell CM, Cranor ML, Rosen PP: Pseudoangiomatous stromal hyperplasia (PASH). A mammary stromal tumor with myofibroblastic differentiation. Am J Surg Pathol 19:270–277, 1995.
3. Arias-Stella J Jr, Rosen PP: Hemiangiopericytoma of the breast. Mod Pathol 2:98–103, 1988.
4. Berg JW, DeCosse JJ, Fracchia AA: Stromal sarcoma of the breast. Cancer 13:418–424, 1962.
5. Callery CD, Rosen PP, Kinne DW: Sarcoma of the breast. A study of 32 patients with reappraisal of classification and therapy. Ann Surg 201:527–541, 1985.
6. Gutman H, Pollock RE, Ross MI, et al: Sarcoma of the breast: Implications for extent of therapy. The MD Anderson experience. Surgery 116:505–509, 1994.
7. Rosen PP: Sarcoma. In Rosen's Breast Pathology, 2nd ed. Philadelphia, Lippincott-Raven, 2001, pp 813–864.
8. Tavassoli F: Mesenchymal lesions. In *Pathology of the Breast*, 2nd ed. Norwalk, CT: Appleton Lange, 1999, pp 675–731.
9. Yu GH, Fishman SJ, Brooks JSJ: Cellular angiolipoma of the breast. Mod Pathol 6:497–499, 1993.
10. Lugo M, Reyes JM, Putony PB: Benign chondrolipomatous tumors of the human female breast. Arch Pathol Lab Med 101:149–151, 1977.
11. Gultekin SH, Hoda SA, Cody HS: Schwannoma of the breast. South Med J 89:288–289, 1996.

12. Uzoaru I, Firfer B, Ray V, et al: Malignant granular cell tumor. Arch Pathol Lab Med 116:206–208, 1992.
13. Rosen PP, Ernsberger D: Mammary fibromatosis. A benign spindle-cell tumor with significant risk for local recurrence. Cancer 63:1363–1369, 1989.
14. Aaron AD, O'Mara JW, Legendre KE, et al: Chest wall fibromatosis associated with silicone breast implants. Surg Oncol 5:93–99, 1996.
15. Ng WH, Lee JS, Poh WT, Wong CY: Desmoid tumor (fibromatosis) of the breast. A clinician's dilemma—a case report and review. Arch Surg 132:444–446, 1997.
16. Taccagni G, Rovere E, Masullo M, et al: Myofibrosarcoma of the breast. Review of the literature on myofibroblastic tumors and criteria for defining myofibroblastic differentiation. Am J Surg Pathol 21:489–496, 1997.
17. Chen KTK: Rare variants of benign vascular tumors of the breast. Surg Pathol 4:309–316, 1991.
18. Hoda SA, Cranor ML, Rosen PP: Atypical hemangiomas of the breast. Am J Surg Pathol 16:553–560, 1992.
19. Pendlebury SC, Bilous M, Langlands AO: Sarcomas following radiation therapy for breast cancer: A report of three cases and a review of the literature. Int J Radiat Oncol Biol Phys 31:405–410, 1995.
20. Parham DM, Fisher C: Angiosarcomas of the breast developing post radiotherapy. Histopathology 31:189–195, 1997.
21. Fineberg S, Rosen PP: Cutaneous angiosarcoma and atypical vascular lesions of the skin and breast after radiation therapy for breast carcinoma. Am J Clin Pathol 102:757–763, 1994.
22. Donnell RM, Rosen PP, Lieberman PH, et al: Angiosarcoma and other vascular tumors of the breast. Pathologic analysis as a guide to prognosis. Am J Surg Pathol 5:629–642, 1981.
23. Britt LD, Lambert P, Sharma R, Ladaga LE: Angiosarcoma of the breast. Initial misdiagnosis is still common. Arch Surg 130:221–223, 1995.
24. Bonetti F, Colombari R, Manfrin E, et al: Breast carcinoma with positive results for melanoma marker (HMB-45). Am J Clin Pathol 92:491–495, 1989.

CHAPTER 13

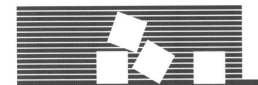

Iatrogenic Lesions of the Breast

Nancy S. Hardt

INTRODUCTION

Iatrogenic lesions of the breast, those that result from health care providers' diagnostic and therapeutic interventions, constitute a colorful and intriguing area of breast pathology. The changes are observable at the gross, sub-gross, and histologic levels. Diagnostic procedures including needle biopsy and excisional biopsy create characteristic changes that may challenge subsequent interpretation of mastectomy specimens. Injected materials (adventitious pigment, paraffin, silicone) and implanted biomaterials are commonly encountered. Recently, the removal of breast prostheses has created demand for identification of the manufacturer of such devices.

LESIONS RESULTING FROM DIAGNOSTIC OR THERAPEUTIC INTERVENTIONS

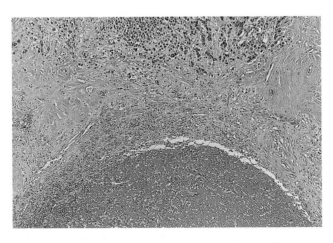

Figure 13–1. Trauma following needle biopsy. After needle biopsy, various tissue reactions may be seen, ranging from the tidy circumscribed hematoma (as shown in this figure) to chronic inflammation characterized by histiocytes in a fibrotic matrix. When biopsy-related fibrosis occurs in a background of benign epithelial changes, stromal desmoplasia associated with tumor may be in the differential diagnosis.

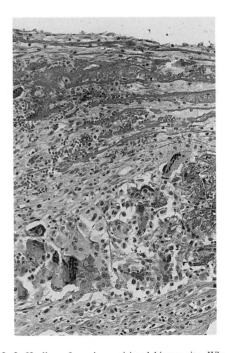

Figure 13–2. Healing of a prior excisional biopsy site. When mastectomy occurs after excisional biopsy, depending on the interval between biopsy and surgery, a variety of healing changes may be observed in the breast. In this figure the surgical cavity is lined by granulation tissue, and just deep to the granulation tissue, giant cells or multinucleated histiocytes are present. Contrast this appearance with the multinucleated histiocytes containing foreign material shown subsequently in the figures on breast prostheses.

163

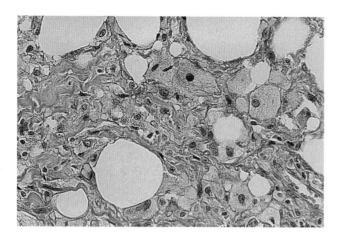

Figure 13–3. Fat necrosis. Fat necrosis may occur in the breast of any post-traumatic or postoperative patient. Note the very fine granularity of the histiocytes, and the contrasting large size of the "empty" vacuoles. Contrast this appearance to histiocytes containing foreign material related to breast implants in the figures shown subsequently.

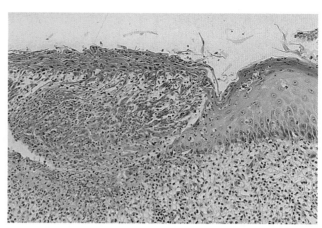

Figure 13–5. Histologic section of healing after laser therapy. Laser therapy to the skin produces sloughing of the epidermis and superficial dermis. Re-epithelialization occurs from the edges and from the deep dermal skin appendages. In this 33-year-old woman who had a breast tattoo removed with laser therapy, biopsy of the healing area revealed necrosis of the epidermis and superficial dermis with early re-epithelialization and numerous polymorphonuclear leukocytes, raising the question of secondary infection of the superficial wound.

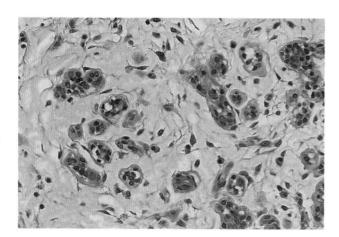

Figure 13–4. Epithelial and stromal changes following radiation therapy and chemotherapy. Radiation therapy or chemotherapy may be followed by breast biopsy or mastectomy. It is important to distinguish between epithelial changes resulting from therapy and tumor. After radiation therapy, fibrosis of the mammary stroma may result in the trapping of epithelial elements in the lobule in a benign process called "pseudoinfiltration." On low power the lobule is usually recognizable. If one uses high power to look carefully at the nuclei, occasional enlarged and hyperchromatic nuclei may be seen, sometimes projecting into the lumen of the duct. These cells are usually present in small numbers, with the rest of the duct retaining polarity and cohesion, and they are interpreted as benign. The figure is from a 38-year-old woman who underwent radiation therapy for poorly differentiated carcinoma with a palpable axillary component. The mass continued to enlarge during radiation therapy, and surgical excision was performed. In addition to necrotic tumor in the axilla, changes noted in the accompanying breast parenchyma were attributed to the radiation therapy.

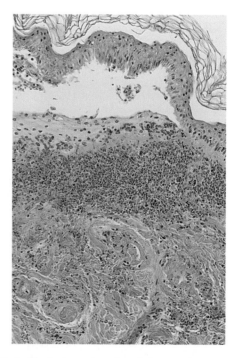

Figure 13–6. Histologic section of warfarin necrosis. Three to 4 days after the initiation of warfarin therapy, some patients develop blisters and blackening of the skin associated with necrosis, requiring resection. For unknown reasons, the breast is a frequent site for necrosis. Histologic hallmarks of warfarin necrosis include thrombosis of small veins and inflammation surrounding and traversing vessel walls. The etiology of the necrosis is uncertain, but some postulate that a temporary hypercoagulable state occasionally occurs after the onset of therapy and before anticoagulation is adequate.

LESIONS RESULTING FROM INJECTION

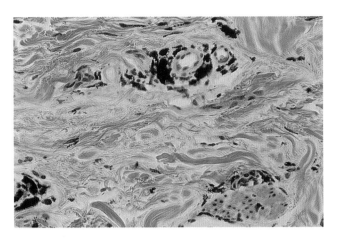

Figure 13–7. Tattoo. The breast is a favored site for tattoos in women. Tattoos are the result of injection of "adventitious pigment" consisting of granules of varying size that localize to the superficial dermis. The granules are most often found around blood vessels or interspersed among collagen bundles in the dermis. Accompanying the pigment, there is frequently a perivascular infiltrate consisting of lymphocytes and histiocytes. The granules are usually intracellular, but may occasionally be too big to be accommodated by a single histiocyte.

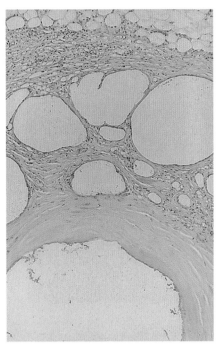

Figure 13–8. Histologic section of paraffin injection. Since early last century, well before breast implants were available, paraffin injection was performed for augmentation of the breast. Most often available in Asia, the materials injected were not of pharmaceutical grade and were not controlled. Paraffin was selected because it was thought that it would remain liquid at body temperature. The paraffin was mixed with various oils or petroleum jelly to make it easier to inject. This practice is known to have continued until shortly after World War II.

After paraffin injection, the foreign material elicited a brisk granulomatous response, resulting almost invariably in an unacceptably firm breast with an uneven cobblestone texture. Some women developed draining sinuses. Most of these women underwent subcutaneous mastectomy and reconstruction. Resected tissue was remarkable for dense fibrosis in spheres and surrounding empty spaces. Any remaining paraffin was removed in the deparaffinization step of tissue processing, leaving only the resulting granulomas and dystrophic calcification.

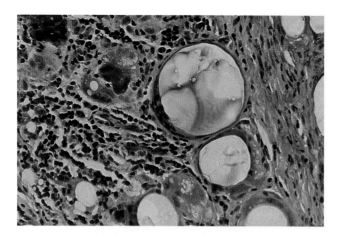

Figure 13–9. Photomicrograph of silicone fluid injection. Injected medical-grade silicone fluid was used for breast augmentation during the 1950s and 1960s. Currently, silicone fluid injection is not Food and Drug Administration approved; consequently, patients in the United States desiring this procedure travel to Mexico and Asia. In addition, silicone fluid has been injected, sometimes intentionally and sometimes inadvertently, into skeletal muscle. As with paraffin, granulomas result and the firm masses and associated fibrosis result in a less than optimal cosmetic result. Liquid silicone may track along anatomic planes of least resistance when pressure is applied. Occasionally, therefore, soft tissue deposits of silicone are found in sites outside the breast. Histologically, silicone granulomas have varying degrees of concentric fibrosis with central multinucleated giant cells surrounding refractile water-clear foreign material with a tendency to remain in rims of the vacuoles or strands in the tissue resected. Some of the silicone is removed during tissue processing.

In this figure, note the difference between fat necrosis, the paraffin granuloma, the nonspecific giant cell response to tissue cavitation in the postbiopsy changes shown in the previous figures, and a silicone granuloma. All have histiocytes and concentric fibrosis, but there the similarities end. The multinucleated giant cells in wound healing have limited quantities of cytoplasm unless suture material is present, whereas the macrophages are simple foamy macrophages. The silicone-related processes have unique-appearing macrophages whose multiple vacuoles vary in size. Some vacuoles contain rims of refractile foreign material. Multinucleated giant cells surround larger droplets of silicone, and stranding of the water-clear foreign material may be observed in the cytoplasm of these aggregates.

TISSUE REACTIONS RESULTING FROM PROSTHESES

As shown in Table 13–1, several manufacturers account for the vast majority of breast prostheses observed in the course of surgical pathology practice at the University of Florida. Each manufacturer chose its own style of implant to produce, and in some cases, styles evolved over the years. This evolution has resulted in a wide variety of implants that may be encountered in the laboratory as a consequence of surgical explantation.

Note that there are many reasons for breast prosthesis removal, including staged reconstruction, revision for unsatisfactory cosmetic result, suspicion of rupture, or the presence of local or systemic symptoms. Implants in place for >8 years are more likely to rupture than those implanted for a lesser amount of time. Further, textured implants were not manufactured until rather recently; therefore, many of those represented in this database are of shorter duration of implantation than the smooth implants.

Silicone gel breast prostheses were introduced in 1963 after the silicone gel was placed in a shell also composed of silicone elastomer. The rubbery elastomer is a more highly cross-linked silicone polymer preparation than the gel and silicone liquid contents. Surgeons noted undesirable contractures of the specialized scar around the implants, called the implant-related capsule. Hence, manu-

Table 13–1
BREAST IMPLANTS BY MANUFACTURERS

	Silicone Gel Implants			Saline Implants			Bilumen Implants			Grand Total
	Intact	Ruptured	Total	Intact	Ruptured	Total	Intact	Ruptured	Total	
Dow Corning										
Smooth	51	116	167	0	0	0	0	5	5	172
Textured MSI	1	1	2	0	0	0	0	0	0	2
McGhan										
Smooth	24	41	65	2	0	2	6	3	9	76
Textured Biocell	11	4	15	49	11	60	1	1	2	77
Heyer-Schulte										
Smooth	6	41	47	2	0	2	1	3	4	53
Mentor										
Smooth	7	5	12	12	0	12	3	0	3	27
Textured Siltex	16	2	18	13	9	22	0	0	0	40
Surgitek										
Smooth	23	28	51	3	1	4	14	19	33	88
Textured polyurethane	20	5	25	0	0	0	0	0	0	25
Bioplasty										
Textured	0	2	2	0	0	0	0	0	0	2
Koken										
Smooth	2	2	4	0	0	0	0	0	0	4
										566

1 = one implant; one patient could have multiple implants in the database.

facturers created alternatives to the original smooth silicone elastomer shell. The thinking was that the elastomer texture would modify the structure of the capsule in such a way as to interrupt the myofibroblast's ability to contract concentrically. By the mid-1980s, elastomer shells became available in textures applied as the shell was cast, and one texture, polyurethane foam, was glued onto the silicone elastomer shell. Manufacturers developed their unique textures: Surgitek chose polyurethane, Dow Corning chose MSI, McGhan chose Biocell, and Mentor chose Siltex.

Most types of elastomer shell texture leave a characteristic mirror image on the associated implant-related capsule. In some cases, fragments of the elastomer texture become incorporated into the host tissue, creating unique foreign body responses.

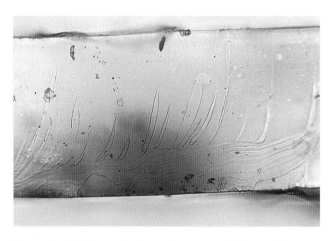

Figure 13–10. Photograph of smooth elastomer shell (neat). Most manufacturers introduced a smooth shell gel-filled implant. The elastomer shell may vary in thickness and in composition in an effort to reduce the phenomenon called "gel bleed," which indicates passage of silicone liquid through an intact elastomer shell.

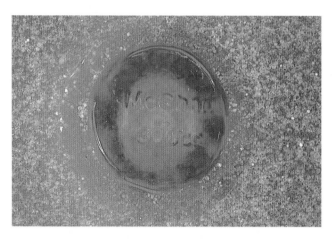

Figure 13–12. Gross photograph of Biocell (McGhan) textured saline-filled tissue expander. Tissue expanders are placed temporarily at the time of mastectomy to allow the soft tissue to be gently stretched to accommodate the final prosthesis. Shown is a textured saline-filled tissue expander with "McGhan" and the size on the patch.

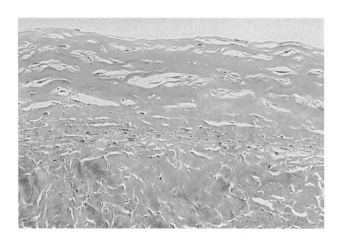

Figure 13–11. Photomicrograph of capsule opposite a smooth-shell, saline-filled implant. When manufactured without texture, the corresponding implant-related capsule is smooth, and if no silicone gel or fluid is present, the implant-related capsule is fairly hypocellular. In this figure, the patient underwent mastectomy for breast cancer, and after two previous unsuccessful reconstructive attempts she was implanted with a smooth-shell, saline-filled implant. Within 2 years contractures were severe and painful, necessitating removal of the implant, which was intact.

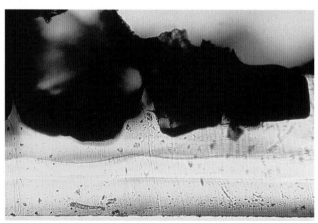

Figure 13–13. McGhan/3M and Biocell texture (neat). Biocell texture consists of cubical indentations in the elastomer shell.

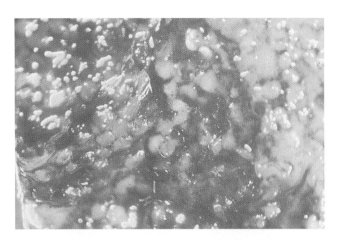

Figure 13–14. Subgross photograph of implant-related capsule opposite a Biocell textured implant. The tissue of the capsule grows to fill in the cubical indentations of the texture, resulting in a cobblestone appearance to the capsule on gross inspection.

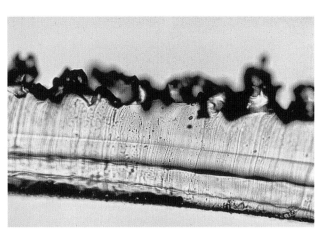

Figure 13–17. Subgross section of Siltex texture (neat). On close inspection, the elastomer texture has bulbous ends.

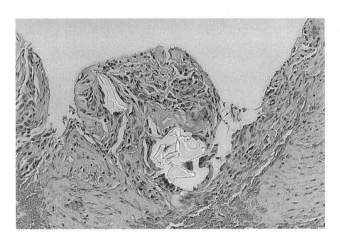

Figure 13–15. Histologic section of implant-related capsule opposite a Biocell textured implant. Histologically, the villous projections noted grossly consist of well-vascularized fibrous tissue with occasional embedded irregular sheets of water-clear foreign material surrounded by multinucleated giant cells. These are fragments of elastomer shell texture incorporated into the capsule.

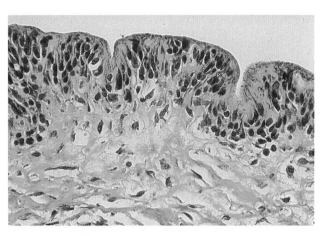

Figure 13–18. Histologic section of implant-related capsule opposite Siltex texture. Although the tissue of the implant-related capsule fills in the irregularities of the implant surface, it is unusual to see fragments of foreign material related to the elastomer shell incorporated into the capsule opposite Siltex texture. The histology of the capsule is structurally and functionally identical to synovium.

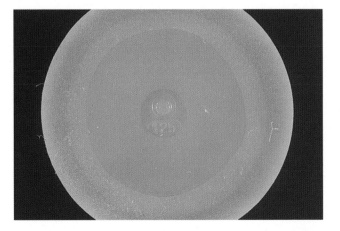

Figure 13–16. Gross photograph of Siltex (Mentor) textured gel-filled implant. This textured gel-filled implant has an opaque appearance. A relatively large back patch covers the majority of the back of the implant. In the center of the back is a circle with a central raised gel-fill point with the size marked in an oval.

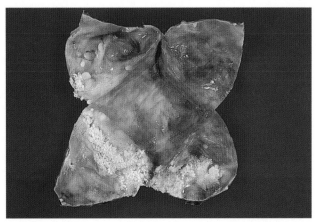

Figure 13–19. Gross photograph of implant-related capsule from a ruptured gel-filled Mentor implant with Siltex texture. The surface of the implant-related capsule is often smooth. In this case, the smooth surface was interrupted by innumerable villous projections.

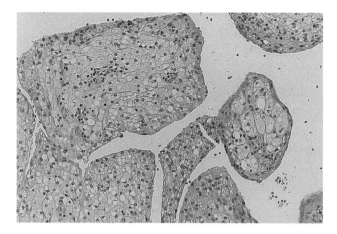

Figure 13–20. Tissue section of the villous projections seen grossly in Figure 13–19. The villous projections consist of back-to-back vacuolated macrophages containing droplets of water-clear refractile foreign material consistent with silicone.

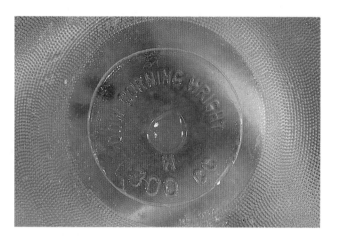

Figure 13–21. Gross photograph of textured MSI (Micro Structured Implant; Dow Corning). Shown is a textured gel-filled implant with "DOW CORNING WRIGHT" on the back patch with central fill point, and the size in cubic centimeters. Note the orderly columns of texture viewed end-on.

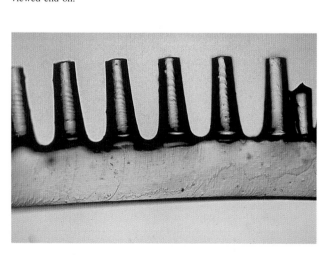

Figure 13–22. Subgross photograph of MSI texture. MSI texture imparts an orderly columnar arrangement to the elastomer texture, as shown in this figure. This particular texture is associated with accumulation of fluid in the capsular space, creating a characteristic appearance on mammography or magnetic resonance imaging of the breast.

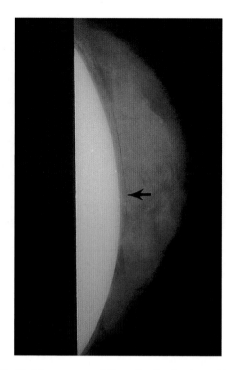

Figure 13–23. Mammogram of Dow Corning implant with MSI texture. Note the raised pillars at the edge of the brightly imaged silicone implant (*arrow*). They are visible due to the presence of intervening fluid in the capsular space. Note also the thin layer of pectoralis muscle overlying the implant and extending between the implant and the fatty breast tissue. This indicates that the implant was placed in a submuscular location.

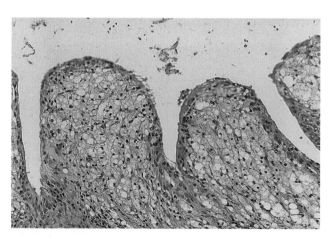

Figure 13–24. Photomicrograph of implant-related capsule opposite MSI texture. The corresponding implant-related capsule demonstrates villous projections; in this case, the stroma is packed with back-to-back histiocytes with vacuoles of foreign material consistent with silicone. This texture is not incorporated into the patient's tissue; however, silicone liquid is evident in spite of a grossly intact elastomer shell.

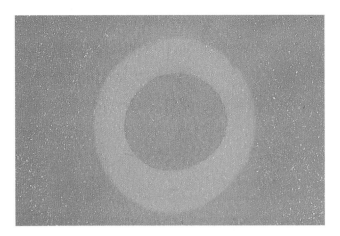

Figure 13–25. Gross photograph of a Surgitek polyurethane foam–covered implant. An opaque-appearing, textured gel-filled implant with an even more opaque white ring identifies a foam-covered Surgitek implant.

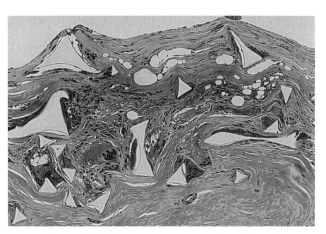

Figure 13–27. Histologic section of an implant-related capsule opposite a polyurethane foam–covered implant. Polyurethane foam is incorporated into the implant capsule, inciting an intense fibrotic reaction. Multinucleated giant cells surround fragments of foam accompanied by histiocytes with varied-size vacuoles containing silicone. Lymphocytes punctuate the scene. Although the implant may be intact to inspection on removal, silicone and polyurethane are invariably present in the capsular tissue. On occasion, foam-covered implants are removed in the surgeon's office, and the capsule remains. Because of the quantity of foam incorporated into the capsule, a contracted mass frequently creates concern for cancer on follow-up mammograms, leading to eventual removal.

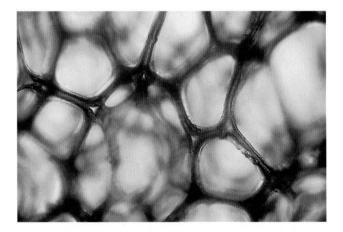

Figure 13–26. Polyurethane foam (neat). Polyurethane is a polymer that when bubbled with gas produces the foam most familiar to us as furniture cushion filling. A thin layer of polyurethane foam is glued to the elastomer shell, usually with a silicone adhesive.

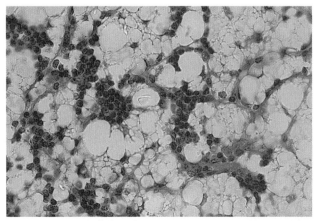

Figure 13–28. Histologic section of polyurethane foam in a regional lymph node. Patients with polyurethane foam–covered implants may note axillary adenopathy, resulting in biopsy. Minute triangular fragments and other irregular fragments of firm foreign material are observed within vacuoles of histiocytes in the lymph node. Other histiocytes have rims of refractile foreign material consistent with silicone.

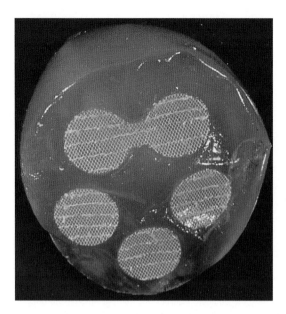

Figure 13–29. Gross photograph of Dow Corning gel-filled implant with Dacron fixation patches. Some implants have fixation patches on the back, designed to prevent rotation of the implant within the implant capsule. The patches are affixed to the surface of the elastomer shell, and are composed of a Dacron mesh. The Dacron mesh is intended to encourage tissue ingrowth. Several manufacturers used fixation patches on the posterior surface of implants. The pattern of fixation patches may lead to the identification of the manufacturer. Five round Dacron back patches, two connected in dumbbell fashion, indicate Dow Corning.

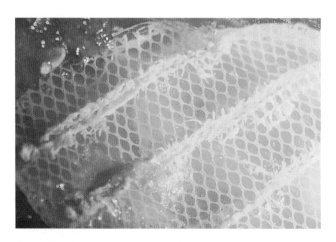

Figure 13–30. Gross photograph of implant-related capsule opposite a gel-filled implant with fixation patches. Early patch patterns covered virtually the entire posterior surface of the implant, resulting in folds of the elastomer shell between patches as the capsule contracted. These folds are frequently the site of implant rupture.

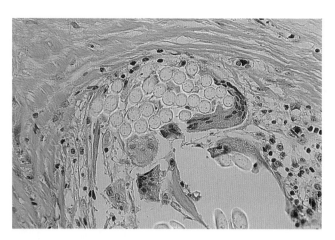

Figure 13–31. Histologic section of implant-related capsule with incorporation of Dacron fibers into the tissue. In this figure, the Dacron is incorporated into the capsule and can be seen resembling multifilament suture. These fibers of Dacron are associated with dense fibrosis and intense histiocytic multinucleated giant cell response.

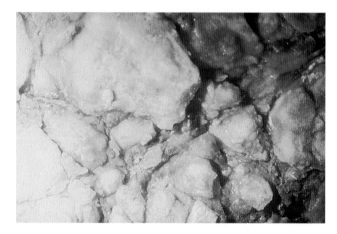

Figure 13–32. Gross photograph of implant-related capsule with "eggshell" dystrophic mineralization associated with a ruptured gel-filled implant with Dacron patches. Most confluent in association with ruptured implants and implants with Dacron patches, surface dystrophic mineralization can be observed in conjunction with intact implants as well. Grossly, the appearance varies from a fine translucent stiff area on the otherwise pliable implant-related capsule to total involvement of the capsule, giving the appearance of cracked eggshells.

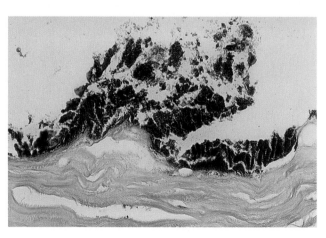

Figure 13–33. Histologic section of implant-related capsule with "eggshell" dystrophic mineralization associated with a ruptured gel-filled implant with Dacron patches. Histologically, the mineralization is most often oriented to the luminal aspect of the capsule, and it may include incorporated extracellular silicone gel droplets.

IDENTIFYING THE MANUFACTURER OF BREAST PROSTHESES

Patients are sometimes unaware of the manufacturer of their implanted device, and the implantation records are frequently unavailable by the time explantation is performed. Textured implants are relatively easy to identify, because histology of the capsule confirms the identification of the texture made on gross inspection, and each manufacturer chose only one texture. However, smooth shell gel-filled implants are particularly hard to differentiate. Careful examination of the back patch and the shell markings allows classification of the majority of implants to the correct manufacturer. Back patches were used to seal the site of gel loading into the elastomer shell.

Back patches frequently have a raised "button" called a fill point. Some surgeons used fine-gauge needles to inject antibiotics, steroids, or other agents into the implant. On gross inspection, a fluid bubble or discoloration within the elastomer shell contents may be observed.

Shell markings are usually 2 to 4 cm from the back patch, oriented at the 12:00, 3:00, 6:00, or 9:00 o'clock positions with reference to the back patch. Shell markings usually consist of numerals, letters, or both. Dr. Michael Middleton, of the University of California at San Diego, has extensive experience identifying implants. His catalog of implants (obtained from the author) assisted in identifying implants from our archives that are illustrated in this chapter.

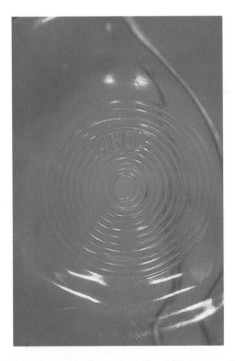

Figure 13–34. Photograph of smooth shell gel-filled implant by Heyer-Schulte, and later, Mentor. This figure shows a single-lumen smooth-shell, gel-filled implant with back patch consisting of concentric ("spiral") rings of raised elastomer. In the center is a raised "button" or gel-fill point. These patches were made by Heyer-Schulte and later Mentor. Note the size indicated in a racetrack-shaped clearing on the patch. Early versions had no embossed size. When Mentor acquired the American company Heyer-Schulte in 1984, an "M" was added to the clearing.

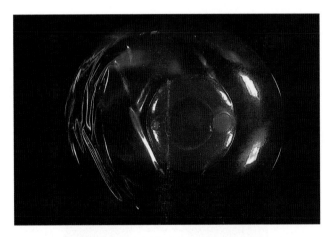

Figure 13–35. Photograph of Dubin type smooth-shell, gel-filled implant by Surgitek, Heyer-Schulte, or McGhan/3M. This distinctive back patch consists of an elastomer disk on which is placed a horizontal bar and a smaller disk, creating overlapping stacked circles. Shell markings are used to distinguish between the three manufacturers. Shell markings consisting of a letter followed by a numeral indicate Heyer-Schulte, whereas numerals at the 6:00 o'clock position facing away from the back patch indicate McGhan, and beveled patch edges with numerals facing toward the back patch indicate Surgitek.

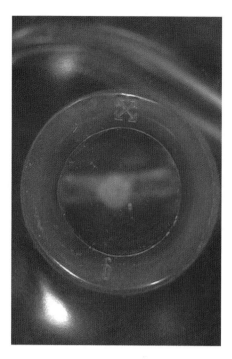

Figure 13–36. Photograph of smooth-shelled implant by Mentor. Smooth shell implants with a symbol consisting of crossed double-head arrows on the edge of the raised back patch with or without a single numeral opposite indicates Mentor.

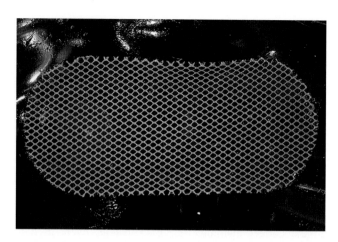

Figure 13–38. Photograph of smooth-shell, gel-filled implant with an eccentrically placed, embedded Dacron-reinforced back patch by Dow Corning. A racetrack-shaped back patch consisting of woven Dacron reinforcement is incorporated into the elastomer shell. This type of patch is not to be confused with the Dacron fixation patch shown earlier (see Fig. 13–29).

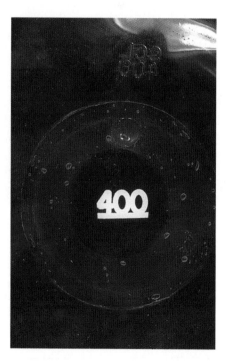

Figure 13–37. Photograph of smooth-shell, gel-filled implant with radiopaque numerals by Surgitek. A smooth-shell, gel-filled implant with a crisp white underlined reversed numeral (which is radiopaque), a beveled back patch, and a raised fill point just above the numeral was made by Surgitek. Just opposite the fill point are shell markings consisting of the letters SCL (*s*trong shell, *c*ohesive gel, *l*ow bleed) and the nonreversed numerals indicating the size in cubic centimeters.

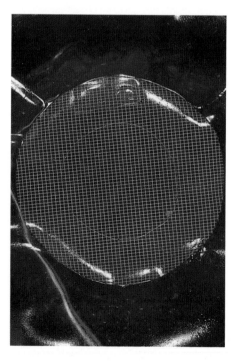

Figure 13–39. Photograph of smooth-shell, gel-filled implant with embedded reinforced back patch by Heyer-Schulte. A smooth shell gel-filled implant with a circular back patch has an embedded rectangular white square mesh pattern as well as a superimposed clear elastomer rectangle shown at the top. This implant was made by Heyer-Schulte.

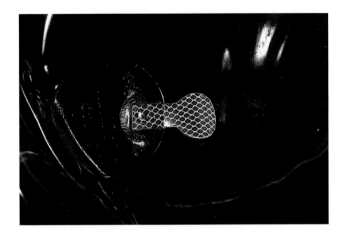

Figure 13–40. Photograph of smooth-shell, gel-filled implant with suture tag by McGhan. A smooth-shell, gel-filled implant with "McGhan" and the size embossed in the center of the back patch has a Dacron-reinforced suture tag in a "keyhole" shape. Other manufacturers used suture tags of slightly different design.

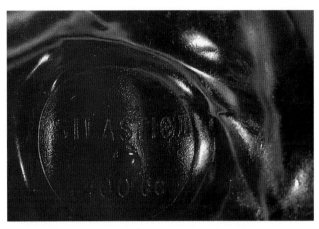

Figure 13–41. Photograph of smooth-shell, gel-filled implant by Dow Corning. A smooth-shell, gel-filled implant with SILASTICII embossed on the patch with a central raised fill point and the implant size below was made by Dow Corning.

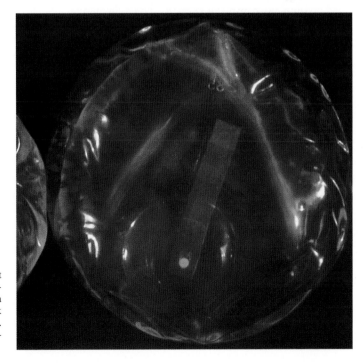

Figure 13–42. Photograph of smooth-shell, double-lumen implant by Surgitek. A double-lumen outer saline–inner gel-filled, smooth-shell implant has an eccentric back patch with beveled edges and a rectangular leaflet Quin-Seal valve that extends beyond the back patch. A white circle with central slit is centered on the patch. Opposite the valve are shell markings with three numerals characteristic of a Surgitek implant.

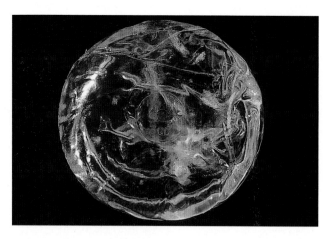

Figure 13–43. Gross photograph of a single-lumen implant with a delaminated elastomer shell by Koken. At first glance, Koken implants appear to be double-lumen implants; however, they are unique single-lumen implants with frequent delamination of the elastomer shell. Koken is a Japanese manufacturer that ceased distribution of implants in 1990. The delaminated shell actually consists of three layers: outer and inner silicone layers (visible in this photograph) and an inner fluorosilicone layer (not seen grossly). Note the appearance of the back patch. The name Koken appears on the patch with the implant size. The patch is viewed through an apparent fenestration in the outer delaminated shell layer.

FOREIGN MATERIAL RELATED TO IMPLANT CONTENTS

In Figures 13–10 through 13–33, foreign material related to implant capsule texture is shown in human tissues. It is well known that the contents of the elastomer shell may also create a tissue reaction, as shown in Figures 13–44 to 13–50. Both ruptured and apparently intact implants impart silicone to the capsular tissue, which occurs in quantities sufficient to recognize them using light microscopy. Analytical chemistry has been used by some authors to definitively identify this foreign material as silicone. Silicone oil presents in tissue as either fine droplets in finely vacuolated histiocytes (which are often back-to-back in tissue) or in larger extracellular and intracellular drops surrounded by multinucleated giant cells, or both.

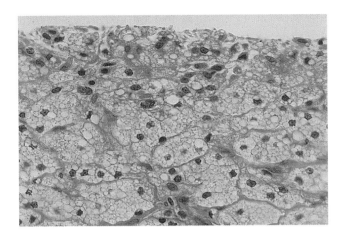

Figure 13–44. Histologic section of silicone liquid in capsule tissue. The contents of a gel-filled implant consist of both slightly and highly cross-linked fragments of silicone elastomer, and it is generally thought that the slightly cross-linked fragments "bleed" through the elastomer shell. Note the variation in size of the intracytoplasmic vacuoles within individual cells, in contrast to the uniform fine vacuoles or single large "empty" vacuoles observed in fat necrosis (compare with Fig. 13–3).

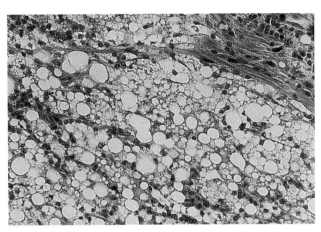

Figure 13–46. Histologic section of silicone in axillary lymph nodes. Silicone and silicone-laden macrophages apparently circulate through the lymphatics to regional lymph nodes. Silicone-laden macrophages may cause axillary lymphadenopathy, prompting biopsy to rule out malignancy. The figure shows the regional lymph node of a patient who developed breast carcinoma after breast augmentation with silicone gel–filled breast implants. Note, in addition to lymphocytes, histiocytes containing vacuoles of refractile foreign material consistent with silicone expanding the lymph node parenchyma.

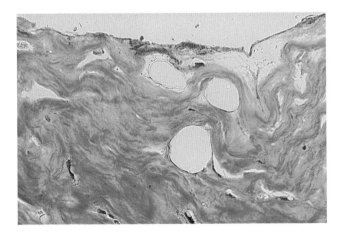

Figure 13–45. Histologic section of silicone gel in tissue. Within vacuoles or extracellular spaces (as shown in this figure), refractile silicone gel has a more stringy or blotchy appearance than the subtle, fine droplets shown in Figure 13–44. The appearance of silicone gel is not restricted to tissues around ruptured implants, and can be seen with apparently intact implants as well.

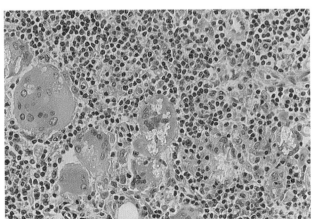

Figure 13–47. Histologic section of silicone rubber related to a joint prosthesis in axillary lymph nodes. This patient developed axillary adenopathy after mastectomy for breast cancer. A biopsy was performed to rule out malignancy. No tumor was seen; however, multinucleated giant cells containing rigid "popcorn"-shaped fragments of refractile foreign material are noted. The patient had never had reconstruction after mastectomy, but she did have a joint prosthesis in her hand. The foreign material is consistent with wear particles from an orthopedic prosthesis.

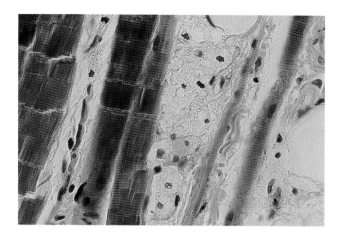

Figure 13–48. Histologic section of silicone fluid in skeletal muscle. After closed capsulotomy, a procedure in which the surgeon forcefully "presses" on a contracted capsule in order to release it, silicone from a ruptured or leaking implant may travel via tissue planes to rest in other tissues of the chest wall. In this figure, skeletal muscle of the chest is infiltrated by macrophages containing fine vacuoles of refractile foreign material.

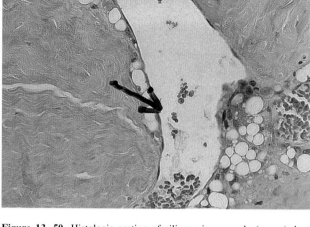

Figure 13–50. Histologic section of silicone in a venule (*arrow*) deep to an implant-related capsule. It is well known that silicone reaches regional lymph nodes, most likely via lymphatic drainage of the breast. Any silicone that is not deposited in lymph nodes may enter the venous circulation via the thoracic duct. On rare occasions, silicone is observed in vascular spaces in the implant-related capsules. Breast capsules are seldom accompanied by other tissues to examine; therefore, the possibility that silicone reaches other tissue sites via the vasculature is not excluded.

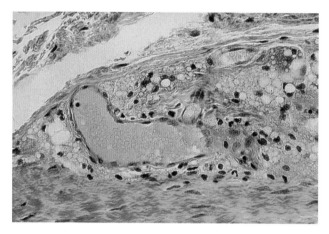

Figure 13–49. Histologic section of venule deep to an implant-related capsule. The stroma deep to the implant-related capsule has a relatively dense vascular network. Surrounding these vessels, tightly packed aggregates of vacuolated histiocytes are frequently observed. The reason for the frequent observation of aggregates around vessels (in this case a vein) is unknown.

CHAPTER 14

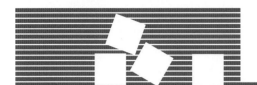

Fine-Needle Aspiration Cytology
Shahla Masood

INTRODUCTION

With remarkable increase in public awareness of breast cancer and advances in radiographic imaging technology, more women seek consultation for the evaluation of their breast lesions. Recognizing that the majority of breast lesions are benign and open biopsies are inconvenient and costly, fine-needle aspiration biopsy (FNAB) remains an increasingly important diagnostic tool in the assessment of the nature of various breast lesions.

FNAB is an accurate, cost-effective, and well tolerated procedure with a reported specificity of 99% and sensitivity of 70% to 99%.[1, 2] This procedure is an attractive alternative to surgical biopsy and may be used as an initial diagnostic method for patients with breast lesions.[3] FNAB provides an opportunity for women to have their breast lesions sampled and examined without significant morbidity and associated costs.[4] In addition, FNAB produces only minimal physical and psychological discomfort to the patient and leaves neither skin deformity nor parenchymal scar. These could interfere with subsequent evaluation during follow-up. Furthermore, the established diagnosis of breast cancer by FNAB provides more flexibility for treatment planning. This is particularly important in respect to a patient's choice in treatment options. FNAB may also serve as a therapeutic procedure if a cyst is encountered. It is an effective tool in the evaluation of local chest wall recurrence, lymph node metastasis, and in inoperable conditions.[5, 6]

FNAB is also considered as the only diagnostic procedure for presurgical chemotherapy regimens[7] and is used effectively in providing prognostic information.[8] The reported morphologic and molecular abnormalities seen in fine-needle aspirates from women who are at increased risk for breast cancer represent an exciting application of this procedure. This could provide an excellent opportu-

nity to better understand the biology of breast cancer, to identify intermediate endpoint biomarkers, and to monitor the effect of potential new agents in breast cancer prevention and treatment.[9–12]

Despite the aforementioned credibility of breast FNAB, limitations exist in the discipline of breast cytopathology. This includes, but is not limited to, the presence of significant diversity in the practice of using this procedure among different institutions. There are also difficulties encountered in the interpretation of a small yet significant number of specific pathologic entities. Criteria that can reliably identify several types of breast lesions, such as atypical hyperplasia, low-grade breast carcinoma, fibro-epithelial tumors, papillary breast lesions, and mucinous tumors of the breast, are not yet well defined. Interestingly, these challenges are not dissimilar to those reported for core needle biopsy.[17] In addition, clinical management of breast lesions also remains controversial. Although several investigators advocate the use of FNAB as an alternative to open biopsy and frozen section,[13, 14] others would limit its use to patients assigned to treatment protocols.[15, 16]

The issues surrounding breast FNAB can be easily resolved by the establishment of a well orchestrated multidisciplinary team of qualified physicians, radiologists, and pathologists who are familiar with the performance and interpretation of breast FNAB. Proficiency in biopsy technique, smear preparation, and the interpretation of cytomorphologic features is the key to a successful FNAB.[18, 19] It should be recognized that breast cytopathology is different from exfoliative cytology, and the interpretation of breast FNAB requires interest, proper training, and familiarity with the merits and pitfalls of the procedure.[20]

INFLAMMATORY BREAST LESIONS

Mastitis and Abscess

Foamy macrophages
Cytophagocytosis
Cell debris in background
Epithelial cells with nuclear enlargement and prominent
  nucleoli
Occasional multinucleated cells

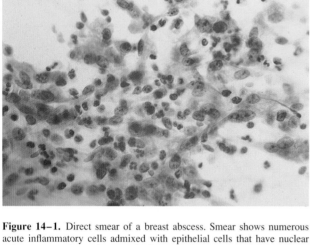

Figure 14–1. Direct smear of a breast abscess. Smear shows numerous acute inflammatory cells admixed with epithelial cells that have nuclear enlargement and prominent nucleoli.

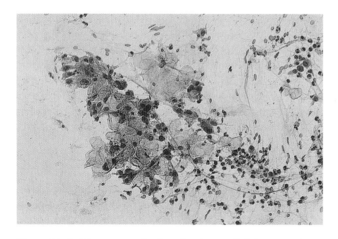

Figure 14–2. Direct smear of subareolar abscess. Cellular smear shows acute inflammatory infiltrate and anucleate squamous cells.

Granulomatous Mastitis

Cellular aspirate
Lymphocytes and plasma cells
Granulomas with epithelioid and multinucleated giant
  cells
Reactive ductal epithelial cells with enlarged nuclei
Clusters of fibroblasts

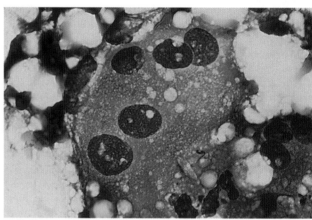

Figure 14–3. Direct smear of granulomatous mastitis. Cellular aspirate demonstrates aggregate of mononuclear inflammatory cells, lymphocytes, and epithelioid cells.

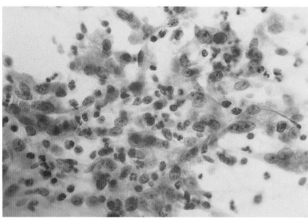

Figure 14–4. Direct smear of the same case as Figure 14–3. Smear shows a multinucleated giant cell.

Fat Necrosis

Foamy or hemosiderin-containing microphages
Inflammatory cells
Multinucleated cells
Fibroblasts
Reactive epithelial cells
Necrotic background

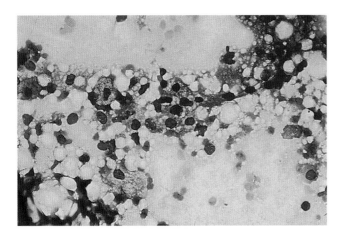

Figure 14–5. Direct aspirate of fat necrosis. Cellular aspirate demonstrates amorphous debris, inflammatory cells, lipid-laden macrophages, and giant cells.

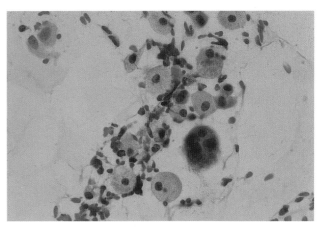

Figure 14–6. Higher magnification of the same case as Figure 14–5. The same features are seen.

NONINFLAMMATORY BENIGN BREAST LESIONS

Fibroadenoma

Cellular aspirate
Stromal fragments
Sheets of nonlayered, ductal epithelial cells forming "antler horns"
Bipolar, naked nuclei
Occasional apocrine cells
Rare multinucleated giant cells

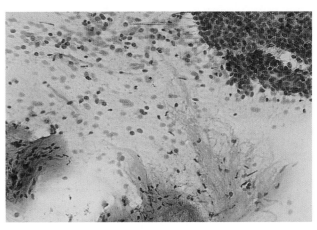

Figure 14–8. Direct smear of fibroadenoma. Both epithelial and stromal elements are seen. Myoepithelial cells with bipolar naked nuclei are present in the background and admixed with epithelial cells.

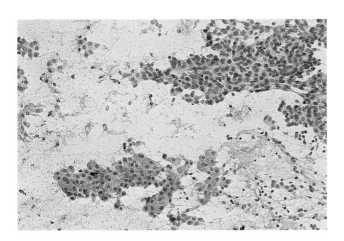

Figure 14–7. Direct smear of fibroadenoma. The aspirate is cellular with a biphasic pattern consisting of epithelial and stromal elements. Epithelial cells are tightly cohesive and uniform, forming an "antler-horn" pattern.

Papilloma

Cellular aspirate
Proteinaceous or bloody background
Foamy or hemosiderin-containing macrophages
Tall columnar cells
Three-dimensional papillary clusters
Presence of myoepithelial cells
Cell balls

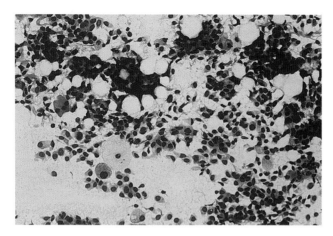

Figure 14–9. Direct aspirate of intraductal papilloma. Cellular aspirate shows isolated and clusters of epithelial and myoepithelial cells, apocrine cells, a few columnar cells, and many foamy microphages.

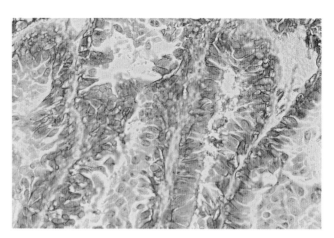

Figure 14–12. Higher magnification of the same case as Figure 14–11. Same features are seen.

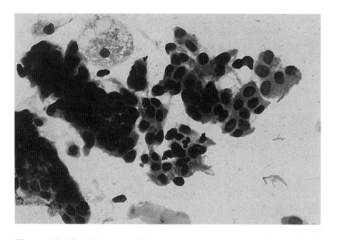

Figure 14–10. Higher magnification of the same case as Figure 14–9. A polymorphic pattern of epithelial cells, myoepithelial cells, apocrine metaplastic cells, and macrophages is seen.

Pregnancy-Associated Lesions

High cell yield
Granular, proteinaceous background
Dispersed cells and loosely arranged cell clusters
Large epithelial cells with uniform nuclei and prominent nucleoli
Abundant, foamy, vacuolated cytoplasm with fraying of cytoplasmic borders
Bipolar, naked nuclei
Foamy macrophages
Occasional multinucleated giant cells

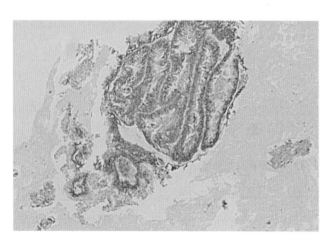

Figure 14–11. Immunochemical stain of smooth muscle actin (SMA) on cell block preparation. A uniform layer of myoepithelial cells is demonstrated by the staining in this papillary lesion.

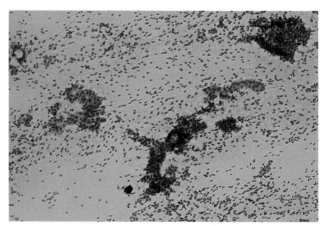

Figure 14–13. Direct smear of pregnancy-associated change. Cellular aspirate shows epithelial cells in loose clusters and dispersed pattern and a proteinaceous background.

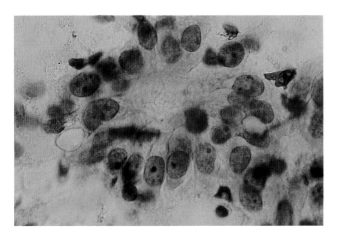

Figure 14–14. Higher magnification of the same case as Figure 14–13. Uniform epithelial cells show granular, vacuolated cytoplasm, indistinct cell borders, and prominent nucleoli.

TREATMENT-INDUCED CHANGES

Granuloma

Epithelial and multinucleated giant cells
Reactive ductal epithelial cells
Clusters of fibroblasts
Lymphocytes and plasma cells

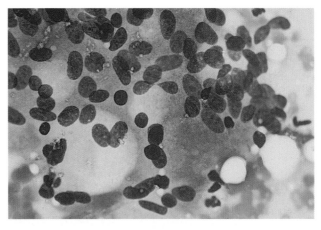

Figure 14–16. Higher magnification of the same case as Figure 14–15. A multinucleate giant cell is demonstrated.

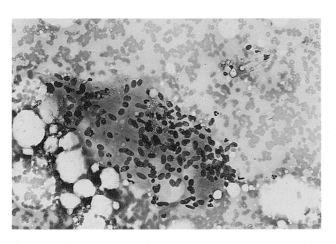

Figure 14–15. Direct smear of breast granuloma. Smear shows epithelioid cells forming ill defined granulomas. A few lymphocytes and plasma cells are also present.

Radiation-Induced Changes

Poor cellularity
Granulation tissue
Fat necrosis
Epithelial atypia and degeneration
Granulomatous reaction
Fibroblastic reaction

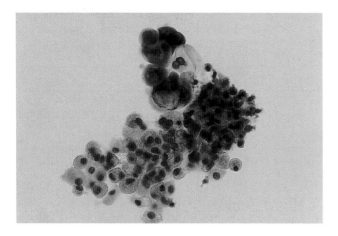

Figure 14–17. Aspirate of radiation-induced changes. Direct smear shows cluster of benign and malignant epithelial cells with degenerative cytoplasmic vacuolization and nuclear condensation. Marked cytologic atypia and macronucleoli are evident among malignant epithelial cells.

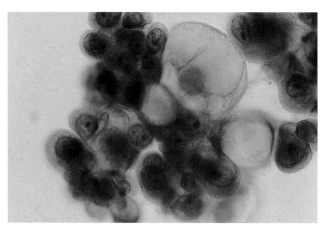

Figure 14–18. Higher magnification of the same case as Figure 14–17. Highly atypical malignant epithelial cells with macronucleoli and cytoplasmic vacuoles are seen.

BENIGN MESENCHYMAL TUMORS

Fibromatosis

Variable cellularity
Pronounced spindle cell proliferation
A few small groups of epithelial cells
Scattered lymphocytes
Amorphous material in the background

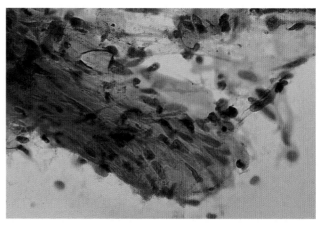

Figure 14–20. Papanicolaou-stained smear of the same case as Figure 14–19. Pronounced spindle cell proliferation is evident.

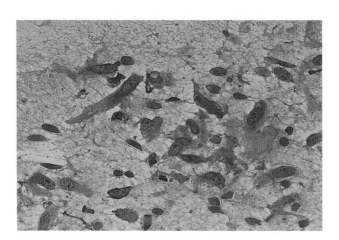

Figure 14–19. Direct smear of breast fibromatosis. Smear shows scattered spindle cells, amorphous material in the background, and a few lymphocytes.

Granular Cell Tumor

Cellular smear
Cohesive clusters of epithelial cells
Abundant granular cytoplasm
Evenly distributed chromatin pattern
Conspicuous nucleoli

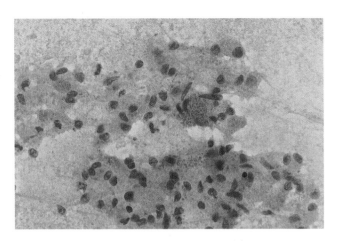

Figure 14–21. Direct smear of granular cell tumor. Clusters of polygonal cells show granular cytoplasm, indistinct cell borders, and conspicuous nucleoli.

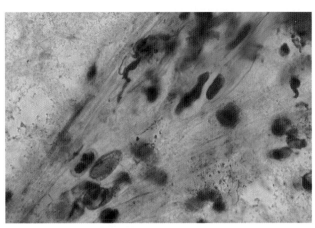

Figure 14–23. Direct smear of neurofibroma. Direct smear demonstrates spindle cells with indistinct borders.

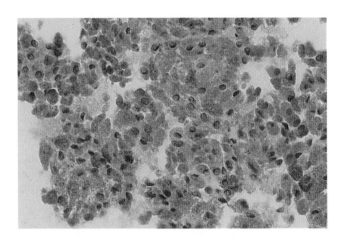

Figure 14–22. Immunostaining for S-100 on cell block preparation. Strongly diffuse cytoplasmic positive staining is demonstrated.

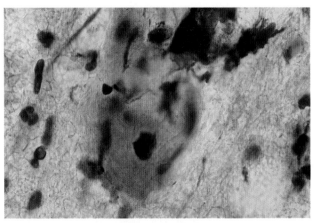

Figure 14–24. Immunostain of neuron-specific enolase on direct smear. Strong expression of neuron-specific enolase is evident.

Neurofibroma

Moderate cellularity
Spindle-shaped cells
Ill defined cytoplasmic borders
Palisading nuclei

FIBROCYSTIC CHANGE, HIGH-RISK AND PREMALIGNANT BREAST DISEASE

Nonproliferative Breast Disease

Low cellularity
Fragments of stromal and/or adipose tissue
Monolayered clusters of uniform cell population with honeycomb pattern
Foam cells, apocrine cells
Myoepithelial cells

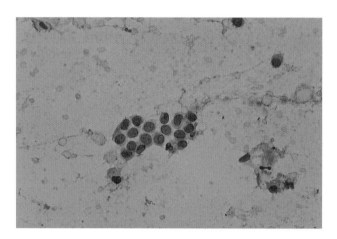

Figure 14–25. Direct smear of nonproliferative breast disease. Paucicellular aspirate shows group of monolayered uniform epithelial cells with honeycomb pattern.

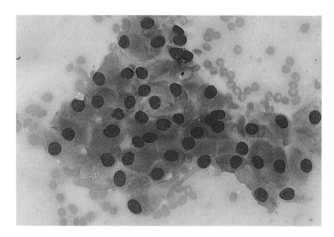

Figure 14–26. Direct smear of nonproliferative breast disease. Group of apocrine cells are seen in the same case as Figure 14–25.

Proliferative Breast Disease without Atypia

Moderate to high cellularity
Conspicuous number of highly cohesive cell clusters

Overriding of nuclei, nuclear enlargement, and occasional micronucleoli
Apocrine cells, histiocytes, calcified particles
Focal loss of polarity
Myoepithelial cells

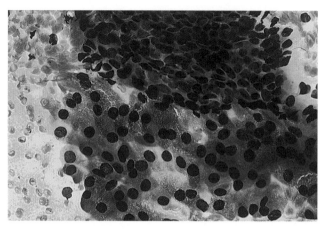

Figure 14–27. Direct smear of proliferative breast disease without atypia. Tightly clustered ductal epithelial cells show overriding of the nuclei and scattered myoepithelial cells. Group of apocrine cells are also seen.

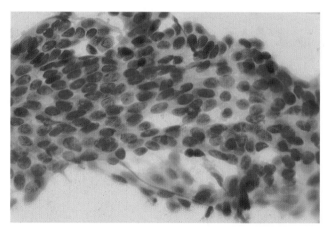

Figure 14–28. Papanicolaou-stained smear of the same case as Figure 14–27. Smear shows tightly cohesive ductal epithelial cells with overriding nuclei and admixed myoepithelial cells.

Proliferative Breast Disease with Atypia

Cellular aspirate
Clustering and crowding of epithelial cells with overriding nuclei
Anisonucleosis and chromatin clumping
Occasional conspicuous nucleoli
Myoepithelial cells within the clusters of atypical cells
Rare apocrine cells and macrophages

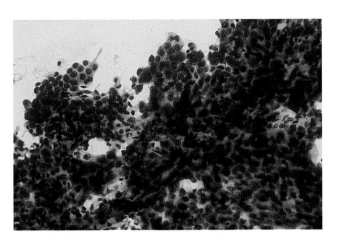

Figure 14–29. Direct aspirate from proliferative breast disease with atypia. Highly cellular aspirate shows clustering and crowding of the epithelial cells. These cells demonstrate loss of polarity and marked nuclear atypia. Myoepithelial cells are seen as dark-stained spindle cells admixed with epithelial cells.

Lobular Neoplasia (Atypical Lobular Hyperplasia/Lobular Carcinoma in Situ)

Variable cellularity
Clustering of epithelial cells
Small cells with inconspicuous nuclei
Cell balls

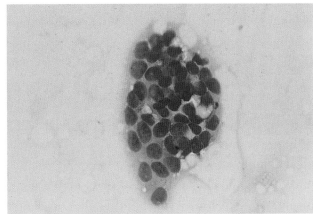

Figure 14–31. Direct smear of lobular neoplasia. A cluster of small cells shows proliferation. The lobular epithelial cells are evenly distributed and uniform.

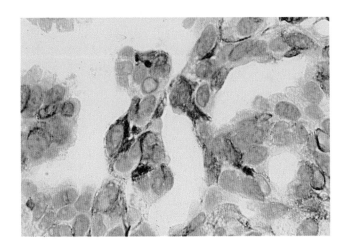

Figure 14–30. Immunostaining of smooth muscle actin (SMA) on cell block preparation. Scattered positive staining with reticular pattern indicates the presence of myoepithelial cells.

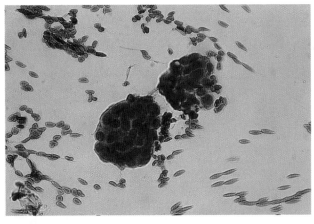

Figure 14–32. Direct smear of lobular neoplasia. Clusters of crowded cells with nuclear enlargement, chromatin clumping, and prominent nucleoli form cell balls.

DUCTAL CARCINOMA IN SITU

Non-Comedo Ductal Carcinoma in Situ

Variable cellularity
Monomorphic population of small to medium-sized epithelial cells
Cell clusters display solid, cribriform, or papillary pattern
Absence of myoepithelial cells

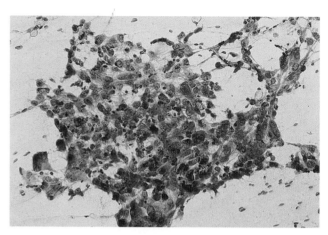

Figure 14–35. Direct smear of comedocarcinoma in situ. Groups of pleomorphic neoplastic epithelial cells show evidence of extensive individual cell necrosis.

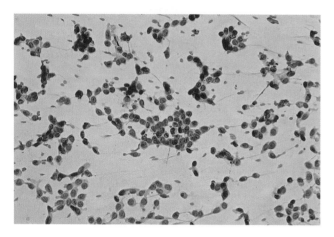

Figure 14–33. Direct smear of non-comedo ductal carcinoma in situ. Aspirate shows cohesive clusters of neoplastic epithelial cells.

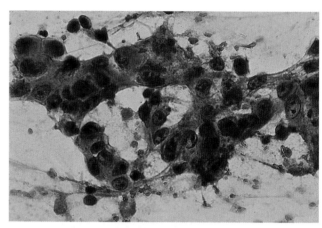

Figure 14–36. Higher magnification of the same case as Figure 14–35. Same features are seen.

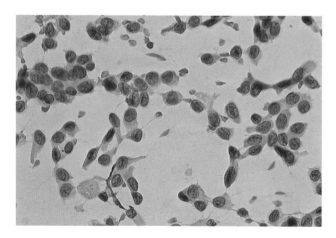

Figure 14–34. Higher magnification of the same case as Figure 14–33. Groups of epithelial cells form cribriform pattern. No myoepithelial cells are present.

Comedocarcinoma in Situ

Highly cellular aspirate
Pleomorphic population of neoplastic epithelial cells
Necrotic background
Individual cell necrosis
Mitoses
Absence of myoepithelial cells

PRIMARY BREAST CARCINOMA

Infiltrating Duct Carcinoma

Cellular aspirate
Variable cell pattern
Necrotic background
Conspicuous loss of cellular cohesion
Pleomorphic, isolated single cells
Occasional small cells with plasmacytoid appearance
Rare multinucleated tumor giant cells
Anisonucleosis

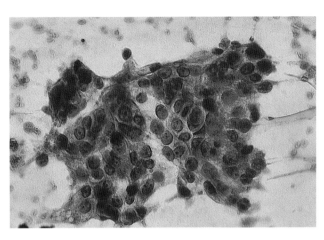

Figure 14–39. Direct smear from infiltrating duct carcinoma, high nuclear grade. Groups of loosely cohesive neoplastic epithelial cells show marked hyperchromasia, anisonucleosis, chromatin clumping, irregular nuclear membranes, and macronucleoli.

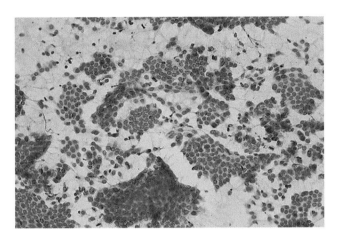

Figure 14–37. Direct smear from infiltrating ductal carcinoma, low nuclear grade. Cellular smear with isolated and clusters of neoplastic epithelial cells with no myoepithelial cells present.

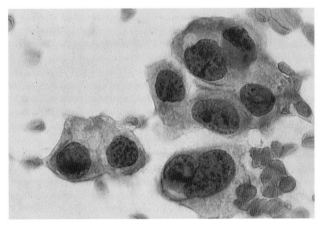

Figure 14–40. Higher magnification of the same case as Figure 14–39. Same features are evident.

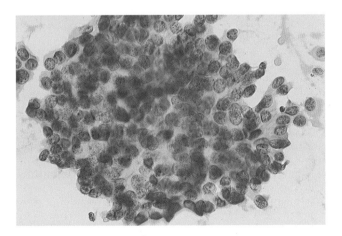

Figure 14–38. Higher magnification of the same case as Figure 14–37. Same features are seen.

Infiltrating Lobular Carcinoma

Low to moderate cell yield
Individual cells, small chains, strands, and small groups
Uniform population of small cells with mild atypia (classic type)
Pleomorphic population of epithelial cells with conspicuous atypia (pleomorphic type)
Small nuclei
Occasional signet ring cells

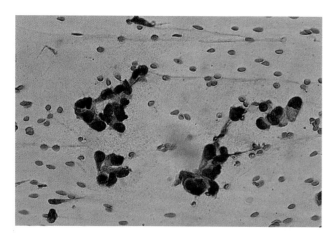

Figure 14–41. Direct smear of infiltrating lobular carcinoma. Moderately cellular aspirate shows uniform population of small cells with hyperchromatic, eccentric nuclei. Occasional signet ring cells are present.

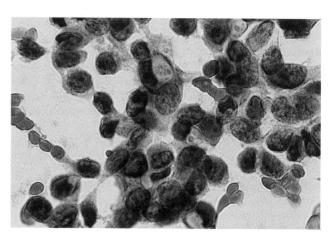

Figure 14–44. Higher magnification of the same case as Figure 14–43. Same features are evident.

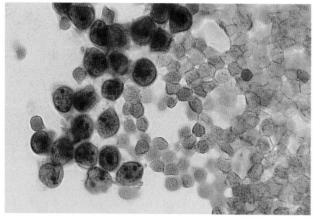

Figure 14–42. Higher magnification of the same case as Figure 14–41. Same features are evident.

Tubular Carcinoma

Variable cellularity
Sheets of epithelial cells forming angulated glandular or
    tubular structures
Nuclear regularity and enlargement
Relatively uniform nuclei
Ground glass nucleus
Cytoplasmic vacuoles

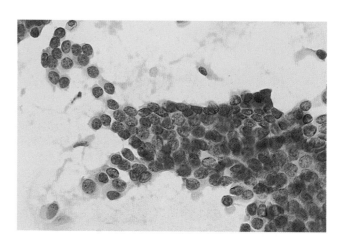

Figure 14–45. Direct smears from tubular carcinoma. Smear shows tubular structure with open lumen and blunted angular structure.

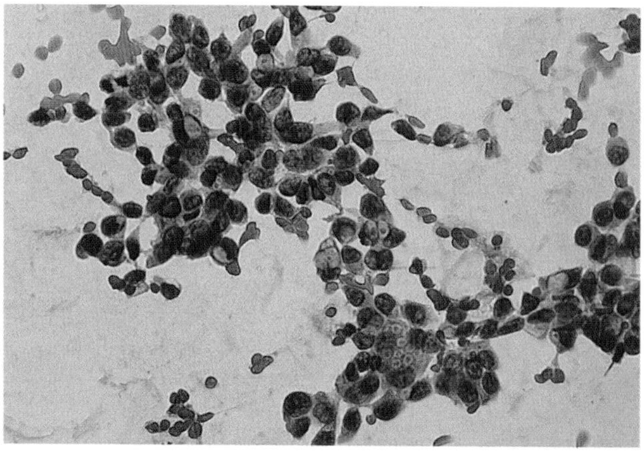

Figure 14–43. Direct smear of pleomorphic lobular carcinoma. Cellular aspirate shows pleomorphic population of neoplastic cells with lobular differentiation.

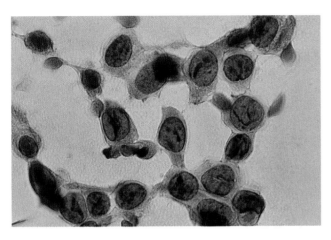

Figure 14–46. Higher magnification of the same case as Figure 14–45. Loosely cohesive neoplastic epithelial cells show uniform nuclei with nuclear grooves and small nucleoli.

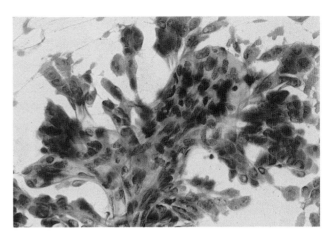

Figure 14–48. Higher magnification of the same case as Figure 14–47. Vascular core is evident with attached papillary fronds resembling a waterfall. Atypical cells show tall columnar appearance.

Infiltrating Papillary Carcinoma

Cell-rich aspirates
Bloody background with hemosiderin-containing macrophages and necrotic debris
Papillary clusters of atypical cells enriched by a fibrovascular core
Large, atypical, naked nuclei
Absence of myoepithelial cells
Tall columnar cells

Mucinous Carcinoma

Variable cellularity
Abundant mucin
Tumor cells isolated and in clusters, often with significant atypia
Occasional signet ring cells
Fragments of stroma with small blood vessels

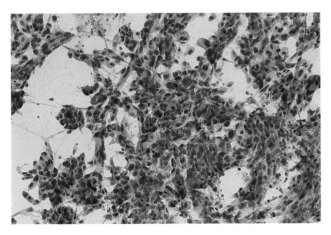

Figure 14–47. Direct smear of infiltrating papillary carcinoma. Cellular smear shows fibrovascular core surrounded by papillary fronds, and monomorphic cell population.

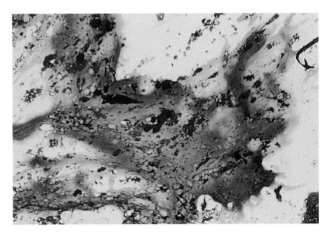

Figure 14–49. Direct smear of mucinous carcinoma. Smear shows abundant extracellular mucin and clustering of epithelial cells.

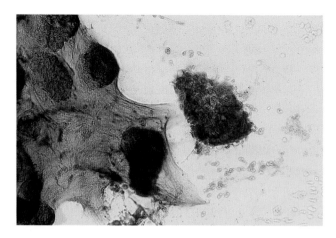

Figure 14–50. Papanicolaou stain of the same case as Figure 14–49. Same features are seen.

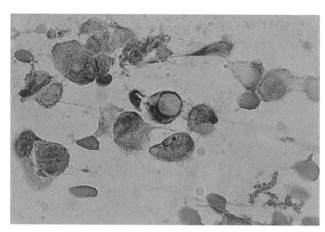

Figure 14–52. Higher magnification of the same case as Figure 14–51. Same features are seen.

Medullary Carcinoma

Cellular smear
Necrotic background
Pleomorphic cells isolated and in syncytial aggregates
Abundant cytoplasm with marked nuclear abnormalities
Bizarre naked nuclei
Occasional multinucleation
Lymphocytes and plasma cells

Signet Ring Cell Carcinoma (Variant of Infiltrating Lobular Carcinoma)

Moderate to rich cellular yield
Small to medium-sized cells, isolated or in clusters
Crescent-shaped nuclei with mucin-filled cytoplasmic vacuoles

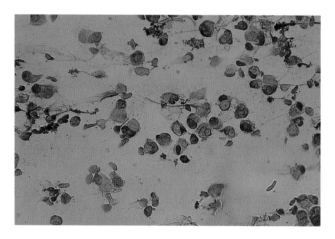

Figure 14–51. Direct smear from signet ring cell carcinoma. Moderate cellular aspirate shows dispersed cell pattern consisting of small cells with crescent-shaped nuclei being compressed to the cell periphery by vacuoles.

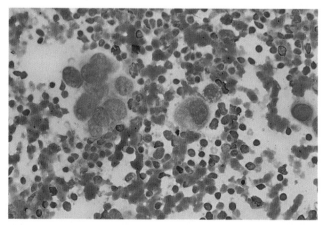

Figure 14–53. Direct smear of medullary carcinoma. Smear shows loose syncytial clusters of neoplastic epithelial cells admixed with lymphocytes and plasma cells.

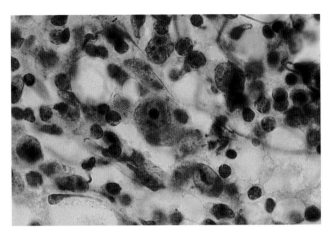

Figure 14–54. Papanicolaou stain of the same case as Figure 14–53. Smear shows highly atypical epithelial cells with marked nuclear abnormality and macronucleoli. Lymphocytes and plasma cells are present.

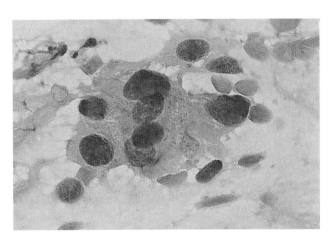

Figure 14–56. Papanicolaou stain of the same case as Figure 14–55. Same features are seen.

Apocrine Carcinoma

Rich tumor cellularity
Atypical cells with abundant glandular cytoplasm
Large irregular nuclei
Marked anisonucleosis
Prominent multiple nucleoli

Secretory Carcinoma

Cellular aspirate
Proteinaceous background
Variable cell arrangement, including "bunches of grapes" or mucous globular structures
Prominent intracytoplasmic vacuoles
Granular cells
Signet ring cells
Variable nuclear atypia
No mitoses or necrosis

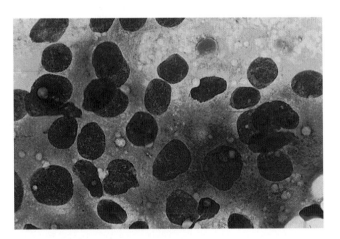

Figure 14–55. Direct smear of apocrine carcinoma. Smear shows granular cell pattern and epithelial cells of various size with abundant cytoplasm.

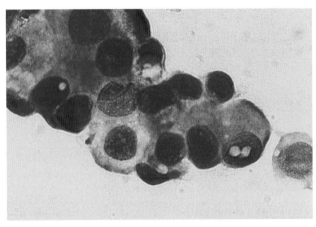

Figure 14–57. Direct smear of secretory carcinoma. Cellular aspirate displays foamy and multivacuolated neoplastic cells that are loosely cohesive and variable in size.

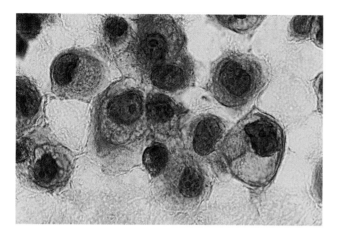

Figure 14–58. Papanicolaou stain of the same case as Figure 14–57. Same features are seen.

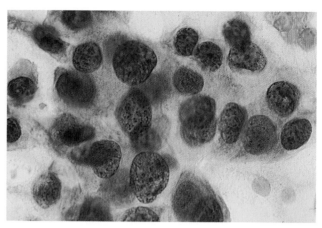

Figure 14–59. Direct imprint of Paget's disease. Smear shows loosely cohesive, variably sized epithelial cells with centrally located nuclei and marked hyperchromasia. Cytoplasm is clear.

Paget's Disease

Variable cellularity
Pleomorphic cell population
Large cells with centrally located nuclei
Frequently positive for hormone receptors

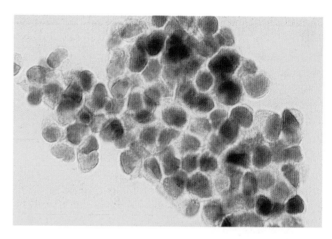

Figure 14–60. Immunostaining of estrogen receptor in Paget's disease. Expression of estrogen receptor is evident by positive nuclear staining.

SARCOMAS OF THE BREAST

Phyllodes Tumor

High cellularity
Biphasic pattern similar to that of fibroadenoma
Cellular stromal components with spindle cells of various sizes and shapes
Variable cytologic atypia and mitotic activity
Macrophages, multinucleated giant cells, and naked nuclei

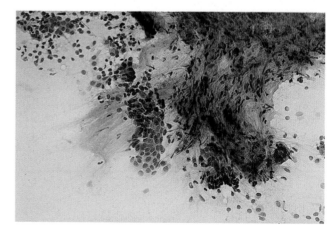

Figure 14–61. Direct smear of phyllodes tumor. Rich cellular aspirate shows biphasic pattern, similar to that of fibroadenoma. The stromal component is cellular with variably sized spindle shaped cells.

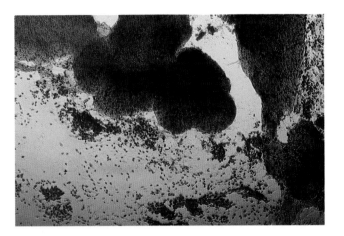

Figure 14–62. Another view of the same case as Figure 14–61. Smear shows marked cellularity of the stroma.

Malignant Phyllodes Tumor

High cellularity
Cells dispersed and in clusters
Lubulated, oval and spindle-shaped nuclei
Prominent nuclei
Rare mitoses

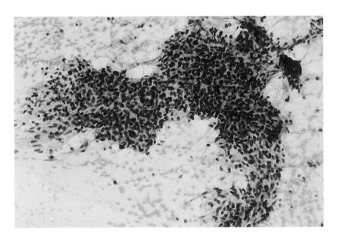

Figure 14–63. Direct smear of malignant phyllodes tumor. Cellular aspirate shows crowded and clustered atypical spindle cells.

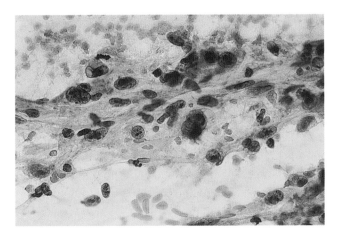

Figure 14–64. Higher magnification of the same case as Figure 14–63. Same features are seen.

Malignant Fibrous Histiocytoma

High cellularity
Pleomorphic cell population
Neoplastic spindle cells
Bizarre tumor giant cells
Mitoses

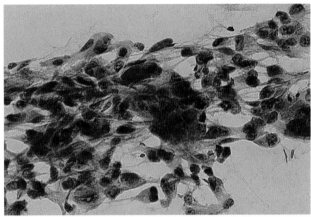

Figure 14–65. Direct smear of malignant fibrous histiocytoma. Cellular aspirate shows loosely cohesive, markedly pleomorphic neoplastic cells and scattered giant cells.

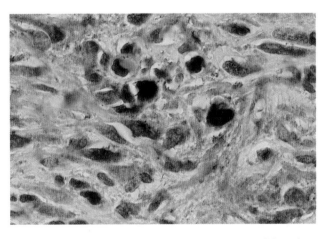

Figure 14–66. Malignant fibrous histiocytoma. Immunostaining of α_1-antichymotrypsin on cell block preparation. Strong positivity is evident.

LYMPHOPROLIFERATIVE DISORDERS

Lymphoma

High cellularity
Variable cell pattern
Monotonous or pleomorphic population of atypical lymphoid cells
Lymphoglandular bodies

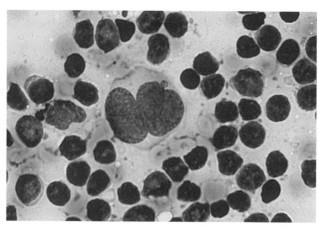

Figure 14-69. Direct smear of Hodgkin's disease. Cellular smear shows pleomorphic population of lymphocytes and plasma cells. A Reed-Sternberg cell is shown.

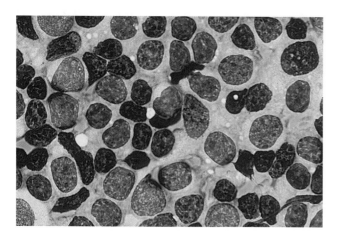

Figure 14-67. Direct smear of lymphoma. Cellular aspirate demonstrates mixed small cleaved and large cell lymphoma.

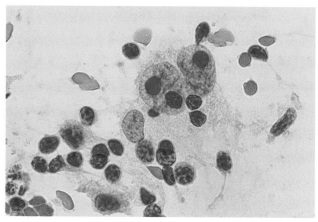

Figure 14-70. Papanicolaou stain of the same case as Figure 14-69. Same features are seen.

Intramammary Lymph Node

Highly cellular
Polymorphic population of mature lymphoid cells
Tingible body macrophages

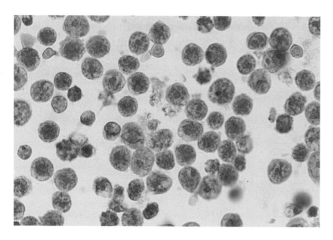

Figure 14-68. Papanicolaou stain of the same case as Figure 14-67. Same features are seen.

Hodgkin's Disease

High cellularity
Polymorphic population of lymphocytes, plasma cells, and eosinophils
Reed-Sternberg cells

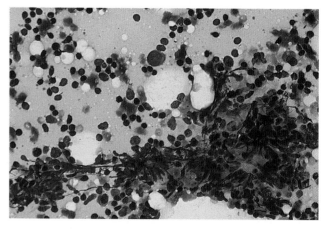

Figure 14-71. Direct smear of intramammary lymph node. Cellular aspirate shows polymorphous population of variably sized lymphocytes.

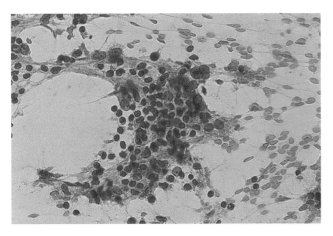

Figure 14–72. Papanicolaou stain of the same case as Figure 14–71. Same features are seen.

METASTATIC CARCINOMA

Cellular aspirate
Variable cellular population
Frequent history of another primary tumor

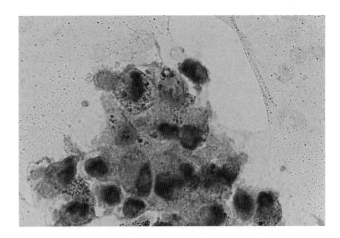

Figure 14–74. Oil-Red O staining of the same case as Figure 14–73. The presence of oil droplets within the neoplastic epithelial cells is evident.

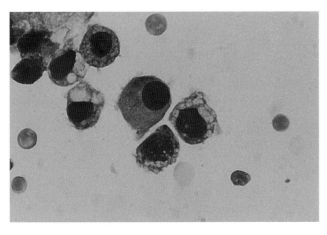

Figure 14–73. Direct smear of metastatic renal cell carcinoma. Smear shows monomorphic population of cells with eccentric nuclei and vacuolated cytoplasm.

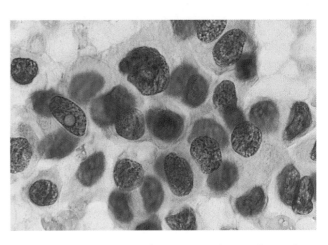

Figure 14–75. Direct smear of metastatic melanoma. Smear shows markedly pleomorphic population of neoplastic cells with hyperchromatic nuclei and macronucleoli.

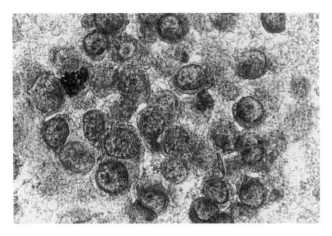

Figure 14–76. HMB-45 immunostaining of the same case as Figure 14–75. The neoplastic cells are positive for HMB-45.

PROGNOSTIC FACTORS

HER-2/neu Expression

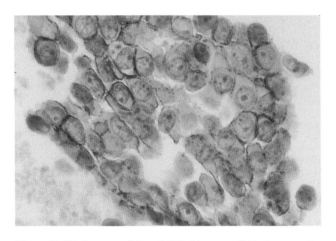

Figure 14–77. Immunostaining of HER-2/neu on cell block preparation of breast fine-needle aspiration biopsy. The HER-2/neu oncogene expression in the neoplastic cells is evident by the cell membrane staining.

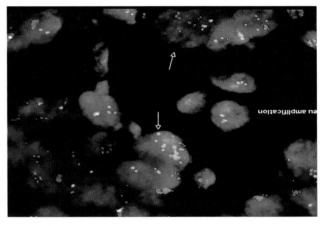

Figure 14–78. Fluorescent in situ hybridization (FISH) of HER-2/neu oncogene on direct smear of breast fine-needle aspiration biopsy. The HER-2/neu oncogene amplification is shown by the arrows.

p53 Expression

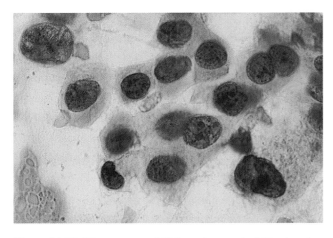

Figure 14–79. Direct smear of high nuclear grade infiltrating duct carcinoma. The marked neoplastic features are evident.

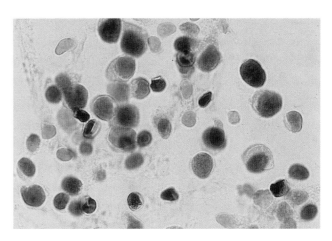

Figure 14–80. Immunochemical staining of p53 protein on direct smear of the same case as Figure 14–79. p53 expression is evidenced by the nuclear staining.

References

1. Silverman JF: Breast. In Bibbo M (ed): Comprehensive Cytopathology. Philadelphia, WB Saunders, 1991, pp 703–770.
2. Masood S: Fine needle aspiration biopsy of non-palpable breast lesions. In Schmidt WA, et al (eds): Cytopathology. 1994 annual. Chicago, ASCP Press 1994, pp 33–63.
3. The uniform approach to breast fine needle aspiration biopsy. National Cancer Institute sponsored conference. Breast J 4:149–168, 1997.
4. Kamisky DB: Aspiration biopsy in the context of the new Medicare fiscal policy. Acta Cytol 28:333–336, 1984.
5. Malberger E, Edonte V, Toledaro O, et al: Fine needle aspiration and cytologic findings of surgical scar lesions in women with breast cancer. Cancer 69:148–152, 1992.
6. Mitnik JS, Vazquez MF, Roses DF, et al: Recurrent breast cancer, stereotaxic localization of fine needle aspiration biopsy. Radiology 182:103–106, 1992.
7. Raqaz J, Baired R, Rebbech P, et al: Neoadjuvant (preoperative) chemotherapy for breast cancer. Cancer 56:719–724, 1985.
8. Masood S: Prognostic factors in breast cancer, use of cytologic preparations. Diagn Cytopathol 13:388–395, 1995.
9. Masood S, Frykberg ER, McLellan GL, et al: Cytologic differentation between proliferative and non-proliferative breast disease in mammographically guided fine needle aspirates. Diagn Cytopathol 7:581–590, 1991.
10. Marshall CJ, Schumann GB, Ward JH, et al: Cytologic identification of clinically occult proliferative breast disease in women with a family history of breast cancer. Am J Clin Pathol 95:157–165, 1991.
11. Fabian C, Kimler B, Brady D, et al: Phase II Chemoprevention trial of DFMO using the random FNA model. Breast Cancer Res Treat 64(1):48, 2000.
12. Masood S, Rasty G: Potential value of cytology in detection of breast cancer precursors by fine needle aspiration biopsy: The "future pap smear for breast cancer." Acta Cytol 43(5):890, 2000.
13. Gupta RK, Naran S, Buchanan A, et al: Fine needle aspiration cytology of the breast: Impact on surgical practice with an emphasis of the diagnosis of breast abnormalities in young women. Diagn Cytopathol 4:206–209, 1988.
14. Gdabett HA, Hsiu IG, Mullen JJ, et al: Prospective evaluation of the role of fine needle aspiration biopsy in the diagnosis and management of patients with palpable solid breast lesions. Ann Surg 56:263–267, 1990.
15. Layfield LJ, Glasgow BJ, Cramer H: Fine needle aspiration in the management of breast masses. Ann Pathol 2:23–62, 1990.
16. Langmur VK, Cramer SF, Hood MG: Fine needle aspiration cytology in the management of palpable, benign and malignant breast disease. Correlation with clinical and mammographic findings. Acta Cytol 33:93–98, 1989.
17. Masood S: Breast fine needle aspiration biopsy. An emerging challenge [editorial]. Breast J 4:137–138, 1998.
18. Frable WJ: Needle aspiration of the breast. Cancer 53:671–676, 1984.
19. Cohn MB, Rodgers C, Hales MS, et al: Influence of training and experience in fine needle aspiration of the breast. Receiver operating characteristics current analysis. Arch Pathol Lab Med 111:518–520, 1987.
20. Masood S: Cytopathology of the Breast. Chicago, ASCP Press, 1996.

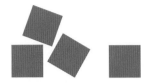

INDEX

A

Abscess
    fine-needle aspiration biopsy of, 180
    subareolar, 27, 180
Acinic cell carcinoma, 49
Adenocarcinoma, 15
Adenoid cystic carcinoma, 49, 148
Adenolipoma, 39, 48
Adenoma. *See specific type, e.g.,* Tubular adenoma.
Adenomyoepithelioma, 49, 54
Adenosis, sclerosing. *See* Sclerosing adenosis.
ADH (atypical ductal hyperplasia). *See* Atypical
    ductal hyperplasia (ADH).
ALH (atypical lobular hyperplasia). *See* Atypical
    lobular hyperplasia (ALH).
Amyloid, 35
Angiogenesis markers, 134
Angiolipoma, 155
Angiosarcoma, 159
    grading of, 160
    low-grade, 158, 159
Apocrine ductal carcinoma in situ, 84
Apocrine metaplasia
    focal, 7
    in lobular carcinoma in situ, 103
    intraductal papilloma with, 69
Aspiration biopsy, fine-needle. *See* Fine-needle aspi-
    ration biopsy.
Atypical ductal hyperplasia (ADH), 77, 95, 96
    clinging carcinoma pattern of, 86
    clinical significance of, 95
    columnar cell type of, 96
    diagnosis of
        core needle biopsy in, 2, 8
        mammography in, 1, 8
    ductal carcinoma in situ compared to, 78, 93
    in pregnancy-like hyperplasia, 96
    intraductal papilloma with, 73
    with micropapillary features, 97
Atypical lobular hyperplasia (ALH), 2, 100, 104.
        See also Lobular neoplasia.
    diagnosis of
        clinical features in, 101
        cytologic features in, 103
        fine-needle aspiration biopsy in, 187
    histologic definitions of, 102
    management of, 108
    risk for subsequent carcinoma in, 106
Atypical vascular lesion, postradiation, 158, 159
"Autoimmune" mastopathy, 29
Axillary lymph node. *See* Lymph nodes, axillary.
Axillary sentinel node biopsy, 127

B

Bcl-2, as prognostic marker, 134
Benign mixed tumor. *See* Pleomorphic adenoma.
Breast prosthesis(es)
    capsule opposite of
        in Biocell texture, 169
        in fixation patches, 172
        in MSI texture, 170
        in polyurethane foam–covered implant, 171
        in Siltex texture, 169
        in smooth saline-filled implant of, 168
        with "egg-shell" dystrophic mineralization, 172
    foreign materials related to, 176–178
    "gel bleed" from, 168
    manufacturer(s) of, 167
        Dow Corning
            smooth-shell gel-filled implant of, 175
            with Dacron patches, 172, 174
            with MSI texture, 170
        Heyer-Schulte
            Dubin-type smooth-shell gel-filled implant
                of, 173
            smooth-shell gel-filled implant of, 173
            with embedded reinforced back patch, 174
        identifying, 173–176
            back patches used for, 173
        Koken, 176
        McGhan/3M
            Dubin-type smooth-shell gel-filled implant
                of, 173
            with Biocell texture, 168, 169
            with suture tag, 175
        Mentor
            ruptured implant of, 169, 170
            smooth-shell gel-filled implant of, 173
            smooth-shell implant of, 174
            with Siltex texture, 169, 170
        Surgitek
            Dubin-type smooth-shell gel-filled implant
                of, 173
            polyurethane foam-covered implant of, 171
            smooth-shell double-lumen implant of, 175
            smooth-shell gel-filled, with radio opaque
                numerals, 174
    ruptured
        Mentor implants as, 169, 170
        villous projections in, 170
        with Dacron patches, 172
    shell of
        smooth elastomer, 168
        texture(s) of
            Biocell, 168, 169

Breast prosthesis(es) (Continued)
  MSI, 170
  Siltex, 169
  tissue reactions resulting from, 166–172
  with Dacron fixation patches, 172, 174
  silicone, 34
    as foreign material, 176–178
    shell of, 166–167
Breasts
  anatomy of, 19–25
  developmental stages of, 20
  in pregnancy
    at term, 22
    fine-needle aspiration biopsy of, 182–183
  minimal changes within "normal," 25
  of elderly women, 24
  of girls, 20
  of males, in situ carcinomas of, 77
  of reproductive-age adult women, 21
  of young women, dense tissue of, 23
  physiologic changes of, 19–25

C

Carcinoma. See specific type, e.g., Medullary carci-
    noma.
  prognostic factors for. See specific factor, e.g.,
    HER = 2/neu.
Cathepsins, as prognostic markers, 134
Cellular fibroadenoma, 39
C-erbB-2 immunostaining, 133, 198
  in comedocarcinoma, 92
C-erbB-3, as prognostic marker, 134
Chemotherapy, epithelial and stromal changes fol-
    lowing, 164
Chest radiographs, in lung cancer, 15
Chondrolipoma, 155
Chromosomal alterations
  in infiltrating lobular carcinoma, 114
  in lobular carcinoma in situ, 107
Clear cell ductal carcinoma in situ, 87
CNB. See Core needle biopsy (CNB).
Coccidioidomycosis, 36
Collagenous spherulosis, 64
  in intraductal papilloma, 70
Colloid carcinoma. See Mucinous carcinoma.
Comedocarcinoma, 81
  c-erbB-2 immunostaining in, 92
  fine-needle aspiration biopsy of, 188
Complex sclerosing lesions, 88
Core needle biopsy (CNB), 1, 2
  epithelial displacement by, 16, 90
  histopathology of, 3
  image guidance of
    radiographic, 1, 2, 5
    ultrasound in, 1, 2, 3, 4
    value of, 13
  of atypical ductal hyperplasia, 2
  of ductal carcinoma in situ, 8
  of focal fibrosis, 6
  of infiltrating duct carcinoma, 9, 11
  of lobular carcinoma in situ, 14
  of lobular neoplasia, 14
  of lymphoma, 15
  of microcalcifications, 2, 3, 5
  of papillary lesions, 2
  of radial scars, 76
  of sclerosing duct papilloma, 75
  specimens from, 5
  vacuum-assisted, 2, 4, 5
Coumarin therapy, 37
Cribriform ductal carcinoma in situ, 78, 80
Cyst(s), inclusion, 32
Cystic hypersecretory ductal carcinoma in situ, 86
Cystosarcoma phyllodes, 39
  benign, 45

Cystosarcoma phyllodes (Continued)
  carcinoma in, 47
  fine-needle aspiration biopsy of, 194–195
  malignant, 46, 47, 195
  metastatic, involving lung, 47
  squamous metaplasia in, 46
  stromal metaplasia in, 47

D

DCIS (ductal carcinoma in situ). See Ductal carci-
    noma in situ (DCIS).
Desmoid tumor, 157, 184
Diabetic mastopathy, 29
Diabetic mellitus, insulin-dependent, 29
Dimorphic ductal carcinoma in situ, 87
Direct excision. See Excisional biopsy.
DNA, as prognostic marker, 134
Duct(s)
  ectasia of, 28, 29, 65
  ruptured, 32
Duct hyperplasia
  intraductal papilloma with, 73
  with lobular involvement, 105
Ductal adenoma, 39, 44
  central sclerosis in, 44, 45
Ductal carcinoma, infiltrating. See Infiltrating duct
    carcinoma (IDC); Infiltrating duct carcinoma
    not otherwise specified (IDC NOS).
Ductal carcinoma in situ (DCIS), 77
  apocrine, 84
  atypical ductal hyperplasia compared to, 78, 93
  clear cell, 87
  cribriform, 78, 80
  cystic hypersecretory, 86
  diagnosis of
    core needle biopsy in, 8
    criteria for, 78
    fine-needle aspiration biopsy in, 188
    mammography in, 1, 8
    microscopic features in, 78
  dimorphic, 87
  estrogen receptor expression in, 92
  grading schemes for, 79, 80
  in cystosarcoma phyllodes, 47
  in fibroadenoma, 42
  infiltrating duct carcinoma compared to, 120
  intracystic papillary, 84
  intraductal hyperplasia compared to, 78
  lobular carcinoma in situ coexisting with, 106
  lobular carcinoma in situ compared to, 93, 106
  margin status in excision of, 91
  microcalcifications in, 90
  microinvasion in, 90
  micropapillary, 82
  mucinous, with prominent signet ring cells, 85
  multicentric, 77
  multifocal, 77
  p53 antigen in, 92
  pseudoinvasion in, 85
  "regressing" high-grade, 82
  reporting recommendations as to, 94
  revertant, 92
  secretory, 87
  solid, 81
  spindle cell, 87
  stratified spindle cell papillary, 83
  types of, 80–88
  with intracytoplasmic lumens, 85
  with lobular involvement, 106
Ductal intraepithelial neoplasia, 77

E

E-cadherin immunostaining, 93
Ectasia, mammary duct, 28, 29, 65

Epithelial lesions
core needle biopsy causing epithelial displacement in, 16, 90
following chemotherapy, 164
nonproliferative and benign proliferative, 57–65
radiation-induced, 164
Estrogen receptor expression, 20, 25, 131
ductal carcinoma in situ and, 92
predictive power of, 132
Excisional biopsy, 1
of radial scar, 3
prior, healing of, 163
reporting guidelines for, 134–135
Extensive intraductal component, 129

F

Fasciitis, nodular, 154
Fat necrosis, 31, 164
fine-needle aspiration biopsy of, 180–181
Fibroadenoma(s), 39
adenosis in, 40
carcinoma in, 42
cellular, 39
diagnosis of
core needle biopsy in, 14
fine-needle aspiration biopsy in, 181
fibrocystic changes in, 40
giant cells in, 41
infarct in, 41
intraductal hyperplasia in, 40
juvenile, 39, 42, 43
leiomyomatous stroma in, 41
lobular carcinoma in situ in, 14, 42
tubular adenoma as, 39, 43, 44
Fibrocystic changes. See Fibrocystic disease.
Fibrocystic disease, 57–65
fine-needle aspiration biopsy of, 186–187
Fibromatosis, 157, 184
Filarial infections, 35
Fine-needle aspiration biopsy, 1, 179–199
limitations of, 1–2, 179
of benign mesenchymal tumors, 184–185
of carcinomas, 189–194
of fibrocystic disease, 186–187
of inflammatory lesions, 180–181
of lymphoproliferative disorders, 196–197
of metastatic carcinoma, 197–198
of noninflammatory benign lesions, 181–183
of sarcomas, 194–195
of treatment-induced changes, 183–184
Focal apocrine metaplasia, 7
Focal fibrosis, 2, 6
Fungal infections, 36

G

Giant cells, in fibroadenoma, 41
Glycogen-rich carcinoma, 148
Granular cell tumor, 156
fine-needle aspiration biopsy of, 184–185
Granuloma
remote suture, 34
silicone, 33
treatment-induced, 183
Granulomatous angiopanniculitis, 32
Granulomatous mastitis
fine-needle aspiration biopsy of, 180
lobular, 31

H

Hamartoma, 39, 48
Hemangioma, 158
Hemorrhagic necrosis, 37

HER-2/neu, 92, 133, 198
Histologic grading
and long-term survival, 123
fixation in, 126
microscopic field diameter in, 125
mitotic count in, 125
Nottingham Histologic Grading Method in, 123
nuclear pleomorphism score in, 124, 125
tubule formation scale and, 124
Histopathologic results, imaging results in concordance with, 2, 6
Hodgkin's disease, 196

I

Iatrogenic lesions, 163–178
fine-needle aspiration biopsy of, 183–184
IDC (infiltrating duct carcinoma). See Infiltrating duct carcinoma (IDC).
IDC NOS (infiltrating duct carcinoma not otherwise specified). See Infiltrating duct carcinoma not otherwise specified (IDC NOS).
"Idiopathic" lobular mastitis, 31
ILC (infiltrating lobular carcinoma). See Infiltrating lobular carcinoma (ILC).
Implants. See Breast prosthesis(es).
Inclusion cysts, 32
Infantile breast bud, 20
Infarction
in fibroadenoma, 41
in intraductal papilloma, 70
Infections, 35–36
Infiltrating apocrine carcinoma, 150, 193
Infiltrating carcinomas. See also specific infiltrating carcinomas, e.g., Infiltrating lobular carcinoma (ILC).
margin status in, 130
prognosis of major types of, 140
Infiltrating cribriform carcinoma, 143
Infiltrating duct carcinoma (IDC)
diagnosis of
core needle biopsy in, 9, 11
fine-needle aspiration biopsy in, 189
mammography in, 9, 10, 11
ductal carcinoma in situ compared to, 120
excision of, 10
histologic grade and long-term survival with, 123
hyalinized stroma in, 130
infiltrating lobular carcinoma compared to, 100–101, 115
metastatic sites in, 115
nipple duct adenoma with, 52
pseudoinvasion in, 120
tumor necrosis in, 131
with intraductal component, 10
Infiltrating duct carcinoma not otherwise specified (IDC NOS), 117, 118, 139
with focal special type features, 119
with focal tubule and single cell cord formation, 118
with medullary carcinoma features, 119
Infiltrating lobular carcinoma (ILC), 100
alveolar variant of, 109, 111, 141
biomarker expression in, 114
chromosomal alterations in, 114
classic, 109, 110, 140, 141
cytology in, 109, 110
diagnosis of
clinical features in, 108
fine-needle aspiration biopsy in, 189–190, 192
histology of, 109
infiltrating duct carcinoma compared to, 100–101, 115
metastatic
axillary lymph nodes involved in, 114
sites in, 115

Infiltrating lobular carcinoma (ILC) *(Continued)*
  pleomorphic, 109, 112, 142, 190
  prognosis in, 101, 113
    markers for, 114
  signet ring cells in, 111, 190, 192
  solid variant of, 109, 111, 141
  tubulolobular, 112, 141
Infiltrating micropapillary carcinoma, 146, 147
Infiltrating papillary carcinoma, 191
Infiltrating syringomatous adenoma of nipple, 49, 53, 54
  nipple duct adenoma compared to, 50t
Inflammatory carcinoma, 151
Inflammatory lesion(s), 26–37
  abscess as
    fine-needle aspiration biopsy of, 180
    subareolar, 27, 180
  duct ectasia as, 28, 29, 65
  fine-needle aspiration biopsy of, 180–181
  mastitis as. *See* Mastitis.
Injection lesions, 165–166
  from paraffin, 33, 165
  from silicone, 33, 166
Intracystic papillary carcinoma, 67, 68, 146
  of male breast, 77
Intracystic papillary ductal carcinoma in situ, 84
Intraductal adenoma(s)
  ductal adenoma as, 39, 44, 45
  pleomorphic adenoma as, 49, 55
Intraductal carcinoma. *See also* Ductal carcinoma in situ (DCIS).
  complex sclerosing lesion involved in, 88
  epithelial displacement by core needle biopsy in, 90
  sclerosing adenoma involved in, 88
  with intraductal papilloma, 74
  with mucocele-like lesions, 86
Intraductal hyperplasia
  ductal carcinoma in situ compared to, 78
  in fibroadenoma, 40
Intraductal papillary lesion(s), 67–76
  intracystic papillary carcinoma as, 67, 68, 146
    of male breast, 77
  intraductal papilloma as. *See* Intraductal papilloma.
  radial scars as. *See* Radial scars.
  sclerosing duct papilloma as, 71, 75
Intraductal papilloma, 68
  calcifications in, 71
  collagenous spherulosis in, 70
  degenerative changes in, 71
  fine-needle aspiration biopsy of, 181, 182
  infarction in, 70
  intraductal carcinoma with, 74
  lobular carcinoma in situ with, 74
  with apocrine metaplasia, 69
  with atypical ductal hyperplasia, 73
  with florid duct hyperplasia, 73
Intramammary lymph node, fine-needle aspiration biopsy of, 196–197

J

Juvenile fibroadenoma, 39, 42, 43

K

Keratin 34βE12 expression, 93
Ki-67 labeling index, 132

L

Lactating adenoma, 39, 44
Lactation

Lactation *(Continued)*
  acute mastitis associated with, 27
  subareolar abscess associated with, 27
Lagios grade, 79
Laser therapy, healing after, 164
LCIS (lobular carcinoma in situ). *See* Lobular carcinoma in situ (LCIS).
Leiomyoma of the nipple, 50, 55
Leiomyomatous stroma, in fibroadenoma, 41
Lipid-rich carcinoma, 148
Lipoma, 155
Liposarcoma, 160
Lobular carcinoma, infiltrating. *See* Infiltrating lobular carcinoma (ILC).
Lobular carcinoma in situ (LCIS), 100, 103, 104. *See also* Lobular neoplasia.
  apocrine metaplasia in, 103
  biomarker expression in, 107
  chromosomal alterations in, 107
  diagnosis of
    clinical features in, 101
    core needle biopsy in, 14
    cytologic features in, 103
    fine-needle aspiration biopsy in, 187
    mammography in, 1
  ductal carcinoma in situ coexisting with, 106
  ductal carcinoma in situ compared to, 93, 106
  extending into interlobular ducts, 104
  histologic definitions of, 102
  in cystosarcoma phyllodes, 47
  in fibroadenoma, 14, 42
  in sclerosing adenosis, 105
  management of, 108
  subsequent carcinoma in
    histologic type of, 107
    risk for, 106
  with intraductal papilloma, 74
Lobular neoplasia, 2. *See also* Atypical lobular hyperplasia (ALH); Lobular carcinoma in situ (LCIS).
  core needle biopsy of, 14
  fine-needle aspiration biopsy of, 187
  mammography of, 14
Lobules
  cancerization of, 88
  unfolded, 58, 59, 60, 105
Lungs
  cancer of, metastasis of, to breast, 15
  cystosarcoma phyllodes metastatic to, 47
Lupus mastitis, 32
Lymph nodes
  axillary
    benign epithelial inclusion in, 127
    cytokeratin-positive fibroblastic reticulum cells in, 127
    metastases to
      extracapsular extension of, 126
      five-year survival in, 126
      in DCIS, 91
      in infiltrating lobular carcinoma, 114
      micro-, 127
      tumor size and, 122
    sentinel node biopsy of, 127
    silicone gel in, 177
  intramammary, fine-needle aspiration biopsy of, 196–197
Lymphocytic mastopathy, 29
Lymphoma
  core needle biopsy of, 15
  fine-needle aspiration biopsy of, 196
Lymphoproliferative disorders, 196–197

M

Male breast, in situ carcinomas of, 77
Malignant fibrous histiocytoma, 195

Mammography, 1, 3
  histopathologic results in concordance with, 2, 6
  of atypical ductal hyperplasia, 1, 8
  of Dow Corning breast prosthesis, 170
  of ductal carcinoma in situ, 1, 8
  of focal fibrosis, 6
  of infiltrating duct carcinoma, 9, 11
    with intraductal component, 10
  of lobular carcinoma in situ, 1
  of lobular neoplasia, 14
  of radial scars, 12, 72
  screening via, 1, 77
Margin status
  in ductal carcinoma in situ, 91
  in infiltrating carcinoma, 130
Mastitis
  acute, 27
  granulomatous ("idiopathic")
    fine-needle aspiration biopsy of, 180
    lobular, 31
  lupus, 32
  plasma cell, 28
  puerperal, 27
  silicone, 33
  tuberculous, 36
Matrix metalloproteinases, 134
Medullary carcinoma, 144
  diagnosis of, 145
  fine-needle aspiration biopsy of, 192–193
  infiltrating duct carcinoma and, 119
Melanoma, metastatic, 197–198
Mesenchymal tumor(s)
  fibromatosis as, 157, 184
  fine-needle aspiration biopsy of, 184–185
  granular cell tumor as, 156, 184–185
  neurofibroma as, 156, 185
Metaplastic carcinoma, 161
  spindle cell type of, 149, 150
Metaplastic matrix-producing carcinoma, 150
Metastasis(es)
  micro-, 127
  occult, 127
  of cystosarcoma phyllodes, to lungs, 47
  of infiltrating duct carcinoma, 115
  of infiltrating lobular carcinoma
    axillary lymph nodes involved in, 114
    sites of, 115
  of lung cancer, to breast, 15
  of melanoma, fine-needle aspiration biopsy of, 197–198
  of renal cell carcinoma, fine-needle aspiration biopsy of, 197
  of sarcoma, 161
  to axillary lymph nodes. *See* Lymph nodes, axillary.
Microcalcifications, 1
  core needle biopsies of, 2, 3, 5
  in ductal carcinoma in situ, 90
  in intraductal papilloma, 71
  in unfolded lobules, 58
Microglandular adenosis, 62, 63, 143
Microinvasion, in ductal carcinoma in situ, 90, 122
Micrometastases, 127
Micropapillary ductal carcinoma in situ, 82
  with infiltrating duct carcinoma not otherwise specified, 146
Microscopic field diameter, 125
Mitotic count, 125
Mitotic index, 125, 132
Mucinous carcinoma, 145, 191–192
Mucinous ductal carcinoma in situ, with prominent signet ring cells, 85
Mucocele-like lesions
  intraductal carcinoma with, 86
  mucinous carcinoma compared, 146
Myoblastoma. *See* Granular cell tumor.
Myoepithelial carcinoma, 50, 55

Myoepitheliosis, 49, 55
Myofibroblastoma, 157

N

Necrosis
  coagulation, 41
  fat, 31, 164, 180–181
  hemorrhagic, 37
  in infiltrating duct carcinoma, 131
  warfarin, 164
Needle biopsy
  core. *See* Core needle biopsy (CNB).
  fine. *See* Fine-needle aspiration biopsy.
  iatrogenic trauma from, 163
Neurofibroma, 156, 185
Nipple
  adenoma of. *See* Nipple duct adenoma.
  infiltrating syringomatous adenoma of, 49, 50t, 53, 54
  leiomyoma of, 50
  Paget's disease of, 77, 151, 194
  tumors of, 49–56
Nipple duct adenoma, 49, 50. *See also* Subareolar papillomatosis.
  adenosis type, 49t, 50
  infiltrating syringomatous adenoma of nipple compared with, 50t
  papillomatosis type, 49t, 51
  proliferative type, 49t, 51
  sclerosing papillomatosis type, 49t, 52
  variants of, 49t
  with infiltrating duct carcinoma, 52
Nodular fasciitis, 154
Non-neoplastic lesions, 26–37
Nonproliferative breast disease, fine-needle aspiration biopsy of, 186–187
Nottingham Histologic Grading Method, 123
Nuclear grade, in ductal carcinoma in situ, 79, 80
Nuclear pleomorphism score, 124, 125

O

Occult metastases, 127
Oophorectomy, 23

P

P53, as prognostic marker, 92, 134, 199
Paget's disease, of nipple, 77, 151
  fine-needle aspiration biopsy of, 194
Papillary apocrine metaplasia, 69
Papilloma, intraductal. *See* Intraductal papilloma.
Paraffin injection, 33, 165
Paraffinoma, 33
Parasitic infection, 35
Periductal sarcoma, 39
Perimenarchal breast tissue, 20
Perineural invasion, 128
Phyllodes tumor. *See* Cystosarcoma phyllodes.
Plasma cell mastitis, 28
Plasminogen activator, 134
Pleomorphic adenoma, 49, 55
Polyurethane foam, for breast prostheses, 171
Postradiation mastopathy, 30
Pregnancy breasts in
  at term, 22
  fine-needle aspiration biopsy of, 182–183
Premenarchal breast tissue, 20
Progesterone receptor expression, 20, 132
Prognosis
  in infiltrating lobular carcinoma, 101, 113, 114
  in major types of infiltrating carcinoma, 140

Prognostic marker(s), 132–134, 198–199
  c-erbB-2 as, 133, 198
    in comedocarcinoma, 92
  HER-2/neu as, 92, 133, 198
  in infiltrating lobular carcinoma, 114
  p53 as, 92, 134, 199
  proliferation markers as, 132
Proliferating cell nuclear antigen, 20
Proliferation markers, 132
Proliferative breast disease, fine-needle aspiration
  biopsy of, 186–187
Prostheses. *See* Breast prosthesis(es).
Protein C deficiency, 37
Pseudoangiomatous stromal hyperplasia, 154
Pseudoinvasion, in ductal carcinoma in situ, 89, 120
"Pseudosarcomatous" fasciitis, 154
Puerperal mastitis, 27

R

Radial scars, 2, 63, 64, 72
  core needle biopsy of, 76
  direct excision of, 3
  mammography of, 12, 72
  tubular carcinoma and, 12, 76
Radiation-induced change(s)
  atypical vascular lesions as, 158, 159
  epithelial and stromal, 164
  fine-needle aspiration biopsy of, 183–184
  mastopathy as, 30
Radiographs
  chest, in lung cancer, 15
  in core needle biopsy guidance, 1, 2, 5
"Regressing" high-grade ductal carcinoma in situ,
  82
Renal cell carcinoma, metastatic, 197
Retraction artifact, 128
Revertant ductal carcinoma in situ, 92
Ruptured ducts, 32

S

Sarcoidosis, 32
Sarcoma
  fine-needle aspiration biopsy of, 194–195
  metastatic, 161
  periductal, 39
Scars, radial. *See* Radial scar(s).
Schwannoma, 156
Sclerosing adenosis, 60, 61, 62
  in fat, 61
  intraductal carcinoma in, 88
  lobular carcinoma in situ in, 105
  tubular carcinoma with, 143
Sclerosing duct papilloma, 71
  core needle biopsy of, 75
Secretory carcinoma, 147
  fine-needle aspiration biopsy of, 193–194
Secretory ductal carcinoma in situ, 87
Signet ring cell(s), mucinous ductal carcinoma in
  situ with, 85
Signet ring cell carcinoma, 111
  fine-needle aspiration biopsy of, 190, 192
Silicone
  breast prostheses from. *See* Breast prosthesis(es).
  injection of, 33, 166
  tissue responses to, 33–34
Skeletal muscle, silicone in, 178
Solid ductal carcinoma in situ, 81

Solid papillary carcinoma, with neuroendocrine fea-
  tures, 147
Spindle-cell ductal carcinoma in situ, 87
Squamous carcinoma, 149
Stratified spindle cell papillary ductal carcinoma in
  situ, 83
Subareolar abscess, 27
  fine-needle aspiration biopsy of, 180
Subareolar papillomatosis. *See also* Nipple duct ade-
  noma.
  variants of, 49t
Surgical biopsy. *See* Excisional biopsy.

T

Tattoos, lesions resulting from, 165
Tavassoli scheme, 79
Tissue expanders, Biocell textured saline-filled, 168
Treatment-induced change(s)
  fine-needle aspiration biopsy of, 183–184
  from chemotherapy, 164
  from radiation. *See* Radiation-induced change(s).
  in DCIS, 91
Tuberculosis, 36
Tubular adenoma, 39, 43
  malignant change in, 44
  tubular carcinoma compared to, 43
Tubular carcinoma, 142
  fine-needle aspiration biopsy of, 190–191
  tubular adenoma compared to, 43
  with adjacent sclerosing adenosis, 143
  with radial scar, 12
Tubulolobular carcinoma, 112
Tumor size
  axillary lymph node metastases and, 122
  measurement of, 121
  relapse-free survival and, 122

U

Ultrasonography, 1
  in core needle biopsy guidance, 1, 2, 3, 4
  of infiltrating duct carcinoma with intraductal
    component, 10
  of intraductal papillary lesions, 69
Unfolded lobules, 58, 59, 60, 105

V

Vacuum-assisted core needle biopsy, 1, 4, 5
Van Nuys scheme, 79
Vascular invasion, 128
Vascular lesion(s)
  postradiation atypical, 158, 159
  silicone causing, 178
  vasculitis as, 37

W

Warfarin necrosis, 164
Weber-Christian disease, 32

X

X-rays
  chest, in lung cancer, 15
  in core needle biopsy guidance, 1, 2, 5